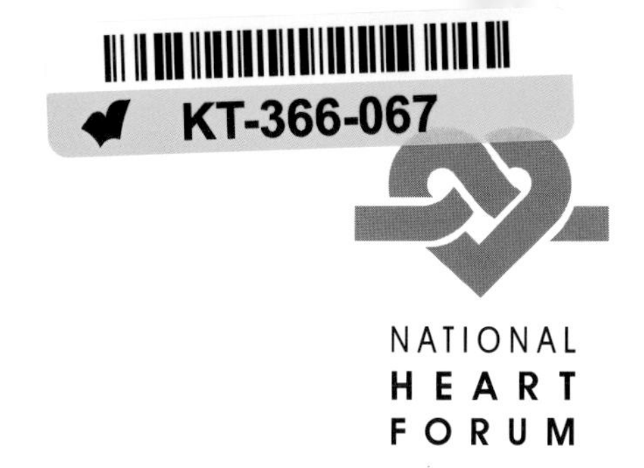

A lifecourse approach to coronary heart disease prevention

Scientific and policy review

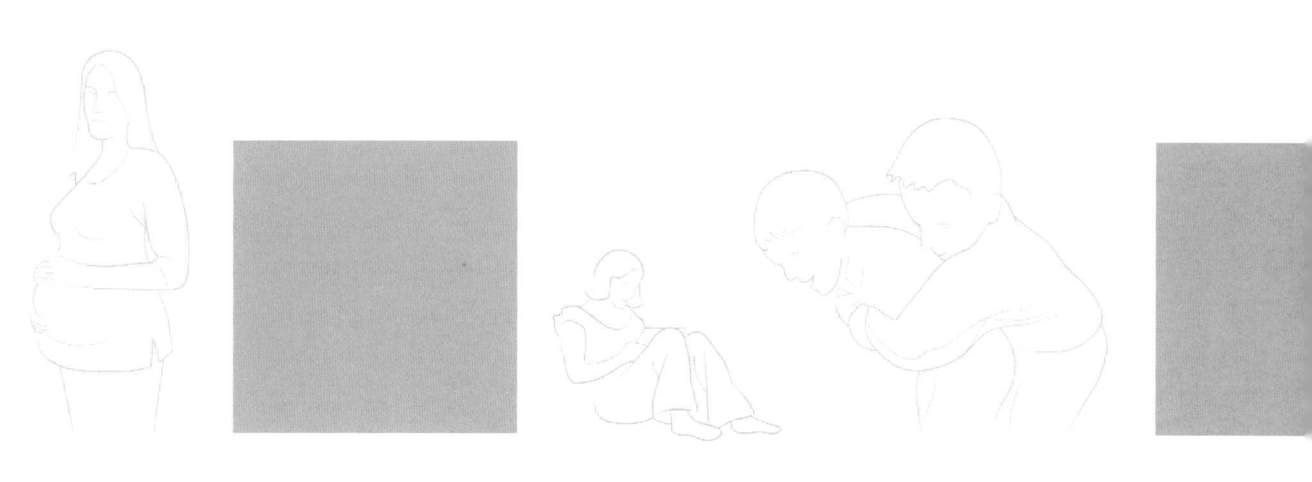

Edited by Dr Alison Giles

London: TSO

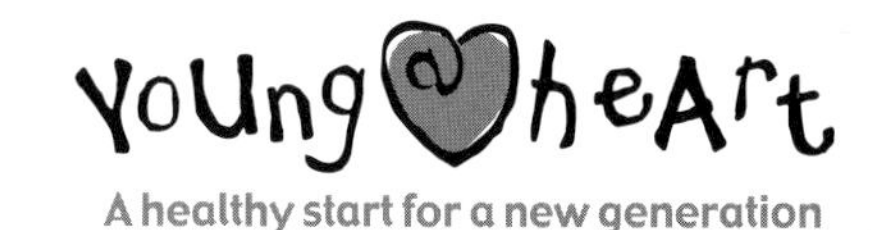

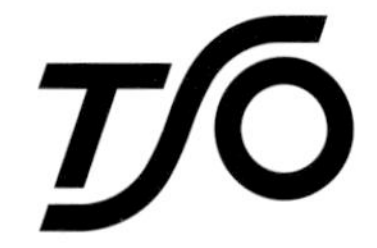

Published by TSO (The Stationery Office) and available from:

Online
www.tso.co.uk/bookshop

Mail, Telephone, Fax & E-mail
TSO
PO Box 29, Norwich, NR3 1GN
Telephone orders/General enquiries: 0870 600 5522
Fax orders: 0870 600 5533
E-mail: book.orders@tso.co.uk
Textphone: 0870 240 3701

TSO Shops
123 Kingsway, London, WC2B 6PQ
020 7242 6393 Fax 020 7242 6394
68-69 Bull Street, Birmingham B4 6AD
0121 236 9696 Fax 0121 236 9699
9-21 Princess Street, Manchester M60 8AS
0161 834 7201 Fax 0161 833 0634
16 Arthur Street, Belfast BT1 4GD
028 9023 8451 Fax 028 9023 5401
18-19 High Street, Cardiff CF10 1PT
029 2039 5548 Fax 029 2038 4347
71 Lothian Road, Edinburgh EH3 9AZ
0870 606 5566 Fax 0870 606 5588

TSO Accredited Agents
(see Yellow Pages)

and through good booksellers

First Published 2003

ISBN 0 11 322526 1

Printed in the United Kingdom by The Stationery Office
N135625 c7 9/03 19585 888215

National Heart Forum
Tavistock House South
Tavistock Square
London WC1H 9LG
www.heartforum.org.uk

Registered Company Number: 2487644
Registered Charity Number: 803286
VAT Number: 564 6088 18

Other publications by the National Heart Forum:

At least five a day: Strategies to increase vegetable and fruit consumption
Coronary heart disease: Are women special?
Coronary heart disease: Estimating the impact of changes in risk factors
Let's get moving: A physical activity handbook for developing local programmes
Looking to the future: Making coronary heart disease an epidemic of the past
Physical activity: An agenda for action
Preventing coronary heart disease in primary care: The way forward
Preventing coronary heart disease: The role of antioxidants, vegetables and fruit
School meals assessment pack
Social inequalities in coronary heart disease: Opportunities for action
Towards a generation free from coronary heart disease: Policy action for children's and young people's health and well-being

For details of how to order these publications, visit the National Heart Forum website on www.heartforum.org.uk

Acknowledgements

The *young@heart* initiative has been generously sponsored by the British Heart Foundation, the Department of Health, the Health Development Agency and the Nuffield Trust.

The National Heart Forum (NHF) is grateful to its member organisations and individual members (see page vii), and the many other people who contributed to the background research and to the young@heart policy summit meeting in June 2001.

Particular thanks are due to:

- those people whose papers form the basis of this report
- the members of the Steering Group and the National Heart Forum project team (see next page)
- participants at the young@heart policy summit meeting in 2001 (see page 367) for their contributions
- the National Children's Bureau, and in particular Gill Frances, for organising the Talkshop and production of the video *A Picture of Health* (see Chapter 15), and the children and young people who took part in these projects
- Bethan Carr, Melanie Morris and Nicola Schmidt for their research assistance on the report
- Rosie Leyden of Wordworks for editorial assistance.

Front cover design by The Creative Element.

Young@heart Steering Group

John Wyn Owen, Nuffield Trust and chair of the young@heart initiative
Professor John Appleby, King's Fund
Dr Charlotte Dargie, University of Cambridge
Dr Maria Duggan, Freelance public health policy consultant
Dr Karen Dunnell, Office for National Statistics
John Garlick, Freelance health policy consultant
Professor Sir Charles George, British Heart Foundation
Professor Desmond Julian, Emeritus Professor of Cardiology, Newcastle upon Tyne
Lady Sylvia Limerick, Community Practitioners' and Health Visitors' Association
Sir Alexander Macara, National Heart Forum
Professor Klim McPherson, National Heart Forum
Margaret Mythen, New Health Network
Professor Roisin Pill, University of Wales College of Medicine
Dr Vivienne Press, British Heart Foundation
Barry Quirk, Lewisham Borough Council
Hamid Rehman, Ethnos Research and Consultancy
Dame Helena Shovelton, Audit Commission
Marilyn Toft, Health Development Agency
Professor David Wood, National Heart Forum

National Heart Forum project team

- Dr Alison Giles
- Jane Landon
- Paul Lincoln
- Louise Sarch

National Heart Forum

The National Heart Forum (NHF) is an alliance of over 45 national organisations concerned with the prevention of coronary heart disease. Members represent the health services, professional bodies, consumer groups and voluntary organisations.

The mission of the National Heart Forum is to work with and through its members to prevent disability and death from coronary heart disease in the UK. In order to achieve this, the NHF operates nationwide and internationally. It has four main objectives:

1. To provide a forum for members for the exchange of information, ideas and initiatives on coronary heart disease prevention

2. To identify and address areas of consensus and controversy, and gaps in research and policy

3. To develop policy based on evidence and on the views of member organisations

4. To stimulate and promote effective action.

The National Heart Forum embraces professional, scientific and policy opinion in current issues in coronary heart disease prevention. It coordinates action to reduce heart disease through information, education, research, policy development and advocacy.

Member organisations

Age Concern England
ASH
ASH Scotland
Blood Pressure Association
British Association for Cardiac Rehabilitation
British Association for Nursing in Cardiac Care
British Association of Sport and Exercise Sciences
British Cardiac Society
British Dietetic Association
British Heart Foundation
British Medical Association
British Nutrition Foundation
CASH (Consensus Action on Salt and Health)
Chartered Institute of Environmental Health
Child Poverty Action Group
Community Practitioners' and Health Visitors' Association
Consumers' Association
CORDA
Coronary Prevention Group
Design and Technology Associates (DATA)
Diabetes UK
Faculty of Public Health Medicine
Health Development Agency
Health Promotion Agency for Northern Ireland
HEART UK (Family Heart Association)
King's Fund
National Association of Governors and Managers
National Heart Research Fund
NHS Confederation
Northern Ireland Chest, Heart and Stroke Association
Nuffield Trust
Primary Care Cardiovascular Society
Royal College of General Practitioners
Royal College of Nursing
Royal College of Paediatrics and Child Health
Royal College of Physicians of London
Royal College of Surgeons of England
Royal Institute of Public Health
Royal Pharmaceutical Society of Great Britain
SHARP (Scottish Heart and Arterial disease Risk Prevention)
Society of Cardiothoracic Surgeons of Great Britain and Ireland
Society of Health Education and Health Promotion Specialists
Society of Occupational Medicine
Sport England
Trades Union Congress
UK Public Health Association

Members

In addition a number of distinguished experts in the cardiovascular field have individual membership.

Professor Raj Bhopal, University of Edinburgh Medical School
Professor George Davey Smith, University of Bristol
Dr Elizabeth Dowler, University of Warwick
Dr Maria Duggan
Dr Karen Dunnell, Office for National Statistics
Professor Shah Ebrahim, University of Bristol
Professor Peter Fentem
Professor Godfrey Fowler
Elaine Fullard
Dr Nicholas Hicks, Milton Keynes Primary Care Trust
Professor Philip James, International Obesity Taskforce
Professor Desmond Julian
Dr John Kemm
Professor Kay Tee Khaw, University of Cambridge
Professor Brian Kirby
Suzi Leather
Sir Alexander Macara
Professor Sir Michael Marmot, University College, London
Professor Klim McPherson, University of Bristol
Professor Jerry Morris, London School of Hygiene and Tropical Medicine
Margaret Mythen, New Health Network
Dr Noel Olsen
Dr Vivienne Press
Professor Peter Quilliam
Dr Mike Rayner, BHF Health Promotion Research Group, Oxford
Lord Nicolas Rea
Dr Jennifer Roberts, London School of Hygiene and Tropical Medicine
Professor Gerry Shaper
Professor Hugh Tunstall-Pedoe, Ninewells Hospital and Medical School
Professor Peter Whincup, St George's Hospital Medical School

Observers

Department of Health
Department of Health, Social Services and Public Safety Northern Ireland
Medical Research Council
The National Assembly for Wales
National Consumer Council
Scottish Consumer Council
The Scottish Executive
The Stroke Association

Contents

Foreword

Young@heart is the National Heart Forum's major policy initiative to tackle the causes of heart disease from its beginnings in early life. Based on evidence from many different sources, young@heart makes the case for a UK-wide national plan to protect children from developing heart disease in later life – and other chronic diseases such as stroke, diabetes and some cancers – and to foster health as well as life expectancy in their adult life.

I have been delighted to be involved in young@heart as chair of the young@heart Steering Group and I applaud and thank all those who have been involved for their dedication and enthusiasm and for bringing a huge wealth of experience and expertise to the initiative.

This report brings together for the first time the comprehensive and unique series of reviews commissioned by the National Heart Forum that have underpinned the young@heart initiative. These reviews document the trends in coronary heart disease risk factors and health inequalities among children and young people and provide clear evidence that the aim of young@heart – *that every child born in the UK today should be able to live to at least the age of 65 free from avoidable coronary heart disease* – can be realised.

Publication of this report could not be more timely for never has the political environment been more conducive to the establishment of a comprehensive national plan that has children and young people's health at the heart: with the Government's commitment to eradicate child poverty and to narrow health inequalities, and its prioritisation of heart disease.

I commend this report to all those with a professional interest in public health and social policy as well as policy-makers and all those concerned with the health and well-being of the young.

John Wyn Owen
Secretary, Nuffield Trust

Introduction

Each year, 121,000 people in the UK die from coronary heart disease (CHD) and of these, 16,500 are aged under 65.[1] The death rate has been falling since the late 1970s but this measure is misleading. The number of heart attacks that occur annually in the UK is estimated to be 275,000, and this figure appears to be rising gradually. Furthermore, 85,000 of these heart attacks occur in people aged under 65. Clearly more needs to be done to prevent the incidence of CHD. On a global scale, results of a World Health Organization study show that CHD incidence rates in the two UK populations included in the study, Belfast and Glasgow, are among the highest in the world.[2]

We often consider the enormous burden of CHD to the NHS and to the economy, but what is commonly overlooked is the human toll. CHD deprives families of able parents and providers and may bring financial hardship with it. About 1.2 million people in the UK have had a heart attack and 2 million people suffer from angina.[1] Many of these people have an impaired quality of life and the majority will require medication for the rest of their lives.

The direct risk factors for CHD are high blood pressure, high blood cholesterol, obesity and type 2 diabetes. The lifestyle risk factors underlying these are, for most people: a poor diet high in saturated fat and salt and low in fruit, vegetables and fibre; a lack of physical activity; and smoking.

There has been increasing concern in recent years regarding the adverse trends in CHD risk factors among adults in the UK. It has been estimated that only 5% of the population of developed countries is at low risk of CHD, with optimum risk factor levels.[3] Since 1997, the government has set in place many policies and initiatives to tackle these trends, although it is too early to know how effective these will be.

The National Heart Forum is concerned about the increase in prevalence of many of the risk factors for CHD among children and young people and yet there has been a lack of urgency on the part of governments and society to address these. Particularly alarming are the sudden rise in obesity among primary and secondary school children and the discovery of type 2 diabetes among teenagers. These developments could halt the current decline in CHD mortality rates and even cause them to rise. They could also result in a new CHD epidemic in 50 years' time, with higher incidence rates and with CHD occurring at an increasingly early age.

Young@heart

It is widely accepted that, in order to reduce the incidence of adult CHD and to reduce health inequalities, a lifecourse approach must be adopted, beginning with the health of the foetus and continuing through childhood and adolescence and into adulthood. This is why, in 2000, the National Heart Forum established its young@heart initiative. The goal of the initiative is:

> **Every child born in the UK today should be able to live to at least the age of 65 free from avoidable coronary heart disease.***

This report sets out a comprehensive review of the literature around the health and well-being of children and young people. The National Heart Forum commissioned the review from leading researchers, to inform its policy development process. In particular the review documents the trends in CHD risk factors among children and young people, and makes recommendations for how the adverse trends might best be tackled.

Key concerns to emerge from the review are:

- **Poor diets among infants, children and young people**
  Chapters 1, 7 and 14 highlight: the continuing low rates of breastfeeding; that infants, children and young people consume low levels of fruit and vegetables and increasing amounts of high-sugar drinks; and that girls are not getting the recommended daily amounts of many essential nutrients. Part of the suggested explanation for these trends is the extensive marketing to children of products containing high levels of fat, sugar and salt.

- **Lack of physical activity among children and young people, particularly among teenage girls**
  Children and young people of all ages are becoming less active (see Chapters 8, 9 and 14). They are being driven by car by their parents rather than walking and cycling (because of distance from schools, and safety concerns); they tend to play indoors (because of the popularity of computer and video games, and again because of safety concerns); and schoolchildren spend less time on physical education at school (due to changes in the curriculum). In particular there is a decline in the amount of activity that girls do as they get older.

---

* This is an adaptation of the Winning Hearts Declaration made in 2000 by the European Heart Network (EHN) at the launch of an initiative to raise awareness among all EU member states of the need for a lifecourse approach to CVD prevention. The National Heart Forum is a member of the EHN and part of the European Heart Health Initiative that is taking forward the EHN initiative at member state level.

- **Persistent rates of smoking among teenagers**
  Smoking rates remain steady among boys and young men and may be increasing among girls and young women (see Chapters 10 and 14).

Evidence from the National Heart Forum's review of the literature informed the development of a National Heart Forum policy framework document, *Towards a generation free from coronary heart disease: Policy action for children's and young people's health and well-being*. This has been the basis of policy advocacy work by the National Heart Forum and others since the launch of the document in 2002.*

The report also contains a broad-ranging synopsis of policies across government, and initiatives in place at the time of publication, that may influence the health and well-being of children and young people (see Chapter 12). Several of these had already been implemented when the young@heart initiative began and the young@heart policy recommendations reflect and build on these.

The National Heart Forum recognises the value of involving children and young people at an early stage in the formulation of policies and initiatives, to ensure that these are effective, appropriate and responsive to children's and young people's needs. To provide a context for the development of the young@heart policy recommendations, the National Heart Forum and the National Children's Bureau (NCB) held a 'talkshop' that brought together 30 NCB young members aged 11-17 years from around the country to explore their attitudes and ideas for a healthy lifestyle and the measures they would like to see put in place to help them remain free from CHD. The outcomes of this event are documented in Chapter 15.

This report therefore brings together a wide range of perspectives in the discussion of the need for a lifecourse approach to CHD prevention. As such it will be of value to the broad public health audience as well as to policy-makers and all those concerned with the health and well-being of infants, children and young people.

We hope that the report is not only stimulating and thought-provoking for the reader, but that it also provides a practical contribution to the development of public health policy and helps to achieve the young@heart goal that 'Every child born in the UK today should be able to live to at least the age of 65 free from avoidable coronary heart disease.'

---

* The key recommendations from *Towards a generation free from coronary heart disease: Policy action for children's and young people's health and well-being* are set out in Part 1 of this report (see page 7). The full policy framework document is available from the National Heart Forum or online at www.heartforum.org.uk/young

References

1 Petersen S, Peto V, Rayner M. 2003. *Coronary Heart Disease Statistics*. London: British Heart Foundation.

2 Tunstall-Pedoe H, Kuulasmaa K, Mahonen M et al for the WHO MONICA Project. 1999. Contribution of trends in survival and coronary-event rates to changes in coronary heart disease mortality: 10 year results from 37 WHO MONICA Project populations. *Lancet*; 353: 1547-57.

3 Beaglehole R. 2001. Global cardiovascular disease prevention: time to get serious. *Lancet*; 358: 661-63.

PART 1

Young@heart key recommendations

Recommendations for policy action for children's and young people's health and well-being

The goal of the National Heart Forum's young@heart initiative is that every child born in the UK today should be able to live to at least the age of 65 free from avoidable coronary heart disease. As part of the young@heart initiative, the National Heart Forum commissioned an extensive review of the research on the early origins of coronary heart disease and the potential for reducing the risk and promoting health from early life and throughout childhood and early adulthood (see Chapters 1-11). It also compiled a synopsis of government policies and initiatives which directly or indirectly affect the heart health of children and young people (see Chapter 12). An expert policy summit meeting in June 2001 brought together contributions from a wide range of experts in public health, health economics, children's welfare and education and from policy-formers in both national and local government (see Appendix). The policy framework document which emerged from the review and summit meeting – *Towards a generation free from coronary heart disease: Policy action for children's and young people's health and well-being*[1] – was launched in the House of Lords in February 2002. This chapter gives a summary of its key recommendations.

The policy framework document proposes a common health-promoting agenda for departments across government and for agencies, partnerships and organisations working at both national and local level across the public and commercial sectors. It puts forward:

- proposals for a **national plan for children's and young people's health and well-being**, with a particular focus on coronary heart disease prevention, and

- recommendations to develop **comprehensive national strategies** for improving nutrition, increasing physical activity, and tackling smoking among children and young people (see Figure 1).

Figure 1 *A national plan for children's and young people's health and well-being*

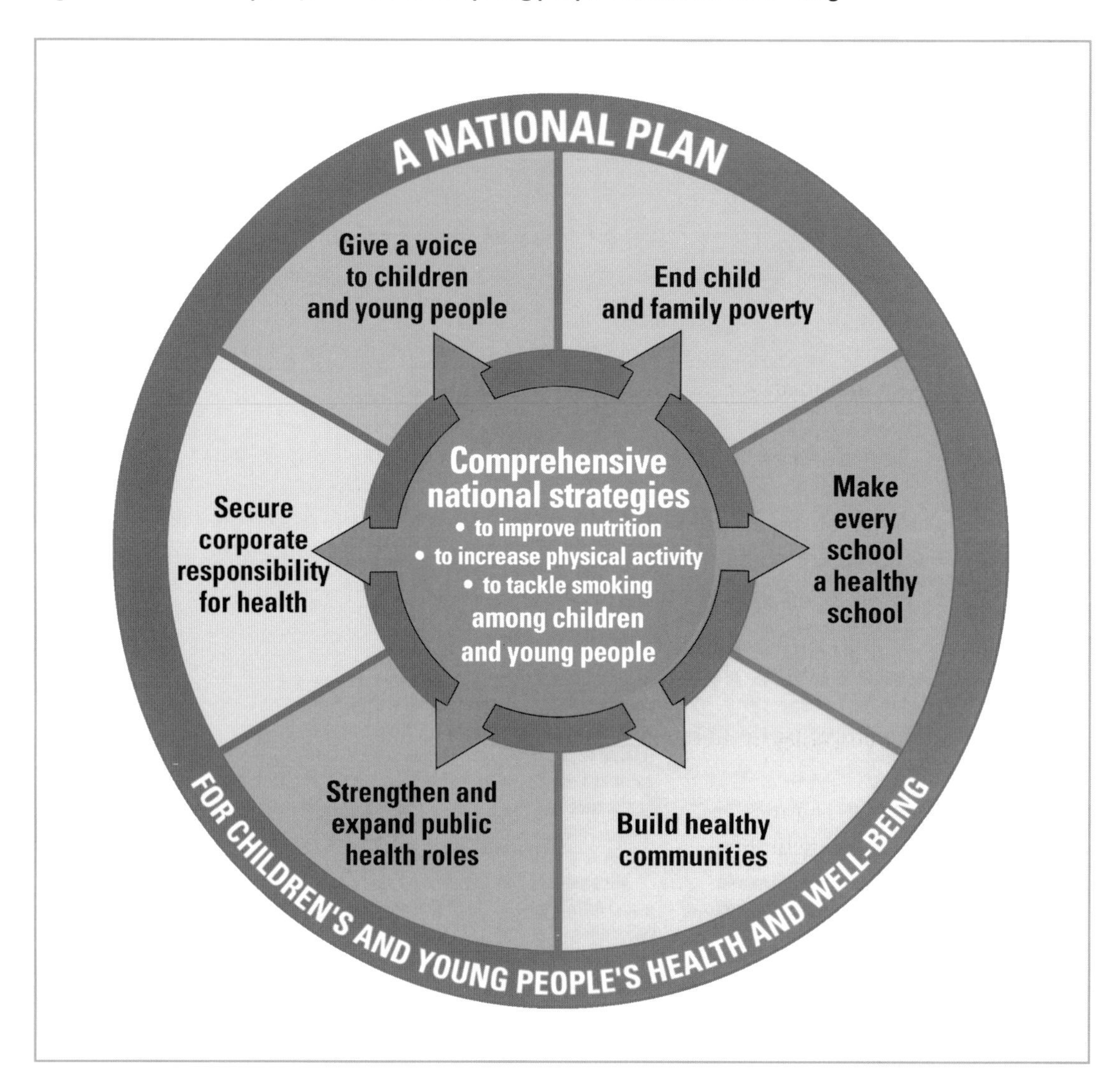

A national plan for children's and young people's health and well-being

A national plan must address all the different direct and indirect influences on children's and young people's health. It must engage the many opportunities for policy action across all sectors, and seek to build health capacity for families, children and young people, in the home, at school and in the community.

The young@heart proposals for a national plan are grouped into six key areas for policy action:

- End child and family poverty
- Make every school a healthy school
- Build healthy communities
- Strengthen and expand public health roles
- Secure corporate responsibility for health, and
- Give a voice to children and young people.

The key recommendations from each of these areas are given on the following pages. Supporting actions for each recommendation are given in the full policy framework document which is available from the National Heart Forum or online at www.heartforum.org.uk

End child and family poverty

The relationship between socioeconomic background, child poverty and long-term ill health is complex. Women from low socioeconomic groups tend to have babies of low birthweight, which is an independent predictor of coronary health disease (CHD). Poor educational attainment is also an independent predictor of CHD, and boys whose fathers are from a low socioeconomic group are unlikely to reach the highest educational level. Under or malnourished children tend to be shorter than their better-off peers and the mechanisms which retard growth appear to increase prevalence of adult hypertension and diabetes.

The key recommendation below, together with the supporting actions described in the policy framework document,[1] reflect the need for income distribution policies which directly tackle family and child poverty, and for investment in targeted services to alleviate the effects of living in poverty.

KEY RECOMMENDATION

1 **The Treasury should undertake a review to reformulate how it calculates minimum income standards and benefit levels, in order to ensure that families can afford the essential requisites to give their children a healthy start in life.**

Make every school a healthy school

A healthy school ethos and environment builds pupils' health, self-esteem and well-being. This in turn can contribute to improved educational attainment and therefore to improved life prospects.

The key recommendations below, together with the supporting actions described in the policy framework document,[1] focus on building and sustaining a whole school approach towards health promotion, linking school policies and culture, the physical environment and the curriculum. In particular, the recommendations focus on actions to strengthen the National Healthy School Standard, actions to curb smoking, and actions to raise the quality and uptake of school meals.

KEY RECOMMENDATIONS

2 **The government should introduce a statutory requirement for all schools to develop and implement health-promoting school policies under the Education Acts.**

3 **The requirements of the National Healthy School Standard should be strengthened and new resources provided to enable and encourage all schools to meet an enhanced national Standard. Meeting the new Standard should be included within the statutory inspection remit of Her Majesty's Inspectorates for Schools.**

4 **Develop and build on existing school-based smoking prevention interventions. These should start in all primary schools and continue into secondary schools and be delivered as part of a statutory provision for school health-based policies under the Education Acts. Interventions should aim to reinforce anti-smoking attitudes and to equip children to understand and resist the influence of the tobacco industry.**

5 **Ensure that the school curriculum and teaching practices support the ethos of a healthy school.**

6 **National targets should be set and monitored to raise the quality and uptake of school meals, with particular emphasis on free school meals.**

Build healthy communities

Access to a healthy diet and opportunities to be physically active are determined by both our physical environment and the organisation of local services. Strategies to tackle social exclusion and to regenerate communities can have an important impact on reducing health inequalities and reducing the avoidable health risks among the most vulnerable groups in society. Social exclusion is strongly linked to a lack of self-esteem and poor mental health among young people.

The key recommendations below, together with the supporting actions described in the policy framework document,[1] reflect the needs of families with babies and young children, especially those living on a low income, and of adolescents. Priority should be given to community level actions that will help tackle food poverty, support active transport plans, raise community participation in sport and recreation, and offer support to young people during adolescence.

KEY RECOMMENDATIONS

7 **There should be government investment and local action to expand the Sure Start programme to provide national coverage for all children under 4 and their families, and strengthen the child health components. These should include nutrition and food skills for parents, particularly on breastfeeding and weaning.**

8 **There should be government investment and local action to ensure national provision of support and mentoring services for teenagers which incorporate a health and well-being element. The Connexions service in England should be expanded and should act as a model for other national services.**

9 **Local Strategic Partnerships in England and Wales, and their equivalents in Scotland and Northern Ireland, should have strong, independent public health input, include plans for children's health and well-being, and reflect the views of children and young people in their development and working practices.**

10 **Develop community forums, with joint funding from health and local authorities, to develop and support local health promotion programmes.**

11 **Increase children's and young people's participation in and access to sport and recreation in the community.**

12 **Make walking and cycling a healthy means of daily travel for more children and young people.**

Strengthen and expand public health roles

Improving children's health and well-being should be a core responsibility shared by all professionals who work with children, young people and families. In order for this to be realised, policies are needed to strengthen public health training, to improve recruitment and retention among key professional groups, and to give a sharper health advocacy focus to existing roles and responsibilities.

The key recommendation below, together with the supporting actions described in the policy framework document,[1] would strengthen existing government initiatives and programmes and support the development of the additional initiatives and programmes recommended by the National Heart Forum.

KEY RECOMMENDATION

13 **Public health training, standards, and recruitment and retention initiatives should be developed to support everyone working with children, young people and families to fulfil a core responsibility for promoting and protecting health.**

Secure corporate responsibility for health

Children and young people are growing up in an increasingly sophisticated commercial environment and are being exposed to it at an ever earlier age via a growing range of media, in the home, at school and in the wider community. The commercial sector is able to influence children's diets by targeting products specifically at them and by branding resources that are freely supplied to schools. The sector is also able to influence children's smoking behaviour through product placement and through exploiting the smoking habits of role models and idols.

The recommendations that follow, together with the supporting actions described in the policy framework document,[1] propose joint working between the commercial sector and government towards good practice, and appropriate regulation, in order to improve children's and young people's diets, to increase support of initiatives to encourage mothers to breastfeed, and to protect children and young people from the influence of the tobacco industry.

KEY RECOMMENDATIONS

14 **There should be a national inquiry to look at the impact of advertising and commercial promotions on family and child health. This should focus in particular on the food and tobacco industries and be the basis for developing appropriate interventions such as advertising regulations.**

15 **Measures should be introduced to limit and control promotions in schools by commercial companies.**

16 **The government should work with the commercial sector to improve the nutritional quality of processed and catered foods and the availability of fruit and vegetables.**

17 **The government should work with food manufacturers and food retailers to improve food labelling and public information about food and healthy eating.**

18 **The government and the health services should ensure that commercial activities do not undermine public health initiatives.**

19 **Ban the promotion of tobacco products.**

Give children and young people a voice

To be effective, appropriate and responsive to children's and young people's needs, policy-making to improve health and well-being has to be informed by children's and young people's views. Engaging children and young people in decisions that influence their lives can also contribute to a sense of citizenship, and help build self-esteem.

The key recommendation below, together with its supporting actions,[1] highlight the need to engage and involve children and young people at the earliest opportunity in the development and implementation of the recommendations made in the policy framework document *Towards a generation free from coronary heart disease: Policy action for children's and young people's health and well-being*[1] and in all other initiatives and decision-making processes that influence their lives and their choices.

KEY RECOMMENDATION

20 All of the policy actions proposed in the young@heart policy framework document[1] should be developed and implemented with a commitment to involving children and young people and taking account of their views, so that national and local policy-making is effective, appropriate and responsive to their needs.

Comprehensive national strategies

The national plan outlined on pages 5-9 draws on recommendations to develop comprehensive national strategies focused on children and young people to improve nutrition, increase physical activity and tackle smoking. These should be developed and implemented across government and across the UK to promote and protect children's and young people's health and well-being.

Improving nutrition

KEY RECOMMENDATIONS

A **Improve nutrition in women before and during pregnancy.**

B **Improve infant and pre-school nutrition.**

C **Improve the quality and uptake of food in schools through a combination of investment in school infrastructure, extending entitlement to free school meals, strengthening the National Healthy School Standard and health-promoting school policies.**

D **Strengthen children's practical understanding about food and nutrition.**

E **Influence the food culture to support a more balanced diet by addressing manufacturing processes and the retailing, marketing and promotion of food as they influence children and young people.**

Increasing physical activity

KEY RECOMMENDATIONS

A **Increase children's and young people's participation in and access to sport and recreation in the community.**

B **Strengthen physical education, sport and active play in schools through a combination of investment, school policies and teaching practices.**

C **Make walking and cycling a healthy means of daily travel for more children and young people.**

Tackling smoking

KEY RECOMMENDATIONS

A Establish a strong national commitment to anti-smoking campaigns and initiatives with a special emphasis in schools.

B Protect unborn babies and young children from the harmful effects of parental smoking.

C Ensure that price and availability are effective disincentives to youth smoking.

D Ban the promotion of tobacco products.

E Help young smokers to stop smoking.

F Create smoke-free environments.

G Recognise the supportive effect of education and welfare policies and initiatives.

References

1 National Heart Forum. 2002. *Towards a Generation Free from Coronary Heart Disease: Policy Action for Children's and Young People's Health and Well-being*. London: National Heart Forum. Available from www.heartforum.org.uk

PART 2

Scientific and policy review

Chapter 1

The foetal and infant origins of coronary heart disease

Professor DJP Barker

MRC Environmental Epidemiology Unit, Southampton General Hospital

This chapter:

- reviews the evidence that cardiovascular disease and type 2 diabetes originate *in utero* in association with altered growth
- demonstrates that people who were small at birth are more vulnerable to the effects of obesity, poor living standards and other adverse influences in adult life, and
- assesses the implications for strategies to prevent coronary heart disease.

Key themes

- People who develop coronary heart disease, hypertension and type 2 diabetes grow differently to other people during foetal life and childhood.
- Slow foetal and infant growth followed by rapid weight gain in early childhood are associated with large increases in disease risk.
- Any effective strategy to prevent coronary heart disease should include:
  - improving body composition and dietary balance among girls and young women
  - protecting the growth of babies *in utero* and during infancy, and
  - preventing rapid weight gain in young children who had low birthweight.

Introduction

The search for biological influences in the adult environment which determine the risk of cardiovascular disease has implicated obesity and cigarette smoking, and evidence on dietary fat has accumulated to the point where a public health policy of reduced intake is prudent. Much, however, remains unexplained. For example, the steep rise in coronary heart disease in many western countries during the 20th century has been associated with rising prosperity, so why, in many countries, do the poorest people in the least affluent places now have the highest rates?

An early clue to the possible importance of the environment in early life came from ecological studies. The geographical distribution of infant mortality in England and Wales in the early years of the last century was found to resemble closely the recent distribution of death rates from coronary heart disease.[1] At that time most deaths in newborn babies were attributed to low birthweight, and one interpretation of the geographical association between coronary heart disease and neonatal mortality (deaths in the first month after birth – see Figure 1) was that harmful influences which act during intra-uterine life, and slow foetal growth, permanently set or 'programme' the body's structure and function in ways which are linked to later coronary heart disease. Since foetal growth is mainly determined by the supply of nutrients, undernutrition was an obvious possible harmful influence. Numerous studies in animals have shown that undernutrition during gestation permanently changes or 'programmes' the body's physiology and metabolism.[2, 3] The geographical association with post-neonatal mortality (deaths from one month to one year) suggested that there was a continuing association between coronary heart disease and undernutrition during infancy.[1]

Figure 1 ***Neonatal mortality in England and Wales, 1911-15, and mortality from coronary heart disease, 1968-78***

Standardised mortality ratio for coronary heart disease 1968-78

150
125
100
75
50

20 30 40 50 60

Neonatal mortality per 1,000 births, 1911-15

London boroughs
County boroughs
Urban districts
Rural districts

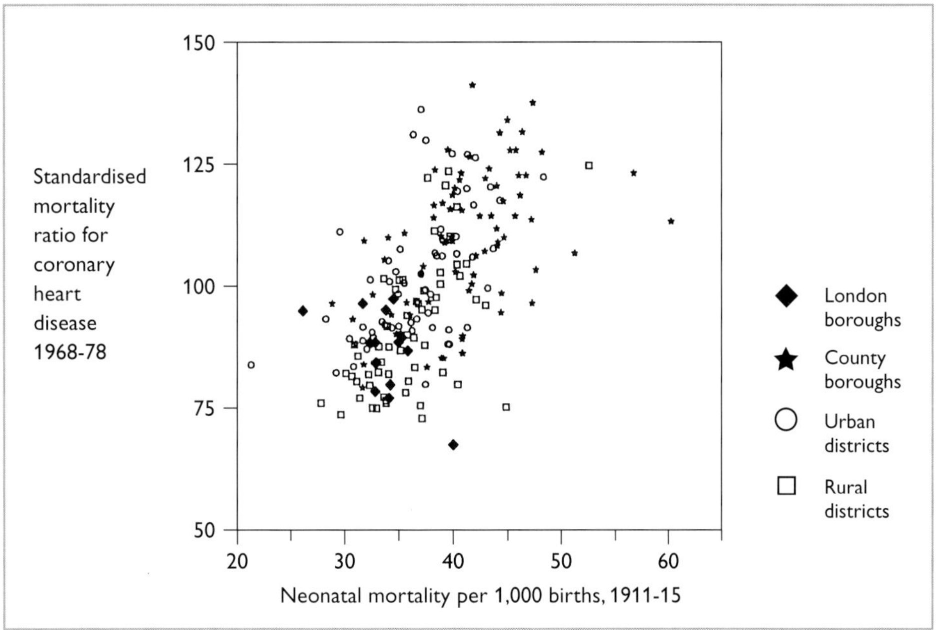

Source: See reference 1.

The undernourished baby

Like other living things humans are 'plastic' during their early development and are readily influenced by the environment. Underlying this is the phenomenon of 'phenotypic plasticity' by which one genotype gives rise to a range of different physiological or morphological states in response to different environmental conditions during development. In foetal life and infancy the tissues and organs of the body go through what are called 'critical' periods of development which often coincide with periods of rapid cell division. 'Programming' describes the process whereby a stimulus or insult at a critical period of development has lasting effects. Rickets has for a long while served as a demonstration that undernutrition at a critical stage of early life leads to persisting changes in the body's structure. Only recently have we realised that some of the persisting effects of early undernutrition become translated into pathology, and thereby determine chronic disease, including coronary heart disease, in later life. That this has gone unremarked for so long is perhaps surprising, given that the heart and blood vessels are 'plastic' during their intra-uterine development, being moulded by the physical and other influences to which they are subjected, and given also the numerous animal experiments showing that undernutrition *in utero* leads to persisting changes in a range of metabolic, endocrine and immune functions known to be important in human disease.[3, 4]

The human foetus adapts to undernutrition by metabolic changes, by redistribution of blood flow and by changes in the production of foetal and placental hormones which control growth.[5] Unlike adaptations made in adult life, foetal adaptations, occurring as they do at the time of the body's most rapid growth, tend to become 'hard-wired' or permanent. The foetus' immediate response to undernutrition is catabolism: it consumes its own substrates to provide energy.[6] One consequence of this may be that the baby sacrifices muscle growth and is born thin. More prolonged undernutrition leads to a slowing in growth. This enhances the foetus' ability to survive by reducing the use of substrates and lowering the metabolic rate. While slowing its rate of growth the foetus may protect tissues that are important for immediate survival, especially the brain. One way in which the brain can be protected is by redistribution of blood flow to favour it.[7] This adaptation is known to occur in many mammals but in humans it has exaggerated costs for growth of the trunk, including the liver and other abdominal viscera, because of the large size of the human brain.

It is becoming increasingly clear that nutrition has profound effects on foetal hormones, and on the hormonal and metabolic interactions between the foetus, placenta and mother on whose coordination foetal growth depends.[6] Foetal insulin and the insulin-like growth factors (IGFs) are thought to have a central role in the regulation of growth and respond rapidly to changes in foetal nutrition. If a mother decreases her food intake, foetal insulin, IGF and glucose concentrations fall, possibly through the effect of decreased maternal IGF. This leads to reduced transfer of amino acids and glucose from mother to foetus, and ultimately to reduced rates of foetal growth.[8] In late gestation and after birth the foetus' growth hormone and IGF axis take over, from insulin, a central role in driving linear growth. Whereas undernutrition leads to a fall in the concentrations of hormones that control foetal growth, it leads to a rise in cortisol, whose main effects are on cell differentiation.[5] One current line of research aims to determine whether the foetus' hormonal adaptations to undernutrition tend, like many other foetal adaptations, to persist after birth and exert lifelong effects on homeostasis and hence on the occurrence of disease.

Animal studies show that a variety of different paths of foetal growth result in similar overall body weight at birth. A foetus that grows slowly throughout gestation may have the same size at birth as a foetus whose growth was arrested for a period and then 'caught up'. Different paths of foetal growth will have different effects on the relative size of different organs at birth, even though overall body weight may be the same. Slowing of growth in late gestation, for example, may be associated with reduced growth of the kidney, whose cells divide rapidly at that time. Animal studies show that blood pressure and metabolism can be permanently changed by levels of undernutrition that do not influence body weight at birth. Preliminary observations point to similar effects in humans,[9] and emphasise the severe limitation of birthweight, unaccompanied by other measures of body size, as a summary of foetal nutritional experience.

Small body size at birth and coronary heart disease

Early epidemiological studies on the intra-uterine origins of coronary heart disease and stroke were based on the simple strategy of examining men and women in middle and late life whose body measurements at birth were recorded. Sixteen thousand men and women born in Hertfordshire during 1911-30 were traced from birth to the present day. Death rates from coronary heart disease fell two-fold between those at the lower and upper ends of the birthweight distribution.[10, 11] A study in Sheffield showed that it was people who were small at birth because they failed to grow, rather than because they were born early, who were at increased risk of the disease.[12] The association between low birthweight and coronary heart disease has been confirmed in studies in Uppsala, Sweden,[13] Helsinki, Finland,[14-16] Caerphilly, Wales,[17] among 80,000 female nurses in the USA,[18] and in a study in South India.[19]

Body proportions at birth and coronary heart disease

The Hertfordshire records and the Caerphilly and Nurses' studies did not include measurements of body size at birth other than weight. The addition of birth length allows a thin baby to be distinguished from a stunted baby with the same birthweight. With the addition of head circumference the baby whose birthweight is low in relation to its head size, which may be a result of 'brain-sparing' redistribution of blood flow, can also be distinguished. Thinness, stunting and a low birthweight in relation to head size are the result of differing foetal adaptations to undernutrition, and other influences, and they have different consequences, both immediately and in the long term.

In South India and Sheffield, higher rates of coronary heart disease were associated with short body length at birth.[19, 20] Thinness at birth, as measured by a low ponderal index (birthweight/length^3), is also associated with coronary heart disease. Table 1 shows findings among 4,630 men born in Helsinki, Finland during 1934-44.[16] While death rates for coronary heart disease were related to low birthweight,[14] there was a much stronger trend with thinness. Interestingly, among women in the same cohort the association between low birthweight and coronary heart disease was similar to that in men, but there was a much stronger association with short body length at birth, and no association with thinness.[15] An inference from this is that at the same levels of maternal nutrition the paths of foetal growth that lead to coronary heart disease differ in girls and boys. Girl foetuses grow more slowly than boys. Slower growing foetuses are in general less vulnerable to undernutrition, and one may speculate that the lower rates of coronary heart disease in women may originate in their slower rates of intra-uterine growth.

Table 1 ***Hazard ratios for coronary heart disease (hospital admissions and deaths) in 4,630 men born in Helsinki in 1934-44, according to body size at birth***

	Hazard ratios (95% confidence interval)	Number of cases/ Number of men
Birthweight (g)		
Up to 2,500	3.63 (2.02 to 6.51)	24/160
– 3,000	1.83 (1.09 to 3.07)	45/599
– 3,500	1.99 (1.26 to 3.15)	144/1,775
– 4,000	2.08 (1.31 to 3.31)	123/1,558
Over 4,000	1.00	21/538
P for trend	0.006	
Ponderal index (kg/m³)		
Up to 25	1.66 (1.11 to 2.48)	104/1,093
25-27	1.44 (0.97 to 2.13)	135/1,643
27-29	1.18 (0.78 to 1.78)	84/1,260
Over 29	1.00	31/578
P for trend	0.0006	

Source: See reference 16.

The associations between body proportions at birth and stroke differ from those for coronary heart disease.[20, 21] Increased risk of stroke is associated with a low ratio of birthweight to head circumference, which may indicate that it is a delayed consequence of brain-sparing adaptations *in utero*.

Small body size in infancy and coronary heart disease

Information routinely recorded in Hertfordshire included the infant's weight at one year. In men, failure of weight gain during the first year of life predicted coronary heart disease and stroke independently of birthweight.[10] Among men who weighed 17 pounds (7.7 kg) or less at age one year, the hazard ratios for coronary heart disease were three times greater than among those who weighed 27 pounds (12.2 kg) or more. Because subsequent studies of the long-term effects of small size at birth have not included data on infant growth, this association between low weight gain in infancy and later coronary heart disease has not been explored. Recently, however, the Hertfordshire findings have been replicated in Helsinki, Finland, where there are two cohorts, an older one born during 1924-33 and a younger one born during 1934-44. Each of the 4,630 men in the younger cohort had his weight and height recorded at birth and at one year, with an average of a further 17 measurements of height and weight between birth and 12 years of age. Table 2 shows that hazard ratios for coronary heart disease fell progressively with increasing weight, height and body mass index at age one year. Small body size at this age predicted coronary heart

Table 2 ***Hazard ratios for coronary heart disease according to body size at one year***

	Hazard ratio (95% confidence interval)	Number of cases/ Number of men
Weight (kg)		
Up to 9	1.82 (1.25 to 2.64)	96/781
– 10	1.17 (0.80 to 1.71)	85/1,126
– 11	1.12 (0.77 to 1.64)	89/1,243
– 12	0.94 (0.62 to 1.44)	49/852
Over 12	1.00	38/619
P for trend	0.0001	
Height (cm)		
Up to 73	1.55 (1.11 to 2.18)	79/636
– 75	0.90 (0.63 to 1.27)	68/962
– 77	0.94 (0.68 to 1.31)	87/1,210
– 79	0.83 (0.58 to 1.18)	64/1,011
Over 79	1.00	59/802
P for trend	0.007	
Body mass index (kg/m^2)		
Up to 16	1.83 (1.28 to 2.60)	72/654
– 17	1.61 (1.15 to 2.25)	89/936
– 18	1.29 (0.91 to 1.81)	83/1,136
– 19	1.12 (0.77 to 1.62)	59/941
Over 19	1.00	54/954
P for trend	0.0004	

Source: See reference 16.

disease independently of size at birth. In a simultaneous analysis with birthweight, the hazard ratio associated with each unit of increase in Z-score for weight between birth and one year was 1.21 (1.08 to 1.36).

Childhood growth

We now know that the path of growth through childhood modifies the risk of coronary heart disease associated with small size at birth and during infancy.[15, 16] Figure 2 shows the growth of 357 men in the 1934-44 Helsinki cohort who were either admitted to hospital with coronary heart disease or died from it. Their growth is expressed as Z-scores. The Z-score for the cohort is set at zero, and a boy maintaining a steady position as large or small in relation to other boys would follow a horizontal path on the figure. Boys who later developed coronary heart disease, however, were small at birth, remained small in infancy but had accelerated gain in weight and body mass index thereafter. In contrast, their heights remained below average.

Figure 2 ***Growth of 357 boys who later developed coronary heart disease in a cohort of 4,630 boys born in Helsinki 1934-44***

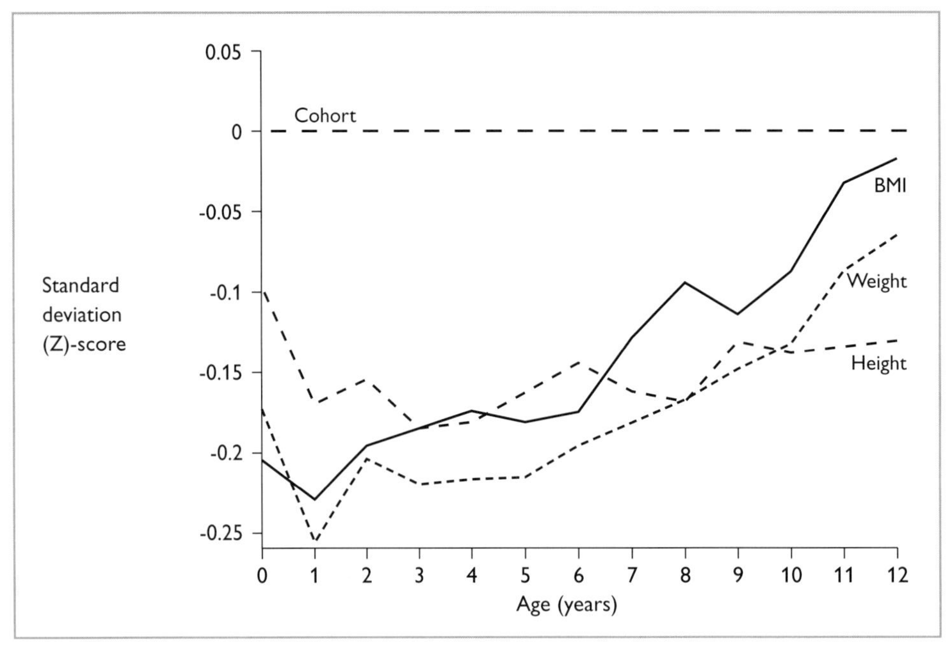

Source: See reference 16.

Figure 3 ***Hazard ratios for coronary heart disease according to ponderal index at birth and body mass index at 11 years in a cohort of 4,630 boys born in Helsinki 1934-44***

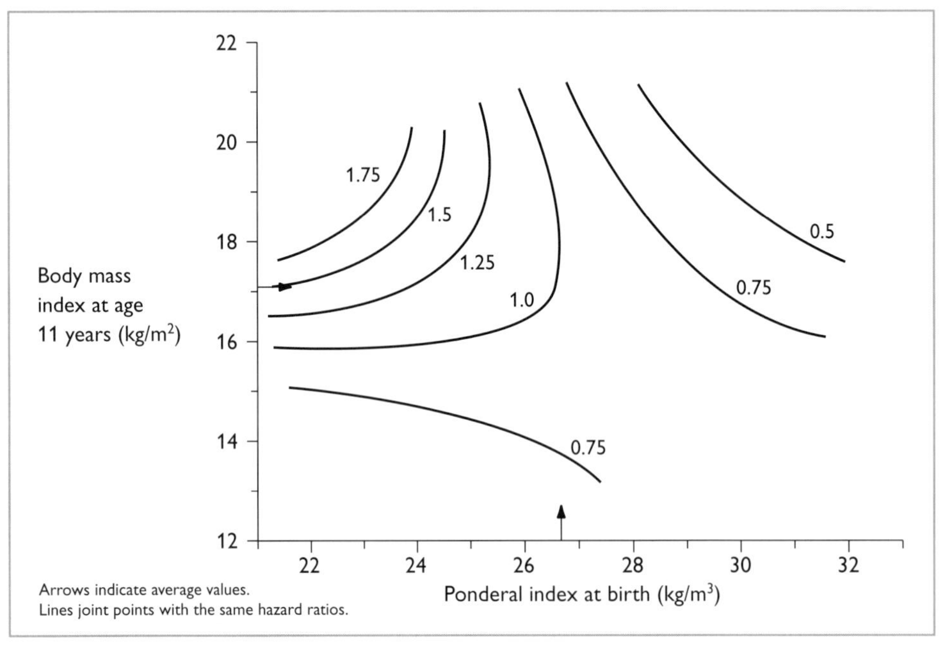

Source: See reference 16.

Table 3 ***Hazard ratios for death from coronary heart disease in 3,639 men born in Helsinki 1924-33 according to ponderal index at birth and body mass index at age 11 years***

Ponderal index (kg/m^3) at birth	Body mass index (kg/m^2) at age 11 years			
	Up to 15.5 (95% CI)	– 16.5 (95% CI)	– 17.5 (95% CI)	Over 17.5 (95% CI)
Up to 25	2.0 (0.8 to 5.4)	2.8 (1.1 to 7.1)	3.1 (1.2 to 8.2)	4.2 (1.5 to 11.6)
– 27	1.2 (0.4 to 3.2)	2.6 (1.0 to 6.7)	3.1 (1.2 to 8.0)	2.3 (0.8 to 6.3)
– 29	1.8 (0.7 to 5.0)	1.3 (0.5 to 3.5)	1.7 (0.6 to 4.4)	2.6 (1.0 to 6.9)
Over 29	1.0	1.3 (0.5 to 3.8)	1.2 (0.4 to 3.4)	1.7 (0.6 to 4.7)

Source: See reference 22.

Figure 3, based on the same data as Figure 2, shows the combined effects of ponderal index at birth and body mass index in childhood. Boys who had a low ponderal index at birth increased their risk of coronary heart disease if they attained even average body mass index in childhood. In contrast, among boys with a high ponderal index no increased risk was associated with a high childhood body mass index.

Table 3 shows deaths from coronary heart disease in the older Helsinki cohort[14] where there was a similar combined effect of low ponderal index and high body mass index at birth on death from coronary heart disease. There are several possible mechanisms by which reduced foetal and infant growth followed by accelerated weight gain in childhood may lead to coronary heart disease. Babies who are thin at birth lack muscle, a deficiency which will persist as the critical period for muscle growth is around 30 weeks *in utero*, and there is little cell replication after birth. If they develop a high body mass index in childhood they may have a disproportionately high fat mass. This may be associated with the development of insulin resistance, as children and adults who had low birthweight but are currently heavy are insulin resistant.

Attributable percentage of cases

The large and detailed data set from Helsinki allows the risk of coronary heart disease associated with poor foetal and infant growth to be quantified.[16] If at birth every boy in this cohort had had a ponderal index above 26kg/m^3, and at one year had been above the cohort average in height (76.2cm) and body mass index (17.7kg/m^2), there would have been a 50% reduction in the number of cases of coronary heart disease occurring before age 65 years. These are modest growth targets. Around three-quarters of all babies born in Southampton today have ponderal indices above 26kg/m^3; and average heights and weights at one year of babies in Britain today are similar to those in the Helsinki cohort. There are obvious reservations about quantifying possible benefit in the UK today from observations made in Finland in the past. Nevertheless, these estimates of risk reduction may be compared with recent estimates that changes in adult lifestyle may reduce the incidence of coronary heart disease by around 8%.[23]

Confounding variables

These observations suggest that influences linked to foetal and infant growth have an important effect on the risk of coronary heart disease and stroke, and that improvement in foetal and infant growth may lead to a substantial reduction in disease incidence. It has been argued, however, that people whose growth was impaired *in utero* and during infancy may continue to be exposed to an adverse environment in childhood and adult life, and it is this later environment that produces the effects attributed to programming.[24-26] There is, however, strong evidence against this. In four of the studies which have replicated the association between birthweight and coronary heart disease, data on lifestyle factors including smoking, employment, alcohol consumption and exercise were collected.[13, 16, 17, 27] The associations between birthweight or infant weight and coronary heart disease remained after allowing for them. In many studies of blood pressure and glucose tolerance, described below, the associations with size at birth have similarly been independent of adult lifestyle.

Effects of adult living standards

Observations on animals show that the environment during development permanently changes not only the body's structure and function but also its responses to environmental influences encountered in later life. Men who had low birthweight are more vulnerable to developing coronary heart disease if they become overweight.[17] Table 4 shows the effect of low income in adult life on coronary heart disease among men in Helsinki.[27] As expected, men who had a low taxable income had higher rates of the disease. The effect of low income, however, was confined to men who had slow foetal growth and were thin at birth, defined by a ponderal index less than $26kg/m^3$. Recent studies in Southampton suggest that this definition includes around one quarter of babies born in Britain today.[28] Men who were not thin at birth were resilient to the effects of low income on coronary heart disease, so that there was statistically significant interaction between the effects of foetal growth and adult income.

The effects of foetal growth on coronary heart disease also interacted with the effects of low social class. Among men with a ponderal index at birth below $26kg/m^3$, low social class was associated with increased hazard ratios for coronary heart disease. Among men in the high ponderal index group, however, there was only a weak trend which became non-significant after adjustment for father's social class. Table 5 is confined to men with a low ponderal index and examines the effect of childhood growth.[27] It shows that the effects of low social class on coronary heart disease were confined to men who were both thin at birth and increased their Z-score for body mass index between 1 and 11 years.

Table 4 ***Hazard ratios for coronary heart disease according to ponderal index at birth (kg/m³) and taxable income in adult life, in men born in Helsinki 1934-44***

Household income in marks per year (£)	Ponderal index 26.0 or below (95% confidence interval) n = 1,475	Ponderal index greater than 26.0 (95% confidence interval) n = 2,154
Over 140,000 (£15,700)	1.00	1.19 (0.65 to 2.19)
111,000-140,000 (£15,700)	1.54 (0.83 to 2.87)	1.42 (0.78 to 2.57)
96,000-110,000 (£12,400)	1.07 (0.51 to 2.22)	1.66 (0.90 to 3.07)
76,000-95,000 (£10,700)	2.07 (1.13 to 3.79)	1.44 (0.79 to 2.62)
75,000 (£8,400)	2.58 (1.45 to 4.60)	1.37 (0.75 to 2.51)
P for trend	<0.001	0.75

Source: See reference 27.

Table 5 ***Hazard ratio for coronary heart disease in men born in Helsinki 1934-44 with a ponderal index at birth below 26kg/m³, according to adult social class and changes in body mass index (BMI) between ages 1 and 11 years***

	Change in Z-score for BMI	
Social class	Decrease (95% confidence interval) n = 536	Increase (95% confidence interval) n = 551
Higher official	0.99 (0.40 to 2.43)	1.00
Lower official	1.03 (0.38 to 2.77)	1.64 (0.67 to 4.03)
Self-employed	0.59 (0.08 to 4.69)	2.36 (0.73 to 7.67)
Labourer	1.76 (0.76 to 4.06)	3.57 (1.72 to 7.41)
P for trend	0.17	<0.001

Source: See reference 27.

One explanation of these findings emphasises the psychosocial consequences of a low position in the social hierarchy, as indicated by low income and social class, and suggests that perceptions of low social status and lack of success lead to changes in neuroendocrine pathways and hence to disease.[29] The findings in Helsinki seem consistent with this. People who are small at birth are known to have persisting alterations in responses to stress, including raised serum cortisol concentrations.[30] Rapid childhood weight gain could exacerbate these effects.

Small body size at birth and hypertension

The trends in coronary heart disease with body size at birth have been found to be paralleled by similar trends in its major biological risk factors – raised blood pressure, impaired glucose tolerance, altered blood lipids and abnormal blood coagulation. An association between low birthweight and raised blood pressure has now been reported in 80 published studies of men, women and children.[31] It has been shown to result from retarded foetal growth rather than premature birth and is not confounded by lifestyle influences. Associations with more precise indices of reduced foetal growth than birthweight have also been described.[32] In different studies babies that are short or thin, have small placentas, or are disproportionately small in relation to the size of their placentas have all been shown to have raised blood pressure.[31-35] These associations between raised blood pressure and differing indices of reduced foetal growth may reflect undernutrition acting at different stages of gestation and programming hypertension through different mechanisms.

Hypertension is associated with the same general pattern of growth as coronary heart disease. Small size at birth is followed by accelerated weight gain. Table 6 is based on 2,997 men and women treated for hypertension in the two Helsinki cohorts[16, 36] and shows the combined effects of birthweight and body mass index at 11 years. The highest risk for hypertension and coronary heart disease occurs among people who had low birthweight but were in the highest body mass index group at 11 years. Similarly to coronary heart disease (see Figure 3), the risk of disease is determined not only by the absolute value of body mass index in childhood but also by the path of growth from birth. It is the tempo of growth as well as the attained body size that determines risk.[36]

A number of possible mechanisms underlying these associations are currently being studied. In children the rise of blood pressure with age is closely related to growth and is accelerated by the adolescent growth spurt. These observations led to the hypothesis that essential hypertension is a disorder of childhood growth,[38] a suggestion which can be reconciled with the association with low birthweight by postulating that accelerated postnatal growth amplifies changes established *in utero*. Studies in Sweden and Finland give support to this.[36, 39] One process which could underlie this is retarded foetal growth which leads to permanently reduced cell numbers in the kidney, in which there is no further cell replication after birth.[40] Subsequent accelerated growth may lead to excessive demand on this limited cell mass. Reduced numbers of nephrons in the kidney may lead to hyperperfusion of each nephron with resulting glomerular sclerosis, further nephron death and a cycle of increasing blood pressure and nephron death.[40] Other mechanisms linking retarded foetal growth and raised blood pressure that are currently under study include reduced elastin deposition in the large arteries during foetal life, with consequent reduced arterial compliance and raised blood pressure,[41] and *in utero* re-setting of the hypothalamic-pituitary-adrenal axis, one of the regulatory mechanisms for blood pressure.[42]

Attributable mortality

The difference in adult systolic blood pressure associated with a 1kg difference in birthweight is around 3.0mm Hg.[31] This is a relatively small effect, although some of

Table 6 ***Odds ratios (95% confidence intervals) for type 2 diabetes and hypertension according to birthweight and body mass index at 11 years: 13,517 men and women born in Helsinki in 1924-44***

	Body mass index at 11 years (kg/m²)			
Birthweight (kg)	Up to 15.7	–16.6	–17.6	Over 17.6
Number of men and women				
– 3.0	991	719	581	560
– 3.5	1,394	1,422	1,264	1,246
– 4.0	827	984	1,122	1,110
Over 4.0	167	254	413	463
Type 2 diabetes (698 cases)				
– 3.0	1.3 (0.6 to 2.8)	1.3 (0.6 to 2.8)	1.5 (0.7 to 3.4)	2.5 (1.2 to 5.5)
– 3.5	1.0 (0.5 to 2.1)	1.0 (0.5 to 2.1)	1.5 (0.7 to 3.2)	1.7 (0.8 to 3.5)
– 4.0	1.0 (0.5 to 2.2)	0.9 (0.4 to 1.9)	0.9 (0.4 to 2.0)	1.7 (0.8 to 3.6)
Over 4.0	1.0	1.1 (0.4 to 2.7)	0.7 (0.3 to 1.7)	1.2 (0.5 to 2.7)
Hypertension (2,997 cases)				
– 3.0	2.0 (1.3 to 3.2)	1.9 (1.2 to 3.1)	1.9 (1.2 to 3.0)	2.3 (1.5 to 3.8)
– 3.5	1.7 (1.1 to 2.6)	1.9 (1.2 to 2.9)	1.9 (1.2 to 3.0)	2.2 (1.4 to 3.4)
– 4.0	1.7 (1.0 to 2.6)	1.7 (1.1 to 2.6)	1.5 (1.0 to 2.4)	1.9 (1.2 to 2.9)
Over 4.0	1.0	1.9 (1.1 to 3.1)	1.0 (0.6 to 1.7)	1.7 (1.1 to 2.8)

Source: See reference 37.

the studies where measurements of size at birth have included placental weight or body length have shown larger associations. In one study the combined effects of birthweight and placental weight ranged over 25mmHg.[33] This is a large effect when compared with the 2mmHg variation in systolic pressure associated with the range of daily sodium intake recorded in 52 countries.[43]

The contrast between the small effects of body size at birth on blood pressure and the large effect on hypertension (Table 6) suggests that lesions that accompany poor foetal growth and tend to elevate blood pressure, such as a reduced number of nephrons, have a small influence on blood pressure within the normal range because counter-regulatory mechanisms maintain normal blood pressure levels. As the lesions progress, however, these mechanisms are no longer able to maintain homeostasis and blood pressure rises. There may be a cycle of rise in blood pressure resulting in further progression of the lesions and further rise in blood pressure.[40] Studies in South Carolina show that among hypertensive patients it tends to be more difficult to control the blood pressures of those with low birthweight by first line medication with diuretics or beta-blocking agents.[44]

Table 7 ***Prevalence of type 2 diabetes and impaired glucose tolerance in men aged 59-70 years***

Birthweight in pounds (kg)	Number of men	% with impaired glucose tolerance or type 2 diabetes (plasma glucose 7.8mmol/l or above)	Odds ratio adjusted for body mass index (95% confidence interval)
5.5 (2.50) or below	20	40	6.6 (1.5 to 28)
– 6.5 (2.95)	47	34	4.8 (1.3 to 17)
– 7.5 (3.41)	104	31	4.6 (1.4 to 16)
– 8.5 (3.86)	117	22	2.6 (0.8 to 8.9)
– 9.5 (4.31)	54	13	1.4 (0.3 to 5.6)
Over 9.5 (4.31)	28	14	1.0
All	370	25	

Source: See reference 45.

Type 2 diabetes

Thirty-eight published studies have now shown associations between low birthweight and altered glucose-insulin metabolism, first reported in Hertfordshire. Table 7 shows the findings among men in Hertfordshire, in whom the prevalence of type 2 diabetes and impaired glucose tolerance fell across the range of birthweight.[45] This association has been confirmed in men and women in other studies.[46-49] Associations with more precise indices of reduced foetal growth, including thinness and shortness at birth, have also been described.[46, 49] These associations are again independent of social class, cigarette smoking, and alcohol consumption. Influences in adult life, however, add to the effects of the intra-uterine environment. The prevalence of impaired glucose tolerance is highest in people who had low birthweight but became obese as adults.[45, 46]

Among the Pima Indians in the US, in whom diabetes in pregnancy is unusually common, young men and women with birthweights over 9.9 pounds (over 4.5 kg) had an increased prevalence of type 2 diabetes.[47] The association between birthweight and diabetes was therefore U-shaped. The increased risk of diabetes among babies with high birthweight was associated with maternal obesity and diabetes. Similar associations between diabetes and high birthweight have been found in the Nurses' Health Study[48] and in India,[50] where babies at increased risk of developing type 2 diabetes were short and fat.

Similarly to coronary heart disease, type 2 diabetes is associated with small size at birth and during infancy followed by accelerated weight gain.[49] Table 6 is based on 698 patients being treated for type 2 diabetes in the two Helsinki cohorts,[16, 36] and shows the combined effects of birthweight and body mass index at 11 years. The highest hazard ratios are among those who had low birthweight but higher body mass index, and again rapid tempo of childhood weight gain increases the risk of later disease independently of the attained body size.

Both insulin resistance and deficiency in insulin production are thought to be important in the pathogenesis of type 2 diabetes.[51] There is evidence that both may be determined in foetal life. Men and women who had low birthweight, or were thin at birth, have a high prevalence of the 'insulin resistance syndrome' in which impaired glucose tolerance, hypertension and raised serum triglycerides occur in the same patient.[52] Findings among men and women who were exposed to the wartime famine in Holland during their intra-uterine lives provide direct evidence that intra-uterine undernutrition is linked to later insulin resistance.[9] Further evidence comes from the observation that mothers who are thin tend to have offspring who are insulin resistant.[53] The association between high birthweight and later type 2 diabetes may be mediated through insulin deficiency rather than resistance.[50] Deficient insulin production may be the consequence of exposure of the foetal endocrine pancreas to raised glucose concentrations.

Size of effect

Table 7 shows that the prevalence of type 2 diabetes and impaired glucose tolerance fell three-fold across the range of birthweight.[45] Findings in Sweden showed a similar fall across the range of ponderal index at birth.[46] After adjustment for body mass index the odds ratio in Table 7 fell six-fold across the range of birthweight. Analysis of the younger Helsinki cohort[16] shows that, if each man and woman had had: a) a birthweight above the median for the cohort, 3.4 kg; b) weight at one year above the median, 10.0 kg; and c) an increase in body mass index between 3 and 12 years below the median increase, 0.5 kg/m^2, there would have been a 62% (95% CI: 43 to 79) reduction in the incidence of type 2 diabetes.

Cholesterol and fibrinogen

The published literature on the association between size at birth and the other biological risk factors for coronary heart disease, raised plasma lipid and fibrinogen concentrations, is limited and smaller than that on the associations between size at birth and blood pressure or glucose-insulin metabolism. In studies in Hertfordshire, low birthweight was associated with low serum HDL cholesterol and raised triglyceride concentrations.[54] In a study in Sheffield in which the birth measurements included abdominal circumference, it was this measurement which most strongly predicted plasma concentrations of total and LDL cholesterol, and apolipoprotein B.[55] A small abdominal circumference predicted raised lipid concentrations in both men and women (see Table 8). Since abdominal circumference at birth reflects, among other things, liver size, and since cholesterol metabolism is regulated by the liver, an inference is that impaired liver growth *in utero* re-sets cholesterol concentration

Table 8 ***Mean serum cholesterol concentrations according to abdominal circumference at birth in men and women aged 50-53 years***

Abdominal circumference in inches (cm)	Number of people	Total cholesterol (mmol/l)	Low density lipoprotein cholesterol (mmol/l)
Up to 11.5 (29.2)	53	6.7	4.5
– 12.0 (30.5)	43	6.9	4.6
– 12.5 (31.8)	31	6.8	4.4
– 13.0 (33.0)	45	6.2	4.0
Over 13.0 (33.0)	45	6.1	4.0
All	217	6.5	4.3
P for trend		0.003	0.0007

Source: See reference 55.

towards a more atherogenic profile. In the Sheffield study a small abdominal circumference also predicted raised plasma fibrinogen concentrations, a measure of blood coagulability that is also controlled by the liver.[56]

Attributable risk

In the Sheffield study the trends in LDL cholesterol concentrations associated with the range of abdominal circumference at birth (see Table 8) were stronger than those associated with the range of adult body mass index.[55] Lowering serum cholesterol concentrations from 6.5 to 6.0mmol/l has been estimated to reduce the risk of coronary heart disease by 30%.[57] The differences in serum cholesterol concentrations associated with the range of abdominal circumference measurements are at least as great.

Mothers and babies today

Hitherto the search for the causes of coronary heart disease, and the way to prevent it, has been guided by a 'destructive' model. The principal causes to be identified are thought to act in adult life and to accelerate destructive processes, for example the formation of atheroma, rise in blood pressure and loss of glucose tolerance. This chapter has summarised the evidence for a new 'developmental' model. The causes to be identified act on the baby and child.

The so-called 'foetal origins' hypothesis resulted from studies of the geographical association between coronary heart disease and poor living standards in England and Wales and the realisation that a poor intra-uterine environment played a major role in this association.[1] Areas of England and Wales with high coronary mortality are characterised historically by poor maternal nutrition and health, reflected in high maternal and neonatal mortality. Today we remain largely ignorant about the impact of maternal nutrition on foetal development.[58] The relatively disappointing effects of dietary interventions in pregnancy on birthweight in humans have led to the erroneous view that foetal nutrition is little affected by maternal nutrition.[6] It is becoming clear, however, that the concept of maternal nutrition must be extended beyond the mother's diet in pregnancy to include her body composition and metabolism both during pregnancy and at the time of conception. Moreover, birthweight is an inadequate summary measure of foetal experience, and we need a more sophisticated view of optimal foetal development which takes account of the long-term sequelae of foetal responses to undernutrition.

Even in the western world, many babies are born thin or stunted. Encouraged by the fashion industry, many young women are unduly thin which, among other effects, may lead to insulin resistance in their babies.[53] Many have diets which are imbalanced according to established criteria, which may be associated with raised blood pressure in their babies.[59, 60] Encouraged by sections of the food industry, others are unduly fat, which leads to a sub-optimal intra-uterine environment which increases the risk of coronary heart disease.[14] If we are to protect babies, we must also protect girls in childhood and adolescence. Body composition is established by childhood growth, and obesity and eating habits are entrained during childhood and adolescence.

Prevention of coronary heart disease

One of the two goals of research into the foetal and infant origins of coronary heart disease is earlier detection and better treatment of disease. The other is prevention of the disease:

1 by improving the body composition and nutrition of girls and young women at the time of conception (that is avoidance of excessive thinness and overweight, and promotion of a balanced diet)

2 by protecting the growth of babies and infants by improving diet during pregnancy and supporting breastfeeding, and

3 by the avoidance of rapid weight gain in childhood among boys and girls who had low birthweight.

There is already sufficient evidence to begin implementing new public health policies without further delay, though a deeper understanding of the biological processes will be needed to refine these policies. Improvements in foetal and infant growth in Britain could lead to a substantial reduction in the incidence of coronary heart disease.

References

1 Barker DJP, Osmond C. 1986. Infant mortality, childhood nutrition and ischaemic heart disease in England and Wales. *Lancet*; 1: 1077-81.

2 McCance RA, Widdowson EM. 1974. The determinants of growth and form. *Proceedings of the Royal Society of London, Series B Biological Sciences*; 185: 1-17.

3 Barker DJP. 1998. *Mothers, Babies and Health in Later Life.* 2nd edition. Edinburgh: Churchill Livingstone.

4 Lucas A, Bock GR, Whelen J (eds.) 1991. Programming by early nutrition in man. In: *The Childhood Environment and Adult Disease.* 1st edition. Chichester: Wiley: 38-55.

5 Fowden AL. 1995. Endocrine regulation of fetal growth. *Reproduction, Fertility and Development*; 7: 351-63.

6 Harding JE. 2001. The nutritional basis of the fetal origins of adult disease. *International Journal of Epidemiology*; 30: 15-23.

7 Rudolph AM. 1984. The fetal circulation and its response to stress. *Journal of Developmental Physiology*; 6: 11-19.

8 Oliver MH, Harding JE, Breier BH, Evans PC, Gluckman PD. 1993. Glucose but not a mixed amino acid infusion regulates plasma insulin-like growth factor-1 concentrations in fetal sheep. *Pediatric Research*; 34; 1: 62-65.

9 Ravelli ACJ, van der Meulen JHP, Michels RPJ, Osmond C, Barker DJP, Hales CN, Bleker OP. 1998. Glucose tolerance in adults after prenatal exposure to famine. *Lancet*; 351: 173-77.

10 Barker DJP, Osmond C, Winter PD, Margetts B, Simmonds SJ. 1989. Weight in infancy and death from ischaemic heart disease. *Lancet*; 2: 577-80.

11 Osmond C, Barker DJP, Winter PD, Fall CHD, Simmonds SJ. 1993. Early growth and death from cardiovascular disease in women. *British Medical Journal*; 307: 1519-24.

12 Barker DJP, Osmond C, Simmonds SJ, Wield GA. 1993. The relation of small head circumference and thinness at birth to death from cardiovascular disease in adult life. *British Medical Journal*; 306: 422-26.

13 Leon DA, Lithell HO, Vagero D, Koupilova I, Mohsen R, Berglund L, Lithell UB, McKeigue PM. 1998. Reduced fetal growth rate and increased risk of death from ischaemic heart disease: cohort study of 15,000 Swedish men and women born 1915-29. *British Medical Journal*; 317: 241-45.

14 Forsen T, Eriksson JG, Tuomilehto J, Teramo K, Osmond C, Barker DJP. 1997. Mother's weight in pregnancy and coronary heart disease in a cohort of Finnish men: follow up study. *British Medical Journal*; 315: 837-40.

15 Forsen T, Eriksson JG, Tuomilehto J, Osmond C, Barker DJP. 1999. Growth in utero and during childhood among women who develop coronary heart disease: longitudinal study. *British Medical Journal*; 319: 1403-07.

16 Eriksson JG, Forsen T, Tuomilehto J, Osmond C, Barker DJP. 2001. Early growth and coronary heart disease in later life: longitudinal study. *British Medical Journal*; 322: 949-53.

17 Frankel S, Elwood P, Sweetnam P, Yarnell J, Davey Smith G. 1996. Birthweight, body-mass index in middle age, and incident coronary heart disease. *Lancet*; 348: 1478-80.

18 Rich-Edwards JW, Stampfer MJ, Manson JE, Rosner B, Hankinson SE, Colditz GA, Willett WC, Hennekens CH. 1997. Birth weight and risk of cardiovascular disease in a cohort of women followed up since 1976. *British Medical Journal*; 315: 396-400.

19 Stein CE, Fall CHD, Kumaran K, Osmond C, Cox V, Barker DJP. 1996. Fetal growth and coronary heart disease in South India. *Lancet*; 348: 1269-73.

20 Martyn CN, Barker DJP, Osmond C. 1996. Mothers' pelvic size, fetal growth, and death from stroke and coronary heart disease in men in the UK. *Lancet*; 348: 1264-68.

21 Eriksson JG, Forsen T, Tuomilehto J, Osmond C, Barker DJP. 2000. Early growth, adult income and risk of stroke. *Stroke*; 31: 869-74.

22 Eriksson JG, Forsen T, Tuomilehto J, Winter PD, Osmond C, Barker DJP. 1999. Catch-up growth in childhood and death from coronary heart disease: longitudinal study. *British Medical Journal*; 318: 427-31.

23 Ebrahim S, Davey Smith G. 1996. *Health Promotion in Older People for the Prevention of Coronary Heart Disease and Stroke*. London: Health Education Authority.

24 Kramer MS, Joseph KS. 1996. Commentary: Enigma of fetal/infant origins hypothesis. *Lancet*; 348: 1254-55.

25 Paneth N, Susser M. 1995. Early origin of coronary heart disease (the 'Barker hypothesis'). *British Medical Journal*; 310: 411-12.

26 Elford J, Whincup P, Shaper AG. 1991. Early life experience and adult cardiovascular disease: longitudinal and case-control studies. *International Journal of Epidemiology*; 20: 833-44.

27 Barker DJP, Forsen T, Uutela A, Osmond C, Eriksson JG. 2001. Size at birth and resilience to effects of poor living conditions in adult life: longitudinal study. *British Medical Journal*; 323: 1273-76.

28 Inskip HM. Unpublished.

29 Marmot M, Wilkinson RG. 2001. Psychosocial and material pathways in the relation between income and health: a response to Lynch et al. *British Medical Journal*; 322: 1233-36.

30 Phillips DIW, Walker BR, Reynolds RM, Flanaghan DEH, Wood PJ, Osmond C et al. 2000. Low birthweight predicts elevated plasma cortisol concentrations in adults from 3 populations. *Hypertension*; 35: 1301-06.

31 Huxley RR, Shiell AW, Law CM. 2000. The role of size at birth and postnatal catch-up growth in determining systolic blood pressure: a systematic review of the literature. *Journal of Hypertension*; 18: 815-31.

32 Barker DJP, Gluckman PD, Godfrey KM, Harding JE, Owens JA, Robinson JS. 1993. Fetal nutrition and cardiovascular disease in adult life. *Lancet*; 341: 938-41.

33 Barker DJP, Bull AR, Osmond C, Simmonds SJ. 1990. Fetal and placental size and risk of hypertension in adult life. *British Medical Journal*; 301: 259-62.

34 Moore VM, Miller AG, Boulton TJC, Cockington RA, Hamilton Craig I, Magarey AM, Robinson JS. 1996. Placental weight, birth measurements, and blood pressure at age 8 years. *Archives of Disease in Childhood*; 74: 538-41.

35 Taylor SJC, Whincup PH, Cook DG, Papacosta O, Walker M. 1997. Size at birth and blood pressure: cross sectional study in 8-11 year old children. *British Medical Journal*; 314: 475-80.

36 Eriksson JG, Forsen T, Tuomilehto J, Osmond C, Barker DJP. 2000. Fetal and childhood growth and hypertension in adult life. *Hypertension*; 36: 790-04.

37 Barker DJP, Eriksson JG, Forsen T, Osmond C. 2002. Fetal origins of adult disease: strength of effects and biological basis. *International Journal of Epidemiology*; 31: 1235-39.

38 Lever AF, Harrap SB. 1992. Essential hypertension: a disorder of growth with origins in childhood? *Journal of Hypertension*; 10: 101-20.

39 Leon DA, Koupilova I, Lithell HO, Berglund L, Mohsen R, Vagero D, Lithell U-B, McKeigue PM. 1996. Failure to realise growth potential in utero and adult obesity in relation to blood pressure in 50 year old Swedish men. *British Medical Journal*; 312: 401-06.

40 Brenner BM, Chertow GM. 1994. Congenital oligonephropathy and the etiology of adult hypertension and progressive renal injury. *American Journal of Kidney Disease*; 23; 2: 171-75.

41 Martyn CN, Greenwald SE. 1997. Impaired synthesis of elastin in walls of aorta and large conduit arteries during early development as an initiating event in pathogenesis of systemic hypertension. *Lancet*; 350: 953-55.

42 Edwards CRW, Benediktsson R, Lindsay RS, Seckl JR. 1993. Dysfunction of placental glucocorticoid barrier: link between fetal environment and adult hypertension? *Lancet*; 341: 355-57.

43 Intersalt Cooperative Research Group. 1988. Intersalt: an international study of electrolyte excretion and blood pressure. Results for 24 hour urinary sodium and potassium excretion. *British Medical Journal*; 297: 319-28.

44 Lackland DT, Egan BM, Syddall HE, Barker DJP. 2002. Associations between birthweight and antihypertensive medication in black and white Americans. *Hypertension*; 39: 179-83.

45 Hales CN, Barker DJP, Clark PMS, Cox LJ, Fall C, Osmond C, Winter PD. 1991. Fetal and infant growth and impaired glucose tolerance at age 64. *British Medical Journal*; 303: 1019-22.

46 Lithell HO, McKeigue PM, Berglund L, Mohsen R, Lithell UB, Leon DA. 1996. Relation of size at birth to non-insulin dependent diabetes and insulin concentrations in men aged 50-60 years. *British Medical Journal*; 312: 406-10.

47 McCance DR, Pettitt DJ, Hanson RL, Jacobsson LTH, Knowler WC, Bennett PH. 1994. Birth weight and non-insulin dependent diabetes: thrifty genotype, thrifty phenotype, or surviving small baby genotype? *British Medical Journal*; 308: 942-45.

48 Rich-Edwards JW, Colditz GA, Stampfer MJ, Willett WC, Gillman MW, Hennekens CH, Speizer FE, Manson JE. 1999. Birthweight and the risk for type 2 diabetes mellitus in adult women. *Annals of Internal Medicine*; 130: 278-84.

49 Forsen T, Eriksson J, Tuomilehto J, Reunanen A, Osmond C, Barker D. 2000. The fetal and childhood growth of persons who develop type 2 diabetes. *Annals of Internal Medicine*; 133: 176-82.

50 Fall CHD, Stein CE, Kumaran K, Cox V, Osmond C, Barker DJP, Hales CN. 1998. Size at birth, maternal weight, and type 2 diabetes in South India. *Diabetic Medicine*; 15: 220-27.

51 DeFronzo RA. 1988. The triumvirate: beta cell, muscle, liver. A collusion responsible for NIDDM. *Diabetes*; 37: 667-87.

52 Barker DJP, Hales CN, Fall CHD, Osmond C, Phipps K, Clark PMS. 1993. Type 2 (non-insulin-dependent) diabetes mellitus, hypertension and hyperlipidaemia (syndrome X): relation to reduced fetal growth. *Diabetologia*; 36: 62-67.

53 Mi J, Law CM, Zhang K-L, Osmond C, Stein CE, Barker DJP. 2000. Effects of infant birthweight and maternal body mass index in pregnancy on components of the insulin resistance syndrome in China. *Annals of Internal Medicine*; 132: 253-60.

54 Fall CHD, Osmond C, Barker DJP, Clark PMS, Hales CN, Stirling Y, Meade TW. 1995. Fetal and infant growth and cardiovascular risk factors in women. *British Medical Journal*; 310: 428-32.

55 Barker DJP, Martyn CN, Osmond C, Hales CN, Fall CHD. 1993. Growth in utero and serum cholesterol concentrations in adult life. *British Medical Journal*; 307: 1524-27.

56 Martyn CN, Meade TW, Stirling Y, Barker DJP. 1995. Plasma concentrations of fibrinogen and factor VII in adult life and their relation to intra-uterine growth. *British Journal of Haematology*; 89: 142-46.

57 Wald NJ, Marmot M, Elliott P (eds.) 1992. Cholesterol and coronary heart disease: to screen or not to screen. In: *Coronary Heart Disease Epidemiology*. Oxford: Oxford University Press: 358-68.

58 Godfrey KM, Barker DJP. 2001. Fetal programming and adult health. *Public Health Nutrition*; 4; 2B: 611-24.

59 Campbell DM, Hall MH, Barker DJP, Cross J, Shiell AW, Godfrey KM. 1996. Diet in pregnancy and the offspring's blood pressure 40 years later. *British Journal of Obstetrics and Gynaecology*; 103: 273-80.

60 Shiell AW, Campbell-Brown M, Haselden S, Robinson S, Godfrey KM, Barker DJP. 2001. High-meat, low-carbohydrate diet in pregnancy: relation to adult blood pressure in the offspring. *Hypertension*; 38: 1282-88.

Chapter 2

Coronary heart disease morbidity by age 53 years in relation to childhood risk factors in the 1946 birth cohort

Professor Michael Wadsworth

Dr Rebecca Hardy

Department of Epidemiology and Public Health, Royal Free and University College London Medical School

This chapter:

- describes the prevalence of ischaemic heart disease morbidity by age 53 years in a nationally representative birth cohort

- shows that the unadjusted childhood risks for heart disease by that age were: poor socioeconomic circumstances, poor height growth by 4 years, and low intake of dietary vitamin C

- shows that other unadjusted risks were parental heart disease, smoking by age 20 years, high body mass index at 43 years, and not taking part in sports at any age, and

- concludes that the independent risk factors were poor home circumstances in early life (represented by crowding at 2 years), smoking by age 20 years, and at 43 years being overweight or obese and not taking part in sport.

Key themes

- Preventive action for reduction of risk of heart disease in the future generation could usefully be taken at the population level by reducing child poverty.
- Preventive action at the individual level in childhood should aim to maximise growth through diet and physical activity, and in adolescence to reduce smoking.
- Preventive action for adults should aim to reduce body mass index and to increase sports activity.

Aim

Increasingly there is evidence that some aspects of cardiovascular disease risk may be found in early life.[1] (See chapter 1.) This chapter reports ischaemic heart disease (IHD) morbidity by age 53 years in a representative national study population on which information on health and development has been collected since birth. The following analysis uses that information to ask whether those with IHD morbidity differ from others in terms of their early life development, nutrition, early smoking habits, and mid-life body size, socioeconomic circumstances and health-related habits.

Methods

The study population is the MRC National Survey of Health and Development, which is a class-stratified sample (N = 5,362) of all births that occurred in England, Wales and Scotland in the week 3-9 March 1946. Information and measurements on health have been collected from this sample in childhood and adolescence (12 times before the age of 20 years), and in adulthood (8 times), most recently at age 53 years. Further details of the study, including information on representativeness and response rates, are given elsewhere.[2,3]

Data on ischaemic heart disease morbidity

Heart disease morbidity was defined as disease classified as ICD9 410-414, that is all forms of ischaemic heart disease. Morbidity information was ascertained from reports to nurses of doctor-diagnosed and treated disease at interviews at ages 36, 43 and 53 years, and from answers to the *Rose angina questionnaire* at ages 43 and 53 years. All reports of hospital in-patient care for ischaemic heart disease were checked with hospitals. The maximum number included in the analysis comprises those who provided information at 36 years, so there is a total of 251 cases and a sample size of 3,322.

Risk factor data

The risk factor data collected for the survey are shown in Table 1.

Table 1 ***Data collected in the MRC National Survey of Health and Development***

Data on early life risk factors	
Prenatal growth	Birthweight.
Postnatal growth	Height at 4 years.
Socioeconomic circumstances	Father's social class (non-manual/manual) when the child was aged 4 years. Crowding in terms of number of persons per room at age 2 years. Low = 0.5 or fewer persons per room. Medium = 1-1.5 persons per room. High = more than 1.5 persons per room.
Diet	Mother's report of one day of diet at age 4 years. The information used here was: – weight of fruit and vegetables consumed – percentage of energy derived from fat – intake of vitamin C in mg per day and – intake of vitamin E in micrograms per day. For more details see Prynne et al, 1999[4].
Data on childhood and adolescent risk factors	
Heart signs	Ascertained by doctors at ages 6, 7, 11 and 15 years.
Body size	Relative weight at 11 and 15 years.
Teachers' assessments of energy	Very energetic/normally energetic/always tired.
Data on early adult risk (20 years)	
Reported smoking	Cigarettes per day at age 20 years. This information is available only for those who responded to a postal questionnaire at this age.
Data on later adult risk (at 43 years)	
Socioeconomic circumstances	Own occupational social class (non-manual/manual).
Body shape	Body mass index (BMI, i.e. kg/m^2), computed from nurse measures of height and weight.
Leg length	Measured standing height minus measured sitting height.
Reported sport participation	In previous 4 weeks – Yes/No.
Reported alcohol consumption	In units.
Data on familial risk	
Parental ischaemic heart disease and parental diabetes	Defined in the same way as for cohort members. Data were derived from cohort members' reports and from parents' death certificates.

Region of residence at birth, and sex, were considered as confounding factors.

Statistical analysis

A model for interval censored data was used with the three time periods of interest being up to 36 years of age, from 36 to 43 years, and from 43 to 53 years. The probability of reporting heart disease conditional on being disease-free at the start of the time period was modelled, and the estimates of effect are expressed in terms of hazard ratios (HR).

Results

The percentage of cohort members reporting heart disease in each time period increased with age (see Table 2). There was little difference between men and women overall, although the incidence was greater for men at younger ages and greater for women at older ages (perhaps because of more deaths among the men). At the oldest ages, the incidence was highest in the North of England and lowest in the Midlands and Wales. At younger ages, incidence was higher in Scotland. Neither sex (P=0.92) nor region of residence at birth (P=0.17) was associated with risk of heart disease.

Table 2 ***Heart disease morbidity within each age group, by sex and region of residence at birth***

	Up to 36 years	36-43 years	43-53 years
Total	27/3,322 (0.8%)	99/2,968 (3.3%)	125/2,507 (5.0%)
Men	18/1,666 (1.1%)	48/1,488 (3.2%)	60/1,290 (4.7%)
Women	9/1,656 (0.5%)	51/1,480 (3.5%)	65/1,217 (5.3%)
Midlands/Wales	10/986 (1.0%)	25/882 (2.8%)	28/748 (3.7%)
South of England	7/1,142 (0.6%)	36/1,038 (3.5%)	41/856 (4.7%)
Scotland	6/373 (1.6%)	15/322 (4.7%)	14/272 (5.2%)
North of England	4/821 (0.5%)	23/726 (3.2%)	42/622 (6.8%)

Analysis of early life factors, adjusted only for period of time (see Table 3), indicated that father's manual social class (HR = 1.64; 95% CI 1.24 to 2.17, P=0.0005), crowding at 2 years (HR = 2.15; 95% CI 1.61 to 2.88 for least versus most crowded, P=0.0001), short height at 4 years (HR = 0.96; 95% CI 0.94 to 0.99 per cm increase in height, P=0.002), and low vitamin C intake at 4 years (HR = 0.95; 95% CI 0.90 to 1.00 per 10mg per day increase in vitamin C, P=0.04) were associated with an increased probability of heart disease in adulthood. Weight of fruit consumed at 4 years also showed some relationship (P=0.06) with heart disease risk, but that was accounted for by vitamin C intake and hence only vitamin C intake was considered in further analyses. The association of the HR of vitamin C intake in fifths with ischaemic heart disease morbidity is shown in Figure 1.

Table 3 ***Estimates of hazard ratio adjusted for period of time (age) only***

Variable	Hazard ratio	(95% confidence interval)	P-value
Birth weight (per kg)	0.88	(0.69 to 1.12)	0.3
Height at 4 years (per cm)	0.96	(0.94 to 0.99)	0.002
Father's social class at 4 years			
Non-manual	1		0.0005
Manual	1.64	(1.24 to 2.17)	
Crowding at 2 years			
Low	1		0.0001
Medium	1.25	(0.90 to 1.74)	
High	2.15	(1.61 to 2.88)	
Weight of fruit consumed at 4 years (per 10g per day)	0.98	(0.95 to 1.00)	0.06
Weight of vegetables consumed at 4 years (per 10g per day)	0.99	(0.97 to 1.02)	0.5
Fat in total calories at 4 years (per %)	1.01	(0.99 to 1.03)	0.5
Vitamin C at 4 years (per 10mg per day)	0.95	(0.90 to 1.00)	0.04
Vitamin E at 4 years (per µg per day)	1.01	(0.87 to 1.18)	0.91
Parental heart disease			
No	1		0.0004
Yes	1.75	(1.28 to 2.39)	
Relative weight at 11 years (per 10%)	1.01	(0.91 to 1.12)	0.9
Relative weight at 15 years (per 10%)	1.03	(0.93 to 1.15)	0.6
Energy at 15 years			
Very energetic	1		0.6
Normally energetic	1.16	(0.63 to 2.14)	
Always tired	1.44	(0.67 to 3.10)	
Heart signs in childhood			
No	1		0.3
Yes	0.83	(0.59 to 1.16)	
Smoker at 20 years			
Never	1		0.0007
Ex-smoker	1.59	(1.00 to 2.52)	
Current smoker	1.84	(1.33 to 2.55)	
BMI at 43 years (per kg/m^2)	1.08	(1.05 to 1.10)	0.0001
Leg length at 43 years (per cm)	0.99	(0.97 to 1.01)	0.4
Social class at 43 years			
Non-manual	1		0.0001
Manual	1.75	(1.34 to 2.27)	
Sports participation at 43 years			
Yes	1		0.0003
No	1.61	(1.24 to 2.08)	
Alcohol intake at 43 years (per 10 units)	1.00	(0.99 to 1.02)	0.9

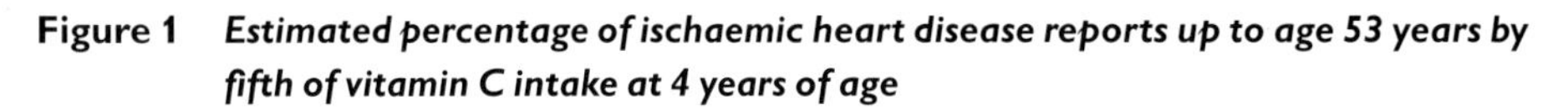
Figure 1 ***Estimated percentage of ischaemic heart disease reports up to age 53 years by fifth of vitamin C intake at 4 years of age***

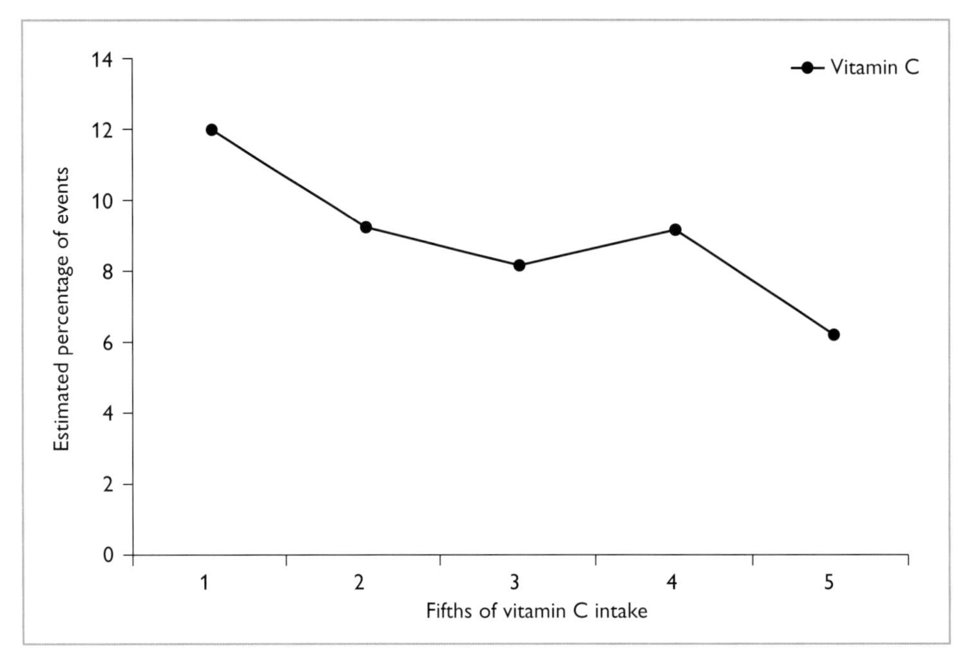

Both crowding (P=0.005) and father's social class (P=0.03) were independently associated with heart disease in adulthood, even after adjustment for the potential confounding factors of sex and region of residence at birth. Height at 4 years and vitamin C intake were confounded by the socioeconomic factors (see Table 4) as well as region of residence at birth.

Having a parent with heart disease was associated with an increased risk of adult heart disease (HR =1.75; 95% CI 1.28 to 2.39, P=0.0004). This effect remained independently associated with the outcome once the early life factors were taken into account as well as after adjustment for sex and region. The effects of both of the early life socioeconomic indicators also remained unchanged in this adjusted model (see Table 5). None of the childhood and adolescent factors considered showed a significant association with heart disease (P>0.1 in all cases).

In an analysis of early adult data, adjusted for period only, smoking behaviour at 20 years was associated with risk of heart disease in later adulthood (P=0.0007). Those who reported being current smokers (HR =1.84; 95% CI 1.33 to 2.55) or ex-smokers (HR =1.59; 95% CI 1.00 to 2.52) were at an increased risk of heart disease compared with those who had never smoked by that age. In the reduced sample of cohort members with data on smoking, the effect of father's social class on heart disease was reduced, and hence crowding was maintained as the early life indicator of early life social conditions. Smoking at 20 years (P=0.002), parental heart disease (P=0.0004),

Table 4 ***Adjusted estimates for early life factors***

Variable	Hazard ratio	(95% confidence interval)	P-value
Father's social class			
Non-manual	1		0.06
Manual	1.37	(0.99 to 1.89)	
Crowding at 2 years			
Low	1		0.003
Medium	1.17	(0.81 to 1.68)	
High	1.87	(1.32 to 2.63)	
Height at 4 years (per cm)	0.98	(0.96 to 1.01)	0.2
Vitamin C at 4 years (per 10mg per day)	0.98	(0.92 to 1.04)	0.5

Weight of fruit intake is not included as it is highly correlated with vitamin C intake. All estimates are adjusted for the other variables listed in the table and period of time.

Table 5 ***Adjusted estimates for early life factors and parental heart disease***

Variable	Hazard ratio	(95% confidence interval)	P-value
Father's social class			
Non-manual	1		0.04
Manual	1.41	(1.02 to 1.95)	
Crowding at 2 years			
Low	1		0.005
Medium	1.18	(0.81 to 1.71)	
High	1.85	(1.29 to 2.66)	
Parental heart disease			
No	1		0.04
Yes	1.68	(1.18 to 2.38)	

All estimates are adjusted for the other variables listed in the table as well as sex, region of residence at birth and period of time.

and crowding at 2 years (P=0.001) remained associated with heart disease in an adjusted model, and these findings were maintained after adjustment for sex and region.

In analyses of the factors from age 43 years, adjusted for period only (see Table 3), high BMI at 43 years (HR =1.08; 95% CI 1.05 to 1.10 per kg/m^2 of BMI, P=0.0001), not participating in sport at 43 years (HR =1.61; 95% CI 1.24 to 2.08, P=0.0003), and being in a manual social class at 43 years (HR =1.75; 95% CI 1.34 to 2.27, P=0.0001) were all associated with an increased risk of heart disease. Adjusted analyses indicated that all three of these factors remained independently associated with heart disease risk after mutual adjustment. The results remained unchanged after further adjustment for sex and region.

Analyses were then performed to ask whether the later life factors confounded the earlier factors. This showed that when BMI, own social class and sports participation at 43 years were added to a model including crowding at 2 years and smoking at 20 years, all factors remained associated with risk of heart disease both before and after additional adjustment for sex and region of residence at birth (see Table 6). (Neither of these were themselves significantly associated with the outcome, although there was some evidence of an effect of region of residence at birth, with those from the Midlands and Wales having a significantly lower risk of heart disease than those from the North of England [P=0.01].) Sports participation was the weakest effect with a P-value of 0.04. The effect of crowding at age 2 years was weaker (P=0.02), with the increased risk being exclusively among the most crowded group.

Table 6 ***Adjusted estimates for early life and later life factors***

Variable	Hazard ratio	(95% confidence interval)	P-value
Crowding at 2 years			
Low	1		0.02
Medium	0.95	(0.64 to 1.41)	
High	1.60	(1.11 to 2.29)	
Parental heart disease			
No	1		0.002
Yes	1.81	(1.25 to 2.62)	
Smoker at 20 years			
Never	1		0.0001
Ex-smoker	2.01	(1.22 to 3.30)	
Current smoker	1.93	(1.33 to 2.78)	
BMI at 43 years (per kg/m^2)	1.07	(1.03 to 1.10)	0.0001
Social class at 43 years			
Non-manual	1		0.02
Manual	1.45	(1.06 to 1.98)	
Sports participation at 43 years			
Yes	1		0.04
No	1.38	(1.01 to 1.89)	

All estimates are adjusted for the other variables listed in the table as well as sex, region of residence at birth and period of time.

The analyses were repeated to assess whether the effects of the early environment were different in the sample with no familial component of risk. In these analyses those who had a parent die under the age of 60 years from heart disease were excluded. In this restricted sample, the results showed very little difference in terms of

Table 7 ***Estimates of hazard ratio adjusted for period of time (age) only, for those with no parental death from heart disease before the age of 60 years***

Variable	Hazard ratio	(95% confidence interval)	P-value
Birth weight (per kg)	0.85	(0.65 to 1.12)	0.3
Height at 4 years (per cm)	0.96	(0.93 to 0.99)	0.009
Father's social class at 4 years			
Non-manual	1		0.01
Manual	1.47	(1.08 to 1.99)	
Crowding at 2 years			
Low	1		0.0001
Medium	1.28	(0.89 to 1.85)	
High	2.21	(1.59 to 3.06)	
Weight of fruit consumed at 4 years (per 10g per day)	0.98	(0.95 to 1.01)	0.1
Weight of vegetables consumed at 4 years (per 10g per day)	0.99	(0.96 to 1.01)	0.3
Fat in total calories at 4 years (per %)	1.01	(0.99 to 1.04)	0.3
Vitamin C at 4 years (per 10mg per day)	0.93	(0.87 to 0.99)	0.02
Vitamin E at 4 years (per µg per day)	1.02	(0.86 to 1.20)	0.9
Relative weight at 11 years (per 10%)	1.02	(0.91 to 1.14)	0.7
Relative weight at 15 years (per 10%)	1.05	(0.93 to 1.18)	0.5
Energy at 15 years			
Very energetic	1		0.5
Normally energetic	1.23	(0.60 to 2.50)	
Always tired	1.63	(0.68 to 3.93)	
Heart signs in childhood			
No	1		0.6
Yes	0.91	(0.63 to 1.30)	
Smoker at 20 years			
Never	1		0.006
Ex-smoker	1.70	(1.03 to 2.80)	
Current smoker	1.73	(1.21 to 2.48)	
BMI at 43 years (per kg/m^2)	1.08	(1.05 to 1.11)	0.0001
Leg length at 43 years (per cm)	0.98	(0.96 to 1.00)	0.08
Social class at 43 years			
Non-manual	1		0.0001
Manual	1.77	(1.33 to 2.37)	
Sports participation at 43 years			
Yes	1		0.009
No	1.46	(1.10 to 1.93)	
Alcohol intake at 43 years (per 10 units)	1.01	(0.99 to 1.02)	0.5

This table excludes survey members who had a parent who died of heart disease at a young age (under 60 years). Forty cases out of the total of 251 were excluded on this basis. The results are not very different to those for the unrestricted sample (see Table 3). A model including social class, crowding, vitamin C intake and childhood height results in the same findings as those for the unrestricted sample as well.

the unadjusted estimated effects (see Table 7), although the power of the analysis was reduced because of the smaller sample size. The effects of vitamin C intake and leg length appear to be slightly stronger in this group. Further multiple regression models were also very similar to those observed for the whole sample and all the same factors reached statistical significance.

Conclusion

This first analysis of heart disease in the 1946 birth cohort showed that factors independently associated with ischaemic heart disease morbidity by age 53 years were from early life (crowding), from early adulthood (smoking), from age 43 years (high BMI, manual social class, no sports participation), and from parental illness. Vitamin C was the dominant factor in the data on diet at 4 years, although its effect was confounded by socioeconomic factors. It may be that the association with parental disease represents a genetic source of risk.

Later born cohorts are likely to have different patterns of risk. High adult body mass is increasing in younger born cohorts, but sports participation seems to be more prevalent, and smoking less prevalent. Although a comparison of data on diet at 4 years used in this analysis with data on diet of 4 year olds in 1992 showed similar intakes of vitamin C, food sources of vitamin C in the most recently born group were limited mostly to drinks, whereas those born in 1946 obtained their vitamin C mostly from fruit and vegetables,[4] i.e. from more complex and mineral-rich sources.

References

1 Barker DJP. 1994. *Mothers, Babies, and Disease in Later Life.* London: British Medical Journal Publishing.

2 Wadsworth MEJ, Mann SL, Rodgers B, Kuh DJL, Hilder WS, Yusuf EJ. 1992. Loss and representativeness in a 43 year follow-up of a national birth cohort. *Journal of Epidemiology and Public Health*; 46: 300-04.

3 Wadsworth MEJ, Kuh DJL. 1997. Childhood influences on adult health: a review of recent work from the British 1946 national birth cohort study. *Paediatric and Perinatal Epidemiology*; 11: 2-20.

4 Prynne CJ, Paul AA, Price GM, Day KC, Hilder WS, Wadsworth MEJ. 1999. Food and nutrient intake in a national sample of 4-year-old children in 1950: comparison with the 1990s. *Public Health Nutrition*; 2: 537-47.

Chapter 3

Physiological measurements in children and young people, and risk of coronary heart disease in adults

Dr Peter McCarron

Department of Epidemiology and Public Health, Queen's University Belfast

Professor George Davey Smith

Department of Social Medicine, University of Bristol

This chapter:

- reviews the coronary risk associated with early life measures of blood pressure, body size, blood lipids, glucose, insulin and also newer circulatory risk factors
- details the tracking of physiological risk factors from childhood into later life and summarises the current trends in these risk factors
- discusses the importance of clustering of these coronary risk factors in early life, and
- outlines the priorities and prerequisites for a future coronary heart disease prevention strategy aimed at young individuals.

Key themes

- A growing body of research indicates that, as in adults, several physiological variables measured in childhood and adolescence are associated with increased risk of coronary heart disease.
- Mildly raised blood pressure, short stature, and overweight (particularly for individuals who remain overweight as adults), and adverse levels of circulatory risk factors (including blood lipids, glucose, and insulin) increase coronary risk. High levels of C-reactive protein and homocysteine also appear to be associated with greater coronary risk.
- Several risk factors track from early life into adulthood. They also cluster in early life and there is a dose-response relationship between the number of early life risk factors and later coronary risk.
- Favourable secular trends have been occurring in blood pressure, height and blood lipids in young individuals, but obesity is increasing among this age group.
- A coronary prevention strategy targeted at young individuals will have to include equitable, population-based interventions to improve nutrition and increase participation in physical activity.
- Improvement in early life coronary risk profile will benefit not only the coronary health of today's children, but possibly also that of future generations.

Introduction

Although death from coronary heart disease (CHD) declined in developed countries during the latter part of the last century[1, 2] it nevertheless remains a major health problem, accounting for 25% of all deaths in the UK.[1] Recent data for England even suggest that CHD prevalence rates in men and women may be increasing,[3] although this may be attributed to declining case fatality. A recent Japanese study has reported an increase in atherosclerotic lesions in young males,[4] while in developing countries CHD is projected to become the leading cause of death by 2020.[5] It is certainly likely that CHD will remain a major health burden for the foreseeable future and will continue to warrant a substantial effort aimed at prevention.

Research to improve understanding of CHD aetiology, and hence to develop interventions to decrease the CHD burden, concentrated until relatively recently on mid-life biological and behavioural factors. Subsequent health interventions have contributed to favourable changes in the distribution of these 'risk factors', which include raised blood pressure, obesity, adverse blood lipid profile, and cigarette smoking in adults, and hence to CHD decline. It has recently been estimated that up to 75% of the CHD burden can be explained by traditional adult risk factors,[6] indicating that other factors are responsible for only 25% of this burden. Newer risk factors have been identified, and a further key development has been research demonstrating that CHD risk begins in early life. Indeed, given that early-life exposures, such as behavioural and socioeconomic risk factors, may strongly influence adult risk factors, and in view of interactions between early-life and adult risk profiles, it is likely that substantially more than 25% of CHD is attributable to factors other than mid-life exposures.

Autopsies of young men who were killed in the Korean and Vietnam wars demonstrated that atherosclerosis, the precursor of CHD, was already present.[7, 8] A limitation precluding generalisation of these findings was that the young men with severe atherosclerosis came from populations with extremely high rates of adult CHD. However, more recently autopsies on population-representative 15-34 year old men and women from across the US who died from external causes have confirmed these findings. In these individuals fatty streaks and fibrous plaques, which are believed to lead to atherosclerosis, were observed in early adolescence and increased in prevalence with age.[9] The earlier observations prompted prospective studies to investigate factors responsible for the development of atherosclerosis in early life.[10, 11]

A different research tradition has developed from the work of Forsdahl, who showed that areas with high infant mortality rates in the early 20th century had high CHD rates subsequently, suggesting that deprivation in early life increased risk of CHD in later life.[12, 13] Research has more recently been undertaken to investigate the foetal origins of CHD risk and has also considered how socially patterned exposures acting in childhood may increase later CHD risk.[12, 14-17] The role of foetal development and childhood socioeconomic circumstances are reviewed elsewhere in this report. (See Chapters 1 and 4.)

Childhood and adolescence also appear to be crucial phases for determining later coronary health.[18] This is important not least because it raises the possibility of developing interventions which can be targeted at prevention or reversal of adverse risk profiles in this age group, thus lessening the future burden of CHD. Such an approach is currently more feasible and likely to be more acceptable than efforts to modify foetal development.

In this review, after briefly summarising the associations between adult physiological risk factors and CHD, the roles of physiological factors measured in childhood and adolescence in determining coronary risk are discussed. These include blood pressure, growth and height, adiposity, blood lipids, glucose and insulin, and also novel risk factors such as homocysteine and C-reactive protein. Findings from the studies which have examined associations between early life factors and risk of CHD are presented. For many studies to date there has not been sufficient time to accrue enough cases to permit robust analysis of the association between early life risk factors and CHD, and so associations between early-life exposures, and both risk factor levels in adulthood, and intermediate outcomes or proxies for CHD (autopsy evidence of fatty streaks, fibrous plaques, coronary artery calcification, arterial distensibility and frank atherosclerosis) are also reviewed. Details of tracking and clustering of risk factors and also current trends in risk factors are discussed. Finally, recommendations for primary prevention are presented.

Blood pressure

Blood pressure in adults and CHD

Observational studies in adults show that both systolic and diastolic blood pressure are positively associated with risk of CHD.[19-24] A meta-analysis of most prospective observational studies showed that risk reductions of up to 37% can be anticipated from a 5-6mmHg lowering of usual diastolic blood pressure.[19] The corresponding figure from randomised trials is 14%,[25,26] and it is not certain whether the discrepancy is due to side effects of antihypertensive drugs, the fact that long-term influences of blood pressure are important, or chance. Importantly, there is no evidence of any threshold below which lower levels of blood pressure are not associated with lower risks of CHD.[21]

Blood pressure in childhood and adolescence, and CHD

The phenomenon of blood pressure tracking from childhood into adulthood,[27-29] with those in the upper segment of the distribution in early life being more likely to have raised blood pressure in later life,[30] suggests that blood pressure in young individuals is likely to be important. Confirmation of this comes from two studies from university settings which have reported on the role of blood pressure in adolescence and later CHD. In the Harvard and Pennsylvania alumni follow-up studies, mildly raised blood pressure was, in a group of male students who were examined between 1916 and 1950 at an average age of 19 years, associated with increased CHD morbidity and mortality over the subsequent 50 years.[31,32] As shown in Table 1, individuals with non-fatal or fatal CHD had mildly elevated blood pressure compared to non-cases and, although no adjustment was made for confounding factors, the findings suggest that even moderately raised blood pressure in early life is deleterious to future coronary health. In a follow-up of Glasgow University students who had detailed medical examinations carried out at a mean age of 20 years from 1948-68[33] both systolic and diastolic blood pressure were positively associated with risk of CHD mortality in men.[34] The hazard ratios (95% confidence interval [95% CI]) per 10mmHg increase in systolic and diastolic blood pressure were, after adjusting for the potential confounders of height, father's social class, cigarette smoking and birth year, 1.15 (95% CI: 1.04 to 1.26) and 1.10 (95% CI: 0.95 to 1.29) respectively. Thus, at a relatively young age and in a population in which the majority (68.5%) were normotensive (blood pressure below 140/90mmHg) with a further 27.6% having a blood pressure over 160/100mmHg, there is already a notable increase in risk of CHD associated with higher blood pressure.

Table 1 ***Comparison of mean systolic and diastolic blood pressure in males attending Harvard and Pennsylvania Universities and risk of non-fatal and fatal CHD***

Condition	Mean systolic blood pressure (sd) mmHg		Mean diastolic blood pressure (sd) mmHg	
	Disease		Disease	
	Present	Absent	Present	Absent
Non-fatal CHD[31]	124.0 (13.0)	120.8 (12.6)	74.7 (9.8)	73.0 (9.1)
Fatal CHD[32]	123.8 (14.8)	120.0 (12.8)	75.3 (10.6)	72.8 (9.2)

sd = standard deviation
Source: See references 31 and 32.

In both the Harvard and Pennsylvania[31, 32] and Glasgow[35] alumni studies, students who were hypertensive had even higher risk of non-fatal and fatal CHD. As shown in Table 2, risks of CHD mortality among Glasgow students examined by category of hypertension,[36] are comparable to men from the Chicago Heart Association Detection Project in Industry (CHADPI)[20] who had a mean age of 29.7 years at baseline, and men in the Multiple Risk Factor Intervention Trial study[21] who had their blood pressure measured when they were on average over 45 years.

The role of measurement error – regression dilution bias

Single exposure measurements are likely to be more spread than long-term average or 'true' values and subsequent misclassification of exposure usually leads to dilution of the measure of effect – regression dilution bias.[19, 37-39] In the follow-up of Glasgow University students, use of the mean of four blood pressure measures, instead of the single baseline measure, elevated the risk of CHD mortality from 1.15 to 1.20 for each 10mmHg rise in systolic blood pressure and from 1.10 to 1.58 for the same rise in diastolic blood pressure,[40] indicating that usual blood pressure is a stronger predictor of future risk than once-off measures, and emphasising the need to properly characterise blood pressure in early adulthood before therapeutic interventions are considered.

Table 2 ***Baseline JNC-VI blood pressure classification, blood pressure category and CHD mortality hazard ratios (HR) (95% CI) for former male Glasgow University students, CHADPI men and MRFIT men***

JNC-VI classification[36]	Blood pressure mmHg	Glasgow[35] HR (95% CI)	Chicago[20] HR (95% CI)	MRFIT[21] HR
Optimal	Below 120/80	1.00	1.39 (0.67 to 2.86)	1.00
Normal	120-129/80-84	1.19 (0.62 to 2.32)	1.00	1.30
High normal	130-139/85-89	1.65 (0.88 to 3.12)	1.37 (0.81 to 2.30)	1.67
Stage 1 HT	140-159/90-99	1.66 (0.88 to 3.13)	1.62 (1.00 to 2.61)	2.56
Stage 2 HT	160-179/100-109	2.73 (1.26 to 5.92)	2.51 (1.44 to 4.37)	4.57*
Stage 3 HT	180/110 or above	2.91 (0.80 to 10.55)	3.60 (1.71 to 7.59)	
Trend across categories		0.002	–	<0.001

* Hazard ratio for stage 2 and stage 3 HT combined

CHADPI = Chicago Heart Association Detection Project in Industry

Sources: See references 20, 21, 35 and 36.

Blood pressure in childhood and adolescence, and intermediate CHD endpoints and other measures of CHD risk

Locality-based cardiovascular disease (CVD) death rates provide a useful marker of CHD risk and have been used, in a manner analogous to the analyses of Forsdahl,[12] to explore the association of risk with various childhood factors. A British school-based study found that mean childhood systolic blood pressure was higher in high CVD mortality towns, particularly after adjustment for height, and that this was unaffected by standardisation for birthweight.[41,42] The blood pressure differences were small but suggest that population differences in blood pressure may be environmentally determined, are established at an early age, and could explain geographical differences in disease rates.

In the Bogalusa Heart Study, a long-term epidemiological study of cardiovascular risk factors from birth up to 38 years in a bi-racial population, there was generally a strong positive correlation between the extent of atherosclerotic lesions in healthy children and adolescents who had been killed in traffic accidents and prior systolic and diastolic blood pressure.[10] These results are corroborated by findings from the multicentre Pathobiological Determinants of Atherosclerosis in Youth (PDAY) study in which hypertensive black men aged 15-34 years had more raised lesions in the abdominal aorta and right coronary artery than normotensive black men, despite having a normal lipoprotein profile.[43] The finding, in the same study, of a lower risk of atherosclerotic change in hypertensive white males aged 15-24 years was considered to be due to the very low prevalence of hypertension in this group and not a real effect of hypertension.

Findings from the follow-up of 1,185 male former medical students attending Johns Hopkins University showed that those who had one casual systolic blood pressure reading of 125mmHg or above had over six times the risk of hypertension in later life compared to those with lower blood pressure.[44] Students whose parents were hypertensive had even more dramatically increased risks – a 10-fold and a greater than 12-fold risk being observed for students with high blood pressure who had one and two hypertensive parents, respectively – suggesting again that CHD risk is strongly related to early life blood pressure and also highlighting the intergenerational – perhaps genetic – component of this risk.

Secular trends in blood pressure

The positive associations between early life factors and later CHD, and other measures of CHD risk, should be considered in the context of trends in these factors in children and adolescents. Two university-based studies have shown quite marked declines over a 20-year period from the late 1940s. In the Queen's University, Belfast, blood pressure declined during the period 1948-70 from 131/78mmHg to 123/72mmHg and from 122/78mmHg to 110/70mmHg in males and females, respectively.[45-47] After adjustment for several confounding variables, similar declines were found among students of Glasgow University over the period 1948-68 as shown in Table 3.[48] In the US there has also been an overall decline in blood pressure among adolescents and young adults between the 1960s and early 1990s[49] and furthermore, it appears that there has been a decline in the US in both systolic and diastolic blood pressure across birth cohorts born between 1887 and 1975 for all ages including 18-24 year olds.[50] Recent data from the 1998 Health Survey for England point to continuing downward trends in blood pressure in a similar age group,[3] but too few data have accumulated as yet to confirm this. A recent review of studies documenting trends in blood pressure in early life showed that declines in blood pressure have been taking place in high-income countries in 5-34 year olds of both sexes and from a range of ethnic groups for at least the last 50 years, indicating that exposures acting in early life are important determinants of blood pressure and blood pressure trends.[51]

There is debate about the possible causes of such trends. Alterations in salt intake may be important. A recent systematic review of trials of salt restriction reported only small reductions in blood pressure.[52] However, in adolescents randomised in infancy to a low or a normal sodium diet, systolic and diastolic blood pressure were lower after 15 years in individuals in the intervention arm compared with the control group, suggesting that sodium restriction in infancy may have greater effects on later blood

Table 3 ***Fully adjusted mean blood pressure for male and female Glasgow University students by year of birth band***

Year of birth	Systolic blood pressure (mmHg)	Diastolic blood pressure (mmHg)
	Male (n = 9,248)	
1925-29	134.5 (133.8 to 135.2)	80.3 (79.8 to 80.8)
1930-34	132.6 (132.1 to 133.2)	78.4 (78.1 to 78.8)
1935-39	131.4 (130.8 to 131.9)	76.3 (75.9 to 76.6)
1940-44	130.0 (129.5 to 130.7)	75.5 (75.1 to 75.9)
1945-50	125.7 (125.0 to 126.3)	74.7 (74.2 to 75.1)
P for trend for 1 year increase	<0.001	<0.001
	Female (n = 3,164)	
1925-29	129.0 (127.5 to 130.5)	79.7 (78.7 to 80.6)
1930-34	128.7 (127.9 to 129.5)	79.6 (79.1 to 80.1)
1935-39	122.9 (121.9 to 123.8)	76.4 (75.8 to 77.0)
1940-44	120.9 (120.1 to 121.8)	76.5 (75.9 to 77.0)
1945-50	120.6 (119.8 to 121.4)	77.0 (76.5 to 77.5)
P for trend for 1 year increase	<0.001	<0.001

* Adjusted for age, height, BMI, smoking, father's social class and age at menarche in females

Source: See reference 48.

pressure than salt reductions in adulthood.[53] Although the results are based on only 40% of subjects initially assigned to the normal sodium group and 31% of those in the low sodium group who participated in the follow-up, and should therefore be interpreted with caution, they are, nonetheless, provocative.

More general alterations in childhood diet may also be important. The declines in blood pressure in Glasgow University students from 1948-68 occurred among individuals who were children at a time when there was a trend towards increasing consumption of vegetables, fruit, and cereals. Fruit and vegetables, unlike other foods, were not rationed during the second world war, resulting in a general improvement in quality of diet across the social spectrum.[54-56] That such changes may have contributed to a progressively more favourable blood pressure profile is supported by an American dietary trial in which there were substantial declines in blood pressure in people assigned diets rich in fruit and vegetables compared with controls on a more typical American diet.[57]

Overall, the findings point to the importance of preventing even mildly raised blood pressure in youth. Empirical support for this notion comes from a recent study in which treated hypertensive men with good blood pressure control who were followed up for 20 years had a significantly increased CHD mortality, compared to non-hypertensive men from the same population,[58] suggesting that preventive measures need to be implemented before middle age if the deleterious effects of raised blood pressure are to be successfully combated. The noted secular declines in blood pressure are welcome, but further efforts are need to understand why these have been taking place and to promote the conditions to sustain them.

Height

Since achieved adult height reflects, in part, the influence of growth, nutrition, infections and socioeconomic circumstances in early life, it is important to explore whether height itself, at different stages of development, is related to CHD risk.

Height in adulthood and CHD mortality

Most large studies have reported inverse relationships between adult height and CHD.[59-73] It is possible that the association between foetal growth and adult height could explain these associations. However, two studies have shown that adjustment for birthweight does not significantly modify the height-mortality relationship.[66, 71] Associations with CHD could also reflect childhood growth and environmental conditions. A further possibility is that they are related to adult socioeconomic position although associations have been shown to persist even after adjustment for socioeconomic position in adult life[59, 61, 71, 72] and also for a wider range of adult cardiovascular risk factors, including cholesterol level, blood pressure, and family history of myocardial infarction.[73, 74] Finally, the early stages of disease could lead to reductions in height and thus generate the inverse association with CHD mortality.[61]

Height in childhood and adolescence, and CHD mortality

The problem of having to adjust for cumulative loss of height with ageing is circumvented in studies in which height was measured in early life. Analyses from the Harvard and Pennsylvania alumni studies found that average height of those with self-reported (but medically confirmed) non-fatal CHD was 68.4 inches compared with 69.3 inches in controls.[32] The age-adjusted CHD attack rate increased with decreasing height from 16 per 1,000 in the tallest group, to 41 per 1,000 in the shortest group. For CHD death the unadjusted odds ratio in those with body height less than 68 inches was 1.3 ($p<0.01$).[31] Although no adjustment was made for other known CHD risk factors in these analyses, it is unlikely that confounding could explain such strong associations.

The association between student height and CHD mortality in former Glasgow University students is shown in Table 4.[75] There was a strong graded inverse risk association, with those in the tallest quintile having less than two-thirds the mortality risk of those in the shortest quintile. Since less than 5% of school leavers entered university in Scotland over the period of this study,[76] and the majority of cohort members will have been in a privileged social position in adult life[77] – a situation

Table 4 ***Hazard ratios for CHD mortality by height in 8,361 Glasgow University male former students***

Mean height (m)	Number of deaths	Age-adjusted HR (95% CI)	Fully adjusted* HR (95% CI)
1.67	67	1.00	1.00
1.72	51	1.11 (0.77 to 1.60)	1.13 (0.78 to 1.62)
1.75	53	0.90 (0.63 to 1.29)	0.94 (0.65 to 1.34)
1.79	42	0.72 (0.49 to 1.06)	0.72 (0.49 to 1.06)
1.84	29	0.62 (0.40 to 0.95)	0.64 (0.41 to 0.99)
HR (95% CI) per 10cm increase in height		0.75 (0.62 to 0.91)	0.76 (0.62 to 0.93)
P for trend **		0.004	0.008

* Adjusted for systolic blood pressure, BMI, father's social class, smoking and quintile of birth year

** Using height as a continuous variable

Source: See reference 75.

which also pertained in the US alumni studies – it is unlikely that these associations are attributable to social patterning of adulthood exposures.

Recent evidence from follow-up of the Boyd Orr Study, originally a detailed dietary survey carried out on 3,762 children in the UK in 1935-37,[78] also reported an inverse relationship between height in childhood and adult CHD mortality, with the influence being restricted to leg length and not being evident for trunk length.[79] The associations were considerably stronger than those seen for adult height and CHD risk and were of greater magnitude for measurements taken among pre-pubertal compared to post-pubertal children. Since leg length is the component of childhood stature responsive to environmental influences, the findings may indicate long-term influences of environmental exposures among young children.[80, 81]

While the evidence that height is inversely related to future CHD risk is robust, there has been little research into the role of height dynamics on health risk. One large Finnish study in which the role of catch-up growth in CHD mortality has been examined found that, in women who were short at birth, CHD risk was greatest in those who were tall in childhood.[82] It was hypothesised that postnatal catch-up growth could be deleterious either because overgrowth of a limited cell mass disrupts cell function, or because large body size imposes an excessive metabolic demand on a limited cell mass.

Height in childhood and adolescence, and intermediate CHD endpoints and other measures of CHD risk

Findings from the 1970 British birth survey revealed that 10 year olds living in areas with high cardiovascular mortality were shorter than those living in other areas.[30] Their mothers were also shorter, suggesting that there are persisting geographical differences in the childhood environment that predispose to differences in cardiovascular mortality. These findings were replicated in a more recent UK study,[42] with little additional effect seen following adjustment for social class and birthweight.

The limited evidence on the relationship between height and intermediate CHD outcomes supports the findings from mortality studies, of taller children having more favourable CHD-risk profiles.[83] In the Bogalusa Heart Study the association of alterations in blood lipids with height change over five years was reported in males aged 8-12 years. Significant negative correlations were observed between height change and changes in levels of serum total cholesterol, high-density lipoprotein cholesterol (HDL cholesterol), and low-density lipoprotein cholesterol (LDL cholesterol) after controlling for a range of confounding variables.[83] The decline in HDL cholesterol noted here appears surprising but may be related to sexual maturation, as shown in earlier studies.[84, 85] Apart from this exception, both greater height *per se*, and growth velocity appeared to confer a better cardiovascular risk profile in adolescents.

Trends in height

Studies of British children illustrate that secular increases in height are still occurring.[86, 87] Such increases may be attributed to a variety of factors including improved nutrition or better environmental circumstances. Whatever their cause, continuing secular trends suggest that the full 'genetic potential' for height has not yet been attained and height remains constrained by environmental factors which may be associated with CHD risk.

Weight and obesity

Indices of body weight and obesity

Body mass index (BMI) is the simplest, most stable measure of adiposity or malnutrition for practical use in epidemiological research.[88, 89] Population mean values for BMI provide a simple measure of adiposity and nutritional status. Although skinfold thickness and densitometry are also measured in cohort studies, BMI is easier to measure and therefore tends to be preferred.

Overweight in adulthood and CHD

In most cohorts in which adequate adjustment is made for the effects of smoking and deaths in the first few years of follow-up, there is a strong positive linear relationship seen between BMI and CHD mortality in both men and women.[90-97] In studies where skinfold measurements have been taken, fat distribution has been found to be more or equally predictive of CVD compared with BMI alone.[98-100]

Overweight in childhood and adolescence and CHD

Weight tracks from childhood into adulthood[10, 101] and small increases in BMI in childhood could therefore predict greater BMI in adulthood as well as greater risk of the accompanying constellation of coronary risk factors.[102, 103] It is important to assess whether associations between childhood BMI and mortality are due to the persistence of overweight into adulthood, or due solely to childhood overweight.

The effect of BMI (and occasionally other measures) in childhood, adolescence, and early adulthood on subsequent morbidity and mortality has been examined in several studies (see Table 5). In the US university alumni studies both fatal and non-fatal CHD were more frequent in those who were overweight when much younger.[31, 32] Using ponderal index – height divided by the cube root of weight – as a measure of relative weight, men with a ponderal index less than 12.9 $m/kg^{\sqrt{3}}$ were 1.3 times more likely to die from CHD, and over 1.7 times more likely to have a non-fatal CHD event than their leaner counterparts.

In a cohort of 717 people in their 40s who were originally weighed between the ages of 9 and 13 years, weight in childhood, relative to age, sex and height, was positively related to non-fatal adult CHD.[104] The highest rates of adult hypertensive vascular disease and 'cardiovascular renal disease' were seen in overweight adults who had been underweight children. Within each adult weight category except the lowest group, those in whom weight had increased most since childhood were at greatest risk. These findings suggest that there is an interaction between childhood and adult overweight and both may be important in the aetiology of adult disease. In a nested case-control study from the 1932 Dutch male cohort, 32-year CHD mortality was increased 2.6-fold in those with a BMI of over 25kg/m^2 compared to 19kg/m^2 when aged 18 years, while those in the leanest group also had an increased risk.[105] In a follow-up study of overweight Swedish children aged two months to 16 years at baseline, overweight persisted into adulthood, and individuals who had CVD by 40 years of follow-up were heavier at puberty and in adulthood and also showed a marked increase in BMI between puberty and age 25 years compared with healthier subjects, suggesting that post-pubertal growth may be more important in determining risk than overweight in early childhood.[106]

A follow-up of the Harvard Growth Study demonstrated that overweight in adolescence predicted CHD mortality in men although adjustment for self-reported adult weight rendered this risk non-significant.[107] In the Boyd Orr cohort, children whose BMI was above the 75th centile had double the risk of CHD mortality compared with thinner individuals.[108] More recently, a prospective follow-up of 3,641 Finnish men born during 1934-44 found that BMI at ages 7, 11, and 15 years was associated with moderately increased risk of coronary death.[109] Data from the

Table 5 ***Studies of the association of BMI in early life and CHD***

Study	Description	Measure(s) of adiposity	Outcome	Main results
Thorne et al, 1968[31]	Cohort study 7,685 former male students at University of Pennsylvania (1931-40) aged under 30 years (mean age 19) who responded to a postal questionnaire in 1962. Self-report information on prevalent, medically confirmed, non-fatal CHD obtained from postal questionnaire.	Ponderal index (height divided by cubed root of weight)	Non-fatal CHD	Two-fold increase in risk in the overweight, ponderal index <12.9 compared to those with a ponderal index of 13.5+.
Paffenbarger et al, 1969[32]	Nested case control study. Cases: 1,146 male Harvard and Pennsylvania University students (1916-50). Cardiovascular risk factors were measured at college entry examination (mean age 19).	Ponderal index	Fatal CHD	Increased risk in those with ponderal index <12.9, odds ratio 1.3; $P<0.01$.
Hoffmans et al, 1989[105]	Nested case control study. Drawn from a cohort of 78,612 Dutch males examined at age 18 years.	BMI four categories: ≤18.99 19-19.99 (reference category) 20-24.99 25+	CHD mortality	'U' shaped relationship. Risk ratios for CHD mortality by BMI group from leanest to most overweight: 1.2, 1.0, 1.3 and 2.6.
Must et al, 1992[107]	Prospective cohort of 508 13-18 year old men and women (15% of those originally studied) who participated in the Harvard Longitudinal Growth Study 1922-35.	BMI. Overweight defined as >75th centile at least twice from 13-18 years.	Incident CHD	Increased relative risk in men for CHD: 2.3 (95% CI 1.4 to 4.1) but not in women. Overweight in adolescence a better predictor than overweight in adulthood.
DiPietro et al, 1994[106]	Prospective cohort of 504 overweight children, aged 2 months to 16 years, who were admitted for investigation of their overweight to hospitals in Stockholm between 1921 and 1947.	BMI	Incident CVD	Subjects with CVD were heavier at puberty and in adulthood than healthier subjects ($P \leq 0.05$). Marked increase in the BMI from post-puberty to age 25 among those who developed CVD ($P \leq 0.001$).
Gunnell et al, 1998[108]	Prospective cohort study of 2,990 girls and boys aged 2-14 years.	BMI Overweight defined as above 75th centile	CHD mortality	Increased relative risk of CHD in both sexes combined: 2.0 (95% CI: 1.0 to 3.9).
Eriksson et al, 1999[109]	Prospective cohort study of 3,641 men measured at 7-15 years.	BMI	CHD mortality	Increased risk of CHD for men in top quartile of BMI vs bottom, 1.53, (P for trend = 0.004).
McCarron et al, 2001[110]	Prospective cohort study of 8,361 men aged 16-30 years at baseline.	BMI at 11 years	CHD mortality	Risk of top quintile of BMI vs bottom, 1.63 (95% CI: 1.08 to 2.45).

Glasgow alumni study are consistent with studies which point to the importance of overweight in early life; former male students in the top quintile of BMI had 1.63 (95% CI: 1.08 to 2.45) times the risk of death from CHD compared with the leanest men in this cohort.[110]

Overweight in childhood and adolescence, and intermediate CHD endpoints and other measures of risk

In the Muscatine study, coronary artery calcification – a marker of atherosclerosis and coronary risk factors in older adults[111] – was more common in young adults who had high BMI during childhood.[112] Similarly in the Bogalusa Heart Study atherosclerotic lesions at autopsy correlated positively with BMI.[10] In the same population, young adults aged 27 to 31 years who had been overweight when 13 to 17 years showed adverse levels of body fatness, systolic and diastolic blood pressure, lipoprotein cholesterol, insulin, and glucose compared to those who had been lean.[113] Clustering of adverse values for the total cholesterol to HDL cholesterol ratio, insulin level, and systolic blood pressure occurred only among the overweight cohort. The finding that excess weight in adolescence persists into young adulthood and has a strong adverse impact on multiple cardiovascular risk factors has been supplemented by recent data which demonstrate that the rate of increase in adiposity is accompanied by concomitant detrimental changes in several coronary risk factors, irrespective of baseline age and adiposity.[114] Two further studies which add to the literature on the importance of the timing of obesity for later coronary risk[115, 116] are consistent with findings which suggest that persistence of overweight into adulthood or thinness in childhood followed by overweight in later life may constitute greater coronary risks than the independent risk of overweight in early life alone.[104-106] Determining the relative importance of overweight at different times in the life course will depend on further studies with good measures of BMI recorded at different stages of childhood and adulthood.

As is the case in adults, fat distribution has also been found to be more strongly associated with cardiovascular risk factors in boys and girls aged 9-17 years than amount of adiposity. Greater deposition of central fat is associated with less favourable levels of plasma lipid and lipoprotein concentrations, and of blood pressure.[117] In the Pathobiological Determinants of Atherosclerosis in Youth (PDAY) Study, post-mortem examinations carried out on men and women aged 15-34 years who died of external causes showed an association between the weight of the abdominal fat pad and the extent of atherosclerotic involvement of the coronary circulation.[118]

Trends in obesity

The prevalence of obesity is increasing in both the US[119, 120] and the UK.[121, 122] Among 3-4 year old children in a representative health authority in England there was a 60% increase in the prevalence of being overweight (having a BMI above the 85th centile) and a 70% increase in the prevalence of obesity (BMI above the 95th centile) between

1989 and 1998.[122] While the factors underlying this increase are complex, changes in diet and decreases in physical activity are both implicated.[123, 124] In addition, children with overweight parents are more likely to be obese themselves,[125] a finding which suggests that weight control in the current generation will have beneficial effects on coronary risk in subsequent generations.

Blood lipid profile

The term adverse blood lipid profile refers to the multiplicity of lipid substances in blood implicated in the pathogenesis of atherosclerosis and CHD.

Blood lipids in adults and CHD

The relationship between a high serum cholesterol concentration and the risk of CHD is unequivocal – a continuous graded association being found between serum cholesterol and long-term risk of CHD.[126-128] Components of total cholesterol have also been investigated, with high levels of LDL cholesterol conferring an increased risk of CHD,[129] while high levels of HDL cholesterol are protective.[130] Fewer studies have been carried out in women, but the available evidence suggests that there is also an inverse gradient for HDL cholesterol, while at any given level LDL cholesterol may be less atherogenic than for men.[131] In trials, lowering LDL cholesterol levels and raising HDL cholesterol levels impeded the progression of atherosclerosis in both men and women[132] and a reduction in cholesterol of 1% has been shown to reduce the risk of CHD by 2-3%.[133, 134]

Blood lipids in children and adolescents, and CHD

As with blood pressure and obesity, serum lipid and lipoprotein levels track from childhood into young adulthood,[135, 136] again highlighting the need for introducing preventive programmes in early life. Since tracking is demonstrated it could be expected that there would be a positive association between early life cholesterol levels and CHD rates, but to date only one study has reported on this. In the Johns Hopkins Precursors Study,[137] serum cholesterol measured at university was a stronger predictor of future CHD mortality risk than has been seen in prospective studies of adults. Table 6 shows the cumulative incidence of cardiac events according to serum cholesterol category in this study. After controlling for other covariates there was an over six-fold greater risk of CHD mortality for those in the highest quartile compared with those in the lowest.

Blood lipids in childhood and adolescence, and intermediate CHD endpoints and other measures of CHD risk

Results from both the Bogalusa Heart Study and the PDAY Study support the inference that plasma lipids in childhood and adolescence are associated with the extent and severity of atherosclerosis in adulthood.[138, 139] In further follow-up, the extent of atherosclerotic lesions in Bogalusa participants generally correlated

Table 6 ***Cumulative incidence of CHD among 1,017 men in the Johns Hopkins Precursors Study after 40 years of follow-up according to baseline serum cholesterol level***

Variable	Number of events	Quartile of cholesterol level (mmol/l)				P for trend
		3.05-4.46	4.47-4.90	4.91-5.39	5.40-8.15	
CHD	97	6.9	11.5	17.5	35.2	<0.001
Myocardial infarction	62	3.4	5.1	7.2	29.2	<0.001
Angina	49	5.7	4.2	13.4	9.2	<0.001

Source: See reference 137.

positively with serum total cholesterol, serum LDL cholesterol, and serum triglyceride concentrations,[10] while in the PDAY Study LDL cholesterol was positively associated, and HDL cholesterol was negatively associated with the extent of fatty streaks and raised lesions in the aorta and right coronary artery.[140]

In a British study in which brachial artery distensibility in 9-11 year old children was used as a measure of cardiovascular risk, there was an inverse association between both total cholesterol and LDL cholesterol and arterial distension.[141] No association was seen with HDL cholesterol and triglyceride levels.

A recent discovery is that aortic fatty streaks progress much faster in children of hypercholesterolaemic mothers than in those of normocholesterolaemic mothers, a finding which was not accounted for by conventional risk factors.[142] The relevance of this finding is that it may give added incentive for tackling risk factors in children and young adults, since it may also lead to lower CHD risk in future generations.

Intervention trials in children and adolescents

Cholesterol-lowering interventions have been tested in children and adolescents but have been heterogeneous in nature. One high-risk intervention trial is the Dietary Intervention Study in Children (DISC) in which there were significant reductions in LDL cholesterol concentration, and no detection of adverse effects, in the treated group relative to the control group.[143] Another large population-based study reported favourable changes in dietary behaviour and other behavioural characteristics but no relative decrease in cholesterol concentrations could be demonstrated, possibly due to design limitations.[144] Such trials are very costly to conduct but the economies of scale from implementation of beneficial interventions on a population-wide basis and the potential for future health service savings are likely to be more economically attractive.

Trends in lipids

Most recent studies have reported trends in adults towards more favourable levels of the blood lipids which are associated with increased CHD risk.[3, 145-148] Over the period 1966-94 the mean serum total cholesterol level among 12-17 year olds in the US showed a small but relatively continuous decline of 0.18 mmol/l, possibly as a result of dietary shifts over this time.[149] Again, fuller understanding of the reason for this decline must be sought to maximise the potential for prevention.

Glucose intolerance and insulin resistance

Glucose intolerance and insulin resistance in adults and CHD

Although not entirely consistent, the available evidence suggests that hyperglycaemia, impaired glucose tolerance, and insulin resistance are all closely related to risk of atherosclerosis and CHD, both through associations with high blood concentrations of glucose or insulin and because of their common clustering with other risk factors such as adverse blood lipid profiles, high blood pressure, and obesity.[150-153]

Cross-sectional studies have shown that hyperinsulinaemia is associated with an adverse pattern of cardiovascular risk factors including obesity, dyslipidaemia and hypertension[154] – syndrome X or insulin resistance syndrome.

Glucose and insulin in children and adolescents, and intermediate CHD endpoints and other measures of CHD risk

In the Bogalusa Heart Study, elevated plasma insulin levels have been shown to track into adulthood[155] and there is also convincing evidence that raised glucose[156] and insulin[157] concentrations in these age groups are positively associated with risk factors for CHD in adulthood. Among individuals who had insulin measured at a mean age of 19 years, follow-up eight years later revealed that, compared with subjects with levels of insulin consistently in the lowest quartile, those with levels always in the highest quartile showed higher levels of several risk factors, including BMI, triglycerides, LDL cholesterol, VLDL cholesterol, glucose, and systolic and diastolic blood pressure, and lower levels of HDL cholesterol.[158] These findings are consistent with those from the developing body of research in adults aimed at improving understanding of the importance of insulin and insulin-related products in CHD risk. Improved understanding of the role of these factors may assist in developing more comprehensive approaches to coronary prevention.

Newer physiological risk factors and CHD

The associations between several 'newer' physiological variables and CHD have been investigated in adults, leading to more recent interest in whether these variables are also risk factors in young individuals.

C-reactive protein (CRP), the major acute phase protein in humans and a predictor of adult cardiovascular risk in prospective studies,[159, 160] has recently been shown to be strongly positively correlated with obesity and also correlated with fibrinogen, HDL cholesterol and systolic blood pressure in a representative sample of 699 British children aged 10-11 years.[161] These findings have since been replicated in the US.[162] In the Third National Health and Nutrition Examination Survey of children aged 8 to 16 years, boys who were overweight (BMI above the 85th centile) were 3.74 (95% CI: 1.66 to 8.43) times more likely to have raised CRP and a similar risk, of 3.17, was reported in girls (95% CI: 1.60 to 6.28).

Several prospective studies have reported associations between elevated plasma homocysteine levels in adulthood and CHD risk.[163] In the Bogalusa Heart Study higher homocysteine levels have been observed among children with a positive family history of CHD.[164] Those children whose parents had unhealthy diets and were from lower socioeconomic position also had higher levels of plasma homocysteine.

These results suggest that, as with other established risk factors, adverse levels of CRP and homocysteine in children are also associated with CHD risk. To date the findings are preliminary and further prospective studies are required to determine whether elevations of these variables are indeed independently related to long-term CHD risk, and if so how they may best be tackled.

Clustering of risk factors and CHD risk

Evidence that CHD risk factors cluster is important and worth emphasising because it reinforces the notion that children and teenagers who are known to have at least one risk factor for CHD may, through the phenomenon of clustering, be at increased coronary risk due to the presence of several other risk factors. Clustering of risk factors also suggests that interventions aimed at one risk factor may have beneficial effects on overall risk factor profile, which will be particularly true if the factor underlying such clustering can be identified and intervened on.

Clustering of risk factors in adults and CHD

In adults there is considerable evidence that the clustering of risk factors – usually defined as having a number of risk factors, including obesity, blood pressure and serum lipids level, above the 75th percentile – is indicative of accelerated rates of atherosclerosis and therefore higher risk of CHD.[165, 166]

Clustering of risk factors in children and adolescents, and intermediate CHD endpoints and other measures of CHD risk

Findings from the Bogalusa Heart Study and elsewhere have demonstrated that clustering of CHD risk factors occurs in childhood and persists into early adulthood.[10, 167, 168] In Bogalusa, participants with several elevated risk factors had adverse patterns of fatty-streak lesions and fibrous plaques in the intimal surface areas of the aorta and coronary arteries.[10] The extent of such pre-atherosclerotic change was dramatic, with the extent of fatty-streak lesions in the coronary arteries 8.5 times greater in persons with three or four risk factors than in those with none, and the extent of fibrous plaques in the coronary arteries 12 times as great. Examined individually, it is clear that risk factors in childhood and adolescence require amelioration to lower the future burden of CHD. However, the stark findings among individuals in whom there are multiple risk factors provide further justification for evaluation of CHD risk and preventive efforts in the young.

Recommendations

The findings presented in this chapter indicate that CHD risk begins in childhood. The upward trend in obesity among young people suggests that the seeds of increased adulthood CHD risk are currently being sown. However, there is also reason for cautious optimism; favourable trends in blood pressure, height, and blood lipids, the demonstrable reversibility of fatty streaks and the encouraging results of some interventions all suggest that preventing CHD is possible and that measures instigated in childhood may be successful in achieving this goal.

Recent national policy initiatives offer the means for implementation of primary prevention interventions. These include the appointment of a minister for Public Health and the requirement of primary care organisations to develop Health Improvement and Modernisation Plans in collaboration with local partners. More specifically the National Service Framework for coronary heart disease[169] and the *NHS Plan*[170] both address the prevention of CHD and set out national quality standards for preventive services. Along with these developments there is also now guidance published by the Health Development Agency aimed at implementing the preventive aspects of the National Service Framework for CHD and detailing specific interventions for children and adolescents.[171]

What should be done? There is currently no role for population-wide screening of children and adolescents. Rather, the goal of primary prevention of CHD is most likely to be achieved through implementation of interventions aimed at improving risk factor profiles across the board. More work is needed to evaluate preventive programmes, but the evidence available at present indicates that improvements in blood pressure, lipid profile, glucose and insulin levels, and weight reduction are likely to be achieved though promotion of better nutrition[172, 173] and increases in physical activity[173] among children and teenagers. Detailed information on possible local interventions to meet dietary and exercise goals is laid out in the Health Development Agency report.[171] Since it is now recognised that coronary risk begins in early life, dietary and physical activity goals have been set for children aged over two years and for teenagers, and include reducing saturated fat and salt intake and increasing the proportion of fruit, vegetables, fish and fibre consumed, and taking one hour of moderate exercise per day (or 30 minutes per day for children who are currently sedentary).

Achieving these goals is, however, a challenge. The Health Development Agency has outlined components which are necessary to increase the effectiveness of any intervention.[171] In broad terms, interventions should be evidence-based, have clear goals and should be long-term rather than short-term in nature. They need to be acceptable to young people and capable of being integrated into everyday life. Family and school involvement can enhance effectiveness of interventions and ideally the whole local community should be considered as the audience for any preventive service. Given the well-recognised social patterning of health, any intervention should, as outlined in the *Independent Inquiry into Inequalities in Health* "be formulated in such a way that by favouring the less well off they will, wherever possible, reduce such inequalities."[174] As a minimum the problems of food poverty, and affordability of, and access to, a healthy diet need to be vigorously addressed, and tackling barriers to adequate exercise for deprived children is also an urgent priority. The finding that adverse social circumstances in childhood are associated with increased CHD risk in adulthood,[175] and that this is not explicable simply in terms of conventional adult risk factors,[176] indicates that further research to uncover the mechanisms of this risk elevation is necessary if interventions are to be developed which comprehensively address the childhood origins of adult CHD risk. Finally, efforts at primary prevention require full government commitment including necessary resources and multi-sectoral cooperation and as a further essential, accountability at national, regional and local levels. Failure to fulfil these prerequisites will result in limited, if any, success in primary preventive efforts.

Conclusions

The evidence that childhood and teenage years are crucial in determining later coronary health is conclusive. Prevention and reduction of coronary risk factors in young people is a major health priority. Programmes to improve diet and exercise among this group need to be developed. If successfully implemented they can not only bring about immediate benefit in risk factor profile, but will also form a solid foundation for sustained coronary health. In addition, bettering diet and exercise may result in the adoption of other healthful behaviours and will lead to a reduction in the risk of other major chronic diseases including type 2 diabetes and cancer. Finally, attempts to prevent CHD by targeting today's children and adolescents may have benefits for the coronary health of subsequent generations.

References

1 Charlton J, Murphy M. 1997. *The Health of Adult Britain 1841-1994.* London: The Stationery Office.

2 Preston SH, Nelson VE. 1974. Structure and change in causes of death: an international summary. *Population Studies*; 28: 19-51.

3 Erens B, Primatesta P. 1999. *Health Survey for England: Cardiovascular Disease.* London: The Stationery Office.

4 Imakita M, Yutani C, Strong JP, Sakurai I, Sumiyoshi A, Watanabe T et al. 2001. Second nation-wide study of atherosclerosis in infants, children and young adults in Japan. *Atherosclerosis*; 155: 487-97.

5 Murray CJ, Lopez AD. The global burden of disease: A comprehensive assessment of mortality and disability from diseases, injury and risk factors in 1990 and projected to 2020. In: Murray CJ, Lopez AD (eds.) 1996. *Global Burden of Disease and Injury Series.* Cambridge, MA: Harvard University Press.

6 Magnus P, Beaglehole R. 2001. The real contribution of the major risk factors to the coronary epidemics: time to end the 'only 50%' myth. *Archives of Internal Medicine*; 161: 2657-60.

7 Enos WF, Holmes RH, Beyer J. 2001. Coronary disease among United States soldiers killed in action in Korea. *Journal of the American Medical Association*; 152: 1090-93.

8 McNamara JJ, Molot MA, Stremple JF, Cutting RT. 1971. Coronary artery disease in combat casualties in Vietnam. *Journal of the American Medical Association*; 216: 1185-87.

9 Strong JP, Malcom GT, McMahan CA, Tracy RE, Newman WP, III, Herderick EE et al. 1999. Prevalence and extent of atherosclerosis in adolescents and young adults: implications for prevention from the Pathobiological Determinants of Atherosclerosis in Youth Study. *Journal of the American Medical Association*; 281: 727-35.

10 Berenson GS, Srinivasan SR, Bao W, Newman WP, III, Tracy RE, Wattigney WA. 1998. Association between multiple cardiovascular risk factors and atherosclerosis in children and young adults. The Bogalusa Heart Study. *New England Journal of Medicine*; 338: 1650-56.

11 Lauer RM, Connor WE, Leaverton PE, Reiter MA, Clarke WR. 1975. Coronary heart disease risk factors in school children: the Muscatine study. *Journal of Pediatrics*; 86: 697-706.

12 Forsdahl A. 1977. Are poor living conditions in childhood and adolescence an important risk factor for arteriosclerotic heart disease? *British Journal of Preventive and Social Medicine*; 31: 91-95.

13 Forsdahl A. 1978. Living conditions in childhood and subsequent development of risk factors for arteriosclerotic heart disease. The cardiovascular survey in Finnmark 1974-75. *Journal of Epidemiology and Community Health*; 32: 34-37.

14 Barker DJP. 1992. *Fetal and Infant Origins of Adult Disease.* London: BMJ Publishing.

15 Barker DJP. 1998. *Mothers, Babies and Health in Later Life.* London: Churchill Livingstone.

16 Davey Smith G, Kuh D. 1993. When is mortality risk determined? Historical insights into a current debate. *Social History of Medicine*; 6: 101-23.

17 Kuh D, Ben-Shlomo Y. 1997. *A Life Course Approach to Chronic Disease Epidemiology.* Oxford: Oxford University Press.

18 McGill HC Jr, McMahan CA, Herderick EE, Malcom GT, Tracy RE, Strong JP. 2000. Origin of atherosclerosis in childhood and adolescence. *American Journal of Clinical Nutrition*; 72: 1307S-15S.

19 MacMahon S, Peto R, Cutler J, Collins R, Sorlie P, Neaton J et al. 1990. Blood pressure, stroke, and coronary heart disease. Part 1, Prolonged differences in blood pressure: prospective observational studies corrected for the regression dilution bias. *Lancet*; 335: 765-74.

20 Miura K, Daviglus ML, Dyer AR, Liu K, Garside DB, Stamler J et al. 2001. Relationship of blood pressure to 25-year mortality due to coronary heart disease, cardiovascular diseases, and all causes in young adult men: the Chicago Heart Association Detection Project in Industry. *Archives of Internal Medicine*; 161: 1501-08.

21 Stamler J, Stamler R, Neaton JD. 1993. Blood pressure, systolic and diastolic, and cardiovascular risks. US population data. *Archives of Internal Medicine*; 153: 598-615.

22 Clausen J, Jensen G. 1992. Blood pressure and mortality: an epidemiological survey with 10 years follow-up. *Journal of Human Hypertension*; 6: 53-59.

23 Antikainen R, Jousilahti P, Tuomilehto J. 1998. Systolic blood pressure, isolated systolic hypertension and risk of coronary heart disease, strokes, cardiovascular disease and all-cause mortality in the middle-aged population. *Journal of Hypertension*; 16: 577-83.

24 Selmer R, Tverdal A. 1996. Changes in blood pressure as a predictor of coronary heart disease and stroke mortality: a 27-year follow up of 15518 men in the City of Bergen, Norway. *Journal of Epidemiology and Biostatistics*; 1: 41-50.

25 Collins R, MacMahon S. 1994. Blood pressure, antihypertensive drug treatment and the risks of stroke and of coronary heart disease. *British Medical Bulletin*; 50: 272-98.

26 Collins R, Peto R, MacMahon S, Hebert P, Fiebach NH, Eberlein KA et al. 1990. Blood pressure, stroke, and coronary heart disease. Part 2, Short-term reductions in blood pressure: overview of randomised drug trials in their epidemiological context. *Lancet*; 335: 827-38.

27 Nelson MJ, Ragland DR, Syme SL. 1992. Longitudinal prediction of adult blood pressure from juvenile blood pressure levels. *American Journal of Epidemiology*; 136: 633-45.

28 Labarthe DR, Eissa M, Varas C. 1991. Childhood precursors of high blood pressure and elevated cholesterol. *Annual Review of Public Health*; 12: 519-41.

29 Yong LC, Kuller LH. 1994. Tracking of blood pressure from adolescence to middle age: the Dormont High School Study. *Preventive Medicine*; 23: 418-26.

30 Barker DJ, Osmond C, Golding J, Kuh D, Wadsworth ME. 1989. Growth in utero, blood pressure in childhood and adult life, and mortality from cardiovascular disease. *British Medical Journal*; 298: 564-67.

31 Thorne MC, Wing AL, Paffenbarger RS Jr. 1968. Chronic disease in former college students. VII. Early precursors in nonfatal coronary heart disease. *American Journal of Epidemiology*; 87: 520-29.

32 Paffenbarger RS Jr, Wing AL. 1969. Chronic disease in former college students. X. The effects of single and multiple characteristics on risk of fatal coronary heart disease. *American Journal of Epidemiology*; 90: 527-35.

33 McCarron P, Davey Smith G, Okasha M, McEwen J. 1999. Life course exposure and later disease: a follow-up study based on medical examinations carried out in Glasgow University (1948-68). *Public Health*; 113: 265-71.

34 McCarron P, Davey Smith G, Okasha M, McEwen J. 2000. Blood pressure in young adulthood and mortality from cardiovascular disease. *Lancet*; 355: 1430-31.

35 McCarron P, Okasha M, McEwen J, Davey Smith G. 2002. Blood pressure in early life and cardiovascular disease mortality. *Archives of Internal Medicine*; 162: 610-11.

36 The Sixth Report of the Joint National Committee on Prevention, Detection, Evaluation, and Treatment of High Blood Pressure. *Archives of Internal Medicine*, 1997; 157: 2413-46.

37 Davis CE, Rifkind BM, Brenner H, Gordon DJ. 1990. A single cholesterol measurement underestimates the risk of coronary heart disease. An empirical example from the Lipid Research Clinics Mortality Follow-up Study. *Journal of the American Medical Association*; 264: 3044-46.

38 Tornberg SA, Jakobsson KF, Eklund GA. 1988. Stability and validity of a single serum cholesterol measurement in a prospective cohort study. *International Journal of Epidemiology*; 17: 797-803.

39 Clarke R, Shipley M, Lewington S, Youngman L, Collins R, Marmot M et al. 1999. Underestimation of risk associations due to regression dilution in long-term follow-up of prospective studies. *American Journal of Epidemiology*; 150: 341-53.

40 Okasha M, McCarron P, McEwen J, Davey Smith G. 1999. Blood pressure during young adulthood and mortality from cardiovascular disease. *Journal of Epidemiology and Community Health*; 53: 656.

41 Whincup PH, Cook DG, Shaper AG, Macfarlane DJ, Walker M. 1988. Blood pressure in British children: associations with adult blood pressure and cardiovascular mortality. *Lancet*; 2: 890-93.

42 Whincup PH, Cook DG, Adshead F, Taylor S, Papacosta O, Walker M et al. 1996. Cardiovascular risk factors in British children from towns with widely differing adult cardiovascular mortality. *British Medical Journal*; 313: 79-84.

43 McGill HC Jr, McMahan CA, Zieske AW, Malcom GT, Tracy RE, Strong JP. 2001. Effects of nonlipid risk factors on atherosclerosis in youth with a favorable lipoprotein profile. *Circulation*; 103: 1546-50.

44 Thomas CB, Duszynski KR. 1982. Blood pressure levels in young adulthood as predictors of hypertension and the fate of the cold pressor test. *Johns Hopkins Medical Journal*; 151: 93-100.

45 Johnston W, Cheeseman EA, Merrett JD. 1957. Observations on routine medical examinations of university entrants in Northern Ireland. *British Journal of Preventive and Social Medicine*; 11: 152-61.

46 Johnston W, Merrett JD. 1962. Further observations on routine medical examinations of university entrants in Northern Ireland. *British Journal of Preventive and Social Medicine*; 16: 76-83.

47 Harland RW. 1980. Sociological, anatomical and physiological changes in first-year students entering Queen's University, Belfast, over thirty years, 1948-77. 1. Preliminary report. *Ulster Medical Journal*; 49: 37-47.

48 McCarron P, Okasha M, McEwen J, Davey Smith G. 2001. Changes in blood pressure among students attending Glasgow University between 1948 and 1968: analyses of cross sectional surveys. *British Medical Journal*; 322: 885-89.

49 Burt VL, Cutler JA, Higgins M, Horan MJ, Labarthe D, Whelton P et al. 1995. Trends in the prevalence, awareness, treatment, and control of hypertension in the adult US population. Data from the health examination surveys, 1960 to 1991. *Hypertension*; 26: 60-69.

50 Goff DC, Howard G, Russell GB, Labarthe DR. 2001. Birth cohort evidence of population influences on blood pressure in the United States, 1887-1994. *Annals of Epidemiology;* 11: 271-79.

51 McCarron P, Davey Smith G, Okasha M. 2002. Secular changes in blood pressure in childhood, adolescence and young adulthood: systematic review of trends from 1948-98. *Journal of Human Hypertension*;16: 677-89.

52 Ebrahim S, Davey Smith G. 1998. Lowering blood pressure: a systematic review of sustained effects of non-pharmacological interventions. *Journal of Public Health Medicine*; 20: 441-48.

53 Geleijnse JM, Hofman A, Witteman JC, Hazebroek AA, Valkenburg HA, Grobbee DE. 1997. Long-term effects of neonatal sodium restriction on blood pressure. *Hypertension*; 29: 913-17.

54 Ministry of Food. 1951. *The Urban Working-class Household Diet 1940-1949. First Report of the National Food Survey Committee.* London: HMSO.

55 Ministry of Food. 1952. *Domestic Food Consumption and Expenditure, 1950* (with a supplement on food expenditure by urban working-class households, 1940-1949). London: HMSO.

56 Baines AHJ, Hollingsworth DF, Leitch I. 1963. Diets of working-class families with children before and after the second world war: with a section on height and weight of children. *Nutrition Abstracts and Reviews*; 33: 653-59.

57 Appel LJ, Moore TJ, Obarzanek E, Vollmer WM, Svetkey LP, Sacks FM et al. 1997. A clinical trial of the effects of dietary patterns on blood pressure. DASH Collaborative Research Group. *New England Journal of Medicine*; 336: 1117-24.

58 Andersson OK, Almgren T, Persson B, Samuelsson O, Hedner T, Wilhelmsen L. 1998. Survival in treated hypertension: follow up study after two decades. *British Medical Journal*; 317: 167-71.

59 Davey Smith G, Hart C, Upton M, Hole D, Gillis C, Watt G et al. 2000. Height and risk of death among men and women: aetiological implications of associations with cardiorespiratory disease and cancer mortality. *Journal of Epidemiology and Community Health*; 54: 97-103.

60 Wannamethee SG, Shaper AG, Whincup PH, Walker M. 1998. Adult height, stroke, and coronary heart disease. *American Journal of Epidemiology*; 148: 1069-76.

61 Leon DA, Davey Smith G, Shipley M, Strachan D. 1995. Adult height and mortality in London: early life, socioeconomic confounding, or shrinkage? *Journal of Epidemiology and Community Health*; 49: 5-9.

62 Hebert PR, Rich-Edwards JW, Manson JE, Ridker PM, Cook NR, O'Connor GT et al. 1993. Height and incidence of cardiovascular disease in male physicians. *Circulation*; 88: 1437-43.

63 Strandberg TE. 1997. Inverse relation between height and cardiovascular mortality in men during 30-year follow-up. *American Journal of Cardiology*; 80: 349-50.

64 Helmert U, Shea S. 1997. Relation between body height and self-reported myocardial infarction in Germany. *Reviews on Environmental Health*; 12: 125-30.

65 Davey Smith G, Shipley MJ, Rose G. 1990. Magnitude and causes of socioeconomic differentials in mortality: further evidence from the Whitehall Study. *Journal of Epidemiology and Community Health*; 44: 265-70.

66 Rich-Edwards JW, Manson JE, Stampfer MJ, Colditz GA, Willett WC, Rosner B et al. 1995. Height and the risk of cardiovascular disease in women. *American Journal of Epidemiology*; 142: 909-17.

67 Reed LJ, Love AG. 1933. Biometric studies on US army officers – somatological norms in disease. *Human Biology*; 5: 61-93.

68 Gertler MM, Woodbury MA, Gottsch LG, White PD, Rusk HA. 1959. The candidate for coronary heart disease. Discriminating power of biochemical hereditary and anthropometric measurements. *Journal of the American Medical Association*; 170: 149-52.

69 Gertler MM, White PD. 1954. *Coronary Heart Disease in Young Adults: A Multidisciplinary Study.* Cambridge, MA: Harvard University Press.

70 Vagero D, Leon D. 1994. Ischaemic heart disease and low birth weight: a test of the fetal-origins hypothesis from the Swedish Twin Registry. *Lancet*; 343: 260-63.

71 Yarnell JW, Limb ES, Layzell JM, Baker IA. 1992. Height: a risk marker for ischaemic heart disease: prospective results from the Caerphilly and Speedwell Heart Disease Studies. *European Heart Journal*; 13: 1602-5.

72 Palmer JR, Rosenberg L, Shapiro S. 1990. Stature and the risk of myocardial infarction in women. *American Journal of Epidemiology*; 132: 27-32.

73 Walker M, Shaper AG, Phillips AN, Cook DG. 1989. Short stature, lung function and risk of a heart attack. *International Journal of Epidemiology*; 18: 602-06.

74 Cook NR, Hebert PR, Satterfield S, Taylor JO, Buring JE, Hennekens CH. 1994. Height, lung function, and mortality from cardiovascular disease among the elderly. *American Journal of Epidemiology*; 139: 1066-76.

75 McCarron P, Okasha M, McEwen J, Davey Smith G. 2002. Height in young adulthood and risk of death from cardiorespiratory disease: a prospective study of male former students of Glasgow University, Scotland. *American Journal of Epidemiology*; 155: 683-87.

76 *Higher Education* (Robbins Report). Cmnd. 2154. 1963. London: HMSO.

77 Office of Population Censuses and Surveys. 1978. *The General Household Survey 1975.* London: HMSO.

78 Gunnell DJ, Frankel S, Nanchahal K, Braddon FE, Davey Smith G. 1996. Lifecourse exposure and later disease: a follow-up study based on a survey of family diet and health in pre-war Britain (1937-1939). *Public Health*; 110: 85-94.

79 Gunnell DJ, Davey Smith G, Frankel S, Nanchahal K, Braddon FE, Pemberton J et al. 1998. Childhood leg length and adult mortality: follow up of the Carnegie (Boyd Orr) Survey of Diet and Health in Pre-war Britain. *Journal of Epidemiology and Community Health*; 52: 142-52.

80 Tanner JM, Hayashi T, Preece MA, Cameron N. 1982. Increase in length of leg relative to trunk in Japanese children and adults from 1957 to 1977: comparison with British and with Japanese Americans. *Annals of Human Biology*; 9: 411-23.

81 Billewicz WZ, Thomson AM, Fellowes HM. 1983. A longitudinal study of growth in Newcastle upon Tyne adolescents. *Annals of Human Biology*; 10: 125-33.

82 Forsen T, Eriksson JG, Tuomilehto J, Osmond C, Barker DJ. 1999. Growth in utero and during childhood among women who develop coronary heart disease: longitudinal study. *British Medical Journal*; 319: 1403-07.

83 Chiang YK, Srinivasan SR, Webber LS, Berenson GS. 1989. Relationship between change in height and changes in serum lipid and lipoprotein levels in adolescent males: the Bogalusa Heart Study. *Journal of Clinical Epidemiology*; 42: 409-15.

84 Lee VA. 1967. Individual trends in the total serum cholesterol of children and adolescents over a ten-year period. *American Journal of Clinical Nutrition*; 20: 5-12.

85 Freedman DS, Cresanta JL, Srinivasan SR, Webber LS, Berenson GS. 1985. Longitudinal serum lipoprotein changes in white males during adolescence: the Bogalusa Heart Study. *Metabolism*; 34: 396-403.

86 Chinn S, Rona RJ. 1984. The secular trend in the height of primary school children in England and Scotland from 1972-1980. *Annals of Human Biology*; 11: 1-16.

87 Kuh DL, Power C, Rodgers B. 1991. Secular trends in social class and sex differences in adult height. *International Journal of Epidemiology*; 20: 1001-09.

88 Rolland-Cachera MF, Sempe M, Guilloud-Bataille M, Patois E, Pequignot-Guggenbuhl F, Fautrad V. 1982. Adiposity indices in children. *American Journal of Clinical Nutrition*; 36: 178-84.

89 Cole TJ. Weight-stature indices to measure underweight, overweight, and obesity. In: Himes JH (ed.) 1991. *Anthropometric Assessment of Nutritional Status*. New York: Wiley-Liss Inc: pp 83-111.

90 Manson JE, Colditz GA, Stampfer MJ, Willett WC, Rosner B, Monson RR et al. 1990. A prospective study of obesity and risk of coronary heart disease in women. *New England Journal of Medicine*; 322: 882-89.

91 Rimm EB, Stampfer MJ, Giovannucci E, Ascherio A, Spiegelman D, Colditz GA et al. 1995. Body size and fat distribution as predictors of coronary heart disease among middle-aged and older US men. *American Journal of Epidemiology*; 141: 1117-27.

92 Selmer R, Tverdal A. 1995. Body mass index and cardiovascular mortality at different levels of blood pressure: a prospective study of Norwegian men and women. *Journal of Epidemiology and Community Health*; 49: 265-70.

93 Jarrett RJ, Shipley MJ, Rose G. 1982. Weight and mortality in the Whitehall Study. *British Medical Journal (Clinical Research Edition)*; 285: 535-37.

94 Hubert HB, Feinleib M, McNamara PM, Castelli WP. 1983. Obesity as an independent risk factor for cardiovascular disease: a 26-year follow-up of participants in the Framingham Heart Study. *Circulation*; 67: 968-77.

95 Rabkin SW, Mathewson FA, Hsu PH. 1977. Relation of body weight to development of ischemic heart disease in a cohort of young North American men after a 26 year observation period: the Manitoba Study. *American Journal of Cardiology*; 39: 452-58.

96 Manson JE, Willett WC, Stampfer MJ, Colditz GA, Hunter DJ, Hankinson SE et al. 1995. Body weight and mortality among women. *New England Journal of Medicine*; 333: 677-85.

97 Phillips A, Shaper AG. 1989. Relative weight and major ischaemic heart disease events in hypertensive men. *Lancet*; 1: 1005-08.

98 Hartz AJ, Rupley DC, Rimm AA. 1984. The association of girth measurements with disease in 32,856 women. *American Journal of Epidemiology*; 119: 71-80.

99 Lapidus L, Bengtsson C, Larsson B, Pennert K, Rybo E, Sjostrom L. 1984. Distribution of adipose tissue and risk of cardiovascular disease and death: a 12 year follow up of participants in the population study of women in Gothenburg, Sweden. *British Medical Journal (Clinical Research Edition)*; 289: 1257-61.

100 Freedman DS, Williamson DF, Croft JB, Ballew C, Byers T. 1995. Relation of body fat distribution to ischemic heart disease. The National Health and Nutrition Examination Survey I (NHANES I) Epidemiologic Follow-up Study. *American Journal of Epidemiology*; 142: 53-63.

101 Power C, Lake JK, Cole TJ. 1997. Measurement and long-term health risks of child and adolescent fatness. *International Journal of Obesity and Related Metabolic Disorders*; 21: 507-26.

102 Guo SS, Chumlea WC. 1999. Tracking of body mass index in children in relation to overweight in adulthood. *American Journal of Clinical Nutrition*; 70: 145S-48S.

103 Vanhala M, Vanhala P, Kumpusalo E, Halonen P, Takala J. 1998. Relation between obesity from childhood to adulthood and the metabolic syndrome: population based study. *British Medical Journal*; 317: 319-20.

104 Abraham S, Collins G, Nordsieck M. 1971. Relationship of childhood weight status to morbidity in adults. *HSMHA Health Report*; 86: 273-84.

105 Hoffmans MD, Kromhout D, Coulander CD. 1989. Body Mass Index at the age of 18 and its effects on 32-year-mortality from coronary heart disease and cancer. A nested case-control study among the entire 1932 Dutch male birth cohort. *Journal of Clinical Epidemiology*; 42: 513-20.

106 DiPietro L, Mossberg HO, Stunkard AJ. 1994. A 40-year history of overweight children in Stockholm: life-time overweight, morbidity, and mortality. *International Journal of Obesity and Related Metabolic Disorders*; 18: 585-90.

107 Must A, Jacques PF, Dallal GE, Bajema CJ, Dietz WH. 1992. Long-term morbidity and mortality of overweight adolescents. A follow-up of the Harvard Growth Study of 1922 to 1935. *New England Journal of Medicine*; 327: 1350-55.

108 Gunnell DJ, Frankel SJ, Nanchahal K, Peters TJ, Davey Smith G. 1998. Childhood obesity and adult cardiovascular mortality: a 57-y follow-up study based on the Boyd Orr cohort. *American Journal of Clinical Nutrition*; 67: 1111-18.

109 Eriksson JG, Forsen T, Tuomilehto J, Winter PD, Osmond C, Barker DJ. 1999. Catch-up growth in childhood and death from coronary heart disease: longitudinal study. *British Medical Journal*; 318: 427-31.

110 Authors' unpublished data.

111 Simons DB, Schwartz RS, Edwards WD, Sheedy PF, Breen JF, Rumberger JA. 1992. Noninvasive definition of anatomic coronary artery disease by ultrafast computed tomographic scanning: a quantitative pathologic comparison study. *Journal of the American College of Cardiology*; 20: 1118-26.

112 Mahoney LT, Burns TL, Stanford W, Thompson BH, Witt JD, Rost CA et al. 1996. Coronary risk factors measured in childhood and young adult life are associated with coronary artery calcification in young adults: the Muscatine Study. *Journal of the American College of Cardiology*; 27: 277-84.

113 Srinivasan SR, Bao W, Wattigney WA, Berenson GS. 1996. Adolescent overweight is associated with adult overweight and related multiple cardiovascular risk factors: the Bogalusa Heart Study. *Metabolism*; 45: 235-40.

114 Srinivasan SR, Myers L, Berenson GS. 2001. Rate of change in adiposity and its relationship to concomitant changes in cardiovascular risk variables among biracial (black-white) children and young adults: The Bogalusa Heart Study. *Metabolism*; 50: 299-305.

115 Freedman DS, Dietz WH, Srinivasan SR, Berenson GS. 1999. The relation of overweight to cardiovascular risk factors among children and adolescents: the Bogalusa Heart Study. *Pediatrics*; 103: 1175-82.

116 Wright CM, Parker L, Lamont D, Craft AW. 2001. Implications of childhood obesity for adult health: findings from thousand families cohort study. *British Medical Journal*; 323: 1280-84.

117 Daniels SR, Morrison JA, Sprecher DL, Khoury P, Kimball TR. 1999. Association of body fat distribution and cardiovascular risk factors in children and adolescents. *Circulation*; 99: 541-45.

118 McGill HC Jr, McMahan CA. 1998. Determinants of atherosclerosis in the young. Pathobiological Determinants of Atherosclerosis in Youth (PDAY) Research Group. *American Journal of Cardiology*; 82: 30T-36T.

119 Ogden CL, Troiano RP, Briefel RR, Kuczmarski RJ, Flegal KM, Johnson CL. 1997. Prevalence of overweight among preschool children in the United States, 1971 through 1994. *Pediatrics*; 99: E1.

120 Shear CL, Freedman DS, Burke GL, Harsha DW, Webber LS, Berenson GS. 1988. Secular trends of obesity in early life: the Bogalusa Heart Study. *American Journal of Public Health*; 78: 75-77.

121 Reilly JJ, Dorosty AR, Emmett PM. 1999. Prevalence of overweight and obesity in British children: cohort study. *British Medical Journal*; 319: 1039.

122 Bundred P, Kitchiner D, Buchan I. 2001. Prevalence of overweight and obese children between 1989 and 1998: population based series of cross sectional studies. *British Medical Journal*; 322: 326-28.

123 Gortmaker SL, Must A, Sobol AM, Peterson K, Colditz GA, Dietz WH. 1996. Television viewing as a cause of increasing obesity among children in the United States, 1986-1990. *Archives of Pediatric and Adolescent Medicine*; 150: 356-62.

124 Morris JN. 1995. Obesity in Britain. Lifestyle data do not support sloth hypothesis. *British Medical Journal*; 311: 1568-69.

125 Lake JK, Power C, Cole TJ. 1997. Child to adult body mass index in the 1958 British birth cohort: associations with parental obesity. *Archives of Disease in Childhood*; 77: 376-81.

126 Keys A. 1980. *Seven Countries: A Multivariate Analysis of Death and Coronary Heart Disease.* Cambridge, MA: Harvard University Press.

127 Verschuren WM, Jacobs DR, Bloemberg BP, Kromhout D, Menotti A, Aravanis C et al. 1995. Serum total cholesterol and long-term coronary heart disease mortality in different cultures. Twenty-five-year follow-up of the seven countries study. *Journal of the American Medical Association*; 274: 131-36.

128 Martin MJ, Hulley SB, Browner WS, Kuller LH, Wentworth D. 1986. Serum cholesterol, blood pressure, and mortality: implications from a cohort of 361,662 men. *Lancet*; 2: 933-36.

129 Stensvold I, Tverdal A, Urdal P, Graff-Iversen S. 1993. Non-fasting serum triglyceride concentration and mortality from coronary heart disease and any cause in middle aged Norwegian women. *British Medical Journal*; 307: 1318-22.

130 Durrington PN. 1993. How HDL protects against atheroma. *Lancet*; 342: 1315-16.

131 Rich-Edwards JW, Manson JE, Hennekens CH, Buring JE. 1995. The primary prevention of coronary heart disease in women. *New England Journal of Medicine*; 332: 1758-66.

132 Kane JP, Malloy MJ, Ports TA, Phillips NR, Diehl JC, Havel RJ. 1990. Regression of coronary atherosclerosis during treatment of familial hypercholesterolemia with combined drug regimens. *Journal of the American Medical Association*; 264: 3007-12.

133 Scandinavian Simvastatin Survival Study Group. 1994. Randomised trial of cholesterol lowering in 4444 patients with coronary heart disease: the Scandinavian Simvastatin Survival Study (4S). *Lancet*; 344: 1383-89.

134 Shepherd J, Cobbe SM, Ford I, Isles CG, Lorimer AR, Macfarlane PW et al. 1995. Prevention of coronary heart disease with pravastatin in men with hypercholesterolemia. West of Scotland Coronary Prevention Study Group. *New England Journal of Medicine*; 333: 1301-07.

135 Webber LS, Wattigney WA, Srinivasan SR, Berenson GS. 1995. Obesity studies in Bogalusa. *American Journal of Medical Science*; 310; Suppl 1: S53-S61.

136 Freedman DS, Shear CL, Srinivasan SR, Webber LS, Berenson GS. 1985. Tracking of serum lipids and lipoproteins in children over an 8-year period: the Bogalusa Heart Study. *Preventive Medicine*; 14: 203-16.

137 Klag MJ, Ford DE, Mead LA, He J, Whelton PK, Liang KY et al. 1993. Serum cholesterol in young men and subsequent cardiovascular disease. *New England Journal of Medicine*; 328: 313-18.

138 Bao W, Srinivasan SR, Wattigney WA, Bao W, Berenson GS. 1996. Usefulness of childhood low-density lipoprotein cholesterol level in predicting adult dyslipidemia and other cardiovascular risks. The Bogalusa Heart Study. *Archives of Internal Medicine*; 156: 1315-20.

139 Pathobiological Determinants of Atherosclerosis in Youth Research Group. 1990. Relationship of atherosclerosis in young men to serum lipoprotein cholesterol concentrations and smoking. A preliminary report from the Pathobiological Determinants of Atherosclerosis in Youth (PDAY) Research Group. *Journal of the American Medical Association*; 264: 3018-24.

140 McGill HC Jr, McMahan CA, Malcom GT, Oalmann MC, Strong JP. 1997. Effects of serum lipoproteins and smoking on atherosclerosis in young men and women. The PDAY Research Group. Pathobiological Determinants of Atherosclerosis in Youth. *Arteriosclerosis, Thrombosis and Vascular Biology*; 17: 95-106.

141 Leeson CP, Whincup PH, Cook DG, Mullen MJ, Donald AE, Seymour CA et al. 2000. Cholesterol and arterial distensibility in the first decade of life: a population-based study. *Circulation*; 101: 1533-38.

142 Napoli C, Glass CK, Witztum JL, Deutsch R, D'Armiento FP, Palinski W. 1999. Influence of maternal hypercholesterolaemia during pregnancy on progression of early atherosclerotic lesions in childhood: Fate of Early Lesions in Children (FELIC) study. *Lancet*; 354: 1234-41.

143 The Writing Group for the DISC Collaborative Research Group. 1995. Efficacy and safety of lowering dietary intake of fat and cholesterol in children with elevated low-density lipoprotein cholesterol. The Dietary Intervention Study in Children (DISC). *Journal of the American Medical Association*; 273: 1429-35.

144 Luepker RV, Perry CL, McKinlay SM, Nader PR, Parcel GS, Stone EJ et al. 1996. Outcomes of a field trial to improve children's dietary patterns and physical activity. The Child and Adolescent Trial for Cardiovascular Health. CATCH collaborative group. *Journal of the American Medical Association*; 275: 768-76.

145 Bild DE, Jacobs DR, Liu K, Williams OD, Hilner JE, Perkins LL et al. 1996. Seven-year trends in plasma low-density-lipoprotein-cholesterol in young adults: the CARDIA Study. *Annals of Epidemiology*; 6: 235-45.

146 National Center for Health Statistics – National Heart, Lung, and Blood Institute Collaborative Lipid Group. 1987. Trends in serum cholesterol levels among US adults aged 20 to 74 years. Data from the National Health and Nutrition Examination Surveys, 1960 to 1980. *Journal of the American Medical Association*; 257: 937-42.

147 Burke GL, Sprafka JM, Folsom AR, Hahn LP, Luepker RV, Blackburn H. 1991. Trends in serum cholesterol levels from 1980 to 1987. The Minnesota Heart Survey. *New England Journal of Medicine*; 324: 941-46.

148 Szklo M, Chambless LE, Folsom AR, Gotto A Jr, Nieto FJ, Patsch W et al. 2000. Trends in plasma cholesterol levels in the atherosclerosis risk in communities (ARIC) study. *Preventive Medicine*; 30: 252-59.

149 Hickman TB, Briefel RR, Carroll MD, Rifkind BM, Cleeman JI, Maurer KR et al. 1998. Distributions and trends of serum lipid levels among United States children and adolescents ages 4-19 years: data from the Third National Health and Nutrition Examination Survey. *Preventive Medicine*; 27: 879-90.

150 Fuller JH, Shipley MJ, Rose G, Jarrett RJ, Keen H. 1983. Mortality from coronary heart disease and stroke in relation to degree of glycaemia: the Whitehall study. *British Medical Journal (Clinical Research Edition)*; 287: 867-70.

151 Ducimetiere P, Eschwege E, Papoz L, Richard JL, Claude JR, Rosselin G. 1980. Relationship of plasma insulin levels to the incidence of myocardial infarction and coronary heart disease mortality in a middle-aged population. *Diabetologia*; 19: 205-10.

152 Jarrett RJ, Keen H, Fuller JH, McCartney M. 1979. Worsening to diabetes in men with impaired glucose tolerance ('borderline diabetes'). *Diabetologia*; 16: 25-30.

153 Marang-van de Mheen PJ, Davey Smith G, Hart CL, Hole DJ, Phillips AN. 2000. The influence of gender, social circumstances and smoking on survival: the Renfrew and Paisley study. *Public Health*; 114: 117-22.

154 Manolio TA, Savage PJ, Burke GL, Liu KA, Wagenknecht LE, Sidney S et al. 1990. Association of fasting insulin with blood pressure and lipids in young adults. The CARDIA study. *Arteriosclerosis*; 10: 430-36.

155 Bao W, Srinivasan SR, Wattigney WA, Berenson GS. 1994. Persistence of multiple cardiovascular risk clustering related to syndrome X from childhood to young adulthood. The Bogalusa Heart Study. *Archives of Internal Medicine*; 154: 1842-47.

156 Urbina EM, Gidding SS, Bao W, Elkasabany A, Berenson GS. 1999. Association of fasting blood sugar level, insulin level, and obesity with left ventricular mass in healthy children and adolescents: The Bogalusa Heart Study. *American Heart Journal*; 138: 122-27.

157 Bao W, Srinivasan SR, Berenson GS. 1996. Persistent elevation of plasma insulin levels is associated with increased cardiovascular risk in children and young adults. The Bogalusa Heart Study. *Circulation*; 93: 54-59.

158 Bao W, Srinivasan SR, Valdez R, Greenlund KJ, Wattigney WA, Berenson GS. 1997. Longitudinal changes in cardiovascular risk from childhood to young adulthood in offspring of parents with coronary artery disease: the Bogalusa Heart Study. *Journal of the American Medical Association;* 278: 1749-54.

159 Kuller LH, Tracy RP, Shaten J, Meilahn EN. 1996. Relation of C-reactive protein and coronary heart disease in the MRFIT nested case-control study. Multiple Risk Factor Intervention Trial. *American Journal of Epidemiology*; 144: 537-47.

160 Ridker PM, Cushman M, Stampfer MJ, Tracy RP, Hennekens CH. 1997. Inflammation, aspirin, and the risk of cardiovascular disease in apparently healthy men. *New England Journal of Medicine*; 336: 973-79.

161 Cook DG, Mendall MA, Whincup PH, Carey IM, Ballam L, Morris JE et al. 2000. C-reactive protein concentration in children: relationship to adiposity and other cardiovascular risk factors. *Atherosclerosis*; 149: 139-50.

162 Visser M, Bouter LM, McQuillan GM, Wener MH, Harris TB. 2001. Low-grade systemic inflammation in overweight children. *Pediatrics*; 107: E13.

163 Stampfer MJ, Malinow MR, Willett WC, Newcomer LM, Upson B, Ullmann D et al. 1992. A prospective study of plasma homocyst(e)ine and risk of myocardial infarction in US physicians. *Journal of the American Medical Association*; 268: 877-81.

164 Greenlund KJ, Srinivasan SR, Xu JH, Dalferes E Jr, Myers L, Pickoff A et al. 1999. Plasma homocysteine distribution and its association with parental history of coronary artery disease in black and white children: the Bogalusa Heart Study. *Circulation*; 99: 2144-49.

165 Truett J, Cornfield J, Kannel W. 1967. A multivariate analysis of the risk of coronary heart disease in Framingham. *Journal of Chronic Diseases*; 20: 511-24.

166 Kleinbaum DG, Kupper LL, Cassel JC, Tyroler HA. 1971. Multivariate analysis of risk of coronary heart disease in Evans County, Georgia. *Archives of Internal Medicine*; 128: 943-48.

167 Webber LS, Voors AW, Srinivasan SR, Frerichs RR, Berenson GS. 1979. Occurrence in children of multiple risk factors for coronary artery disease: the Bogalusa Heart Study. *Preventive Medicine*; 8: 407-18.

168 Khoury P, Morrison JA, Kelly K, Mellies M, Horvitz R, Glueck CJ. 1980. Clustering and interrelationships of coronary heart disease risk factors in schoolchildren, ages 6-19. *American Journal of Epidemiology*; 112: 524-38.

169 Department of Health. 2000. *National Service Framework for Coronary Heart Disease.* Department of Health.

170 Department of Health. 2001. *The NHS Plan: A Plan for Investment, A Plan for Reform.* London: The Stationery Office.

171 Health Development Agency. 2000. *Coronary Heart Disease – Guidance for Implementing the Preventative Aspects of the National Service Framework.* London: Health Development Agency.

172 Department of Health. 1994. *Nutritional Aspects of Cardiovascular Disease: Report of the Cardiovascular Review Group of the Committee on Medical Aspects of Food Policy.* London: HMSO.

173 WHO/FIMS Committee on Physical Activity for Health. 1995. Exercise for health. *Bulletin of the World Health Organization;* 73: 135-36.

174 Department of Health. 1998. *Independent Inquiry into Inequalities in Health.* London: The Stationery Office.

175 Davey Smith G. Socioeconomic differentials. In: Kuh D, Ben Shlomo Y (eds.) 1997. *A Life Course Approach to Chronic Disease Epidemiology*. Oxford: Oxford University Press: pp 242-73.

176 Davey Smith G, Hart C, Blane D, Hole D. 1998. Adverse socioeconomic conditions in childhood and cause specific adult mortality: prospective observational study. *British Medical Journal*; 316: 1631-35.

Chapter 4

Socioeconomic position and coronary heart disease risk factors in children and young people

Dr G David Batty

Epidemiology Unit, London School of Hygiene and Tropical Medicine

Professor David A Leon

Epidemiology Unit, London School of Hygiene and Tropical Medicine

This chapter:

- identifies, through systematic review, UK-based epidemiological studies exploring the relation of indices of socioeconomic position to 11 confirmed or potential CHD risk factors in children or young adults
- outlines the key elements of those studies which met the inclusion criteria
- summarises and critiques the evidence for an association between indices of socioeconomic position and each of these risk factors, and
- advances future research directions.

Key themes

- There was consistent evidence for a relation between indices of socioeconomic position and birthweight, height, obesity (in early adulthood only), cigarette smoking, and some aspects of diet, particularly fat and fibre consumption, such that the most favourable levels of these risk factors were apparent in younger persons from higher social backgrounds. The direction of these relationships was the same as those seen in UK adults.
- Obesity does not appear to show a socioeconomic gradient in children under approximately 15 years of age. The well documented negative association in adults only emerges in later teenage years.
- For physical inactivity/low cardiorespiratory fitness, blood pressure, blood cholesterol, obesity (in childhood) and some emerging CHD risk factors (i.e. C-reactive protein, homocysteine and fibrinogen) there is currently little evidence of a clear association with indices of socioeconomic position.
- While survey data concerning the social patterning of key CHD risk factors in children are available, there is a paucity of published reports.
- In order to establish a firmer evidence base, a priority for future work should be to undertake a consistent set of analyses on the socioeconomic distribution of CHD risk factors in childhood based on existing survey data.

Introduction

Despite the declining incidence of coronary heart disease (CHD) in the latter half of the 20th century, it remains one of the leading causes of death in the UK.[1] Clinically, it is a condition of middle and old age with few cases diagnosed earlier than the fourth decade of life. Following the Framingham study in the 1940s,[2] a series of population-based studies of middle-aged men and women conducted throughout the world have identified several physiological (obesity, hypertension, atherogenic lipid profiles, low cardiorespiratory fitness, and short stature) and behavioural (cigarette smoking, physical inactivity, and diets rich in saturated fats and low in fibre) risk factors for this condition.[3, 4] Additionally, while moderate alcohol consumption – traditionally considered separately from dietary patterns – appears to be cardioprotective, inebriation-inducing quantities ('binge drinking') are associated with an increased risk of cardiovascular events.[5]

Although the studies of middle-aged men and women on which these observations have been based are numerous, far fewer investigations have been conducted to examine whether these CHD risk factors when measured in childhood and early adult life are associated with later disease. Some of these studies are reviewed in this report (see Chapters 1 and 3). Based on these reviews and other reports there are several good reasons to implicate indices measured in infancy, childhood, and early adult life in the development of coronary heart disease. Firstly, there is evidence from a small number of cohort studies that some CHD risk factors measured in childhood and early adulthood are predictive of subsequent CHD events. These include raised blood pressure,[6, 7] adverse lipid profiles,[6, 8] overweight/obesity,[9, 10] short stature,[11] low birthweight,[12] cigarette smoking[6, 13] and physical inactivity.[14] Secondly, from childhood into early adult life several of these risk factors seem to 'track', such that there is a tendency for levels in childhood to be correlated with levels in later life.[15] Thirdly, there are convincing data from autopsy investigations that the natural history of atherosclerosis extends back into teenage years[16, 17] and even to the *in utero* period.[18]

Given that the evidence suggests that unfavourable levels of certain variables in pre- and early adult life may increase the risk of CHD, if successful preventative measures are to be implemented during this period it is necessary, in turn, to understand their determinants. Socioeconomic position – as measured most commonly by occupational social class but also by income and highest educational attainment – has generally been shown to be related to CHD risk factors in a graded fashion in UK adult men[19-22] and women.[22] We examine if this is also the case for children and young adults by reviewing UK-based studies that have related socioeconomic factors to cigarette smoking, birthweight, height, adiposity, dietary characteristics, physical activity/cardiorespiratory fitness, blood pressure, blood cholesterol, and emerging risk factors for CHD (i.e. C-reactive protein, homocysteine and fibrinogen). Inclusion of a risk factor measured in childhood in our review, however, does not imply that there is conclusive evidence linking it to coronary heart disease in later life. This is particularly so with respect to dietary characteristics for which we are unaware of any studies relating early life patterns to adult CHD.[†] However, because this behaviour is linked to several of the risk factors described above – most notably obesity – we nevertheless include it.

This chapter begins with an outline of the aim of this review and a description of the methods used to identify pertinent studies. It continues with a discussion of the relation of a range of indices of socioeconomic position to individual CHD risk factors and concludes by summarising our observations and advancing some directions for future research.

[†] Data on the link between early life dietary characteristics and subsequent CVD are likely to emerge from the Boyd Orr (Carnegie) cohort study (David Gunnell – personal communication) and the 1946 birth cohort study.[23] See Chapter 2 for a preliminary analysis.

Aim of review

The aim of this review is to collate evidence from published sources concerning the association between indicators of socioeconomic position and risk factors for CHD among children and young people in the UK.

Method

We carried out a systematic search of PUBMED as available in electronic form from January 1966 to October 2000 using the following terms for exposure: 'socio-economic', 'socioeconomic'; and for outcome: 'blood pressure', 'cholesterol', 'obesity', 'smoking', 'activity', 'fitness', 'height', 'fat', and 'fibre'. All searches incorporated the term 'child'. The reference sections of identified papers were then examined for additional publications, our own files were searched, and some researchers in the field were contacted for further information. The first of these three approaches was a particularly fruitful source of further information.

To be included in the review, publications had to, firstly, present information on the socioeconomic distribution of one or more of the CHD risk factors described above and, secondly, include study participants from the United Kingdom aged 24 years or less, as consistent with the World Health Organization's definition of the period spanning childhood, adolescence and youth.[24] Where available, we have given emphasis to studies based on nationally representative samples and have included the most recently published data as these are the most relevant with respect to public health action today. We have, however, included results of surveys conducted in previous decades to enable us to explore variation over time in the socioeconomic distribution of CHD risk factors in childhood. Indeed, in some cases, this practice has been essential because of the absence or paucity of contemporary information. It should be noted that associations between socioeconomic position and CHD risk factors in earlier decades are not necessarily a reliable guide as to what may prevail today and in this regard we chose not to review in detail publications reporting data collected before 1950, although earlier papers are sometimes cited in order to place more contemporary work in context.

This review does not claim to be completely comprehensive. In particular, it is likely that we have overlooked some data, particularly if they have been published in limited circulation reports by agencies that have not attracted much attention in the research community – the so called 'grey' literature. Importantly, we are aware of a number of examples of surveys that could be used to explore the socioeconomic distribution of some CHD risk factors in children, where either no such analyses have been carried out or where the results have not been placed in the public domain, possibly because of negative findings.

Measuring socioeconomic position and gradients

The published sources we have reviewed use a wide range of different measures of socioeconomic position including the Registrar General's occupational social class schema, income, educational attainment and aspirations, family size, receipt of state benefits, and housing tenure. Except in surveys of young adults who were employed, these measures relate to parental or household characteristics rather than those of the children themselves. While these different measures can be regarded as inter-related dimensions of socioeconomic position, it is beyond the scope of this review to determine whether any one (or more) particular dimension underlies the reported gradients.

Results

Table 1 on pages 84-89 summarises each major publication identified from the literature search, the study on which the report is based, the study sample, period of and age at measurement, the measure(s) of socioeconomic position used, and what CHD risk factor data were collected. The published reports are grouped together according to the decade in which the risk factor data they refer to were collected, with publications relating to the most recent period (1990-99) described first.

In this review we will principally draw on several well established UK studies which have examined the social patterning in one or more CHD risk factor. These include the MRC National Survey of Health and Development (1946 birth cohort),[56] the National Child Development Study (1958 birth cohort)[57] and the Child Health and Education Study (1970 birth cohort),[58] all of which are on-going longitudinal studies with periodic surveys of their populations. We also review evidence from the National Study of Health and Growth (NSHG)[59, 60] which is based on a series of cross-sectional studies conducted from 1972 until their discontinuation in 1994. In 1995 the Health Survey for England (HSE) included children in its sampling frame for the first time and in so doing replaced the NSHG. A report aggregating data on children for the former surveys from 1995-97 is available[31] and, while results of the 1998 phase for adults have also been published in hard copy,[61] selected data on children can only be accessed over the world wide web[26] at the time of writing. A similar survey of the Scottish population that included children was conducted in 1998[25] and the findings are also described herein. While some of these studies have attempted to examine the dietary characteristics of children, this was done in most depth by investigators on the National Diet and Nutrition Surveys which surveyed pre-school children in 1967/68[51] and in 1992/93,[34] schoolchildren in 1983[43] and in 1997,[27, 28] and young adults in 1997.[27, 28] Findings from the Nine[62] and Ten Towns studies[38] of primary schoolchildren are also reviewed. The former is a cross-sectional survey of children drawn from nine towns which were included in the British Regional Heart Study of adults;[63] the latter is a mixed longitudinal study based on five towns characterised by high adult CVD rates

Table 1 *Overview of publications of UK studies relating indicators of socioeconomic position in children and young adults to CHD risk factors, according to period of data collection*

Study name and reference	Description†	Year of risk factor measurement	Age at risk factor measurement (years)	Indicator of socioeconomic position	Diet	Cigarette smoking	Physical activity/ fitness	Blood pressure	Blood cholesterol	Adiposity	Height
Conducted in 1990 to 1999											
Scottish Health Survey[25]	Nationally representative sample of 3,892 children	1998	2-15	Occupational social class	✓		✓	✓		✓	
Health Survey for England[26]	3,142 children from randomly sampled households	1998	2-15	Occupational social class Household income						✓	
National Diet and Nutrition Survey: Young People Aged 4 to 18 Years[27, 28]	Nationally representative sample of 2,672 young people in Britain	1997	4-18	Occupational social class Household income Receipt of state benefits	✓		✓	✓	✓	✓	✓
Department of Health Ninth National Survey of Smoking among Secondary School Children[29]	2,854 secondary schoolchildren in England and Scotland	1996	11-15	Home amenities (car, PC, dishwasher) Housing tenure Educational aspirations Predicted GCSE exam results		✓					
Teenage Smoking Attitudes in 1996[30]	3,657 secondary schoolchildren in England	1996	11-15	Number of cars in family Housing tenure Educational aspirations Expectation that GCSE exams will be taken Predicted GCSE exam results		✓					

† Study design is cross-sectional unless otherwise stated.

Study name and reference	Description†	Year of risk factor measurement	Age at risk factor measurement (years)	Indicator of socioeconomic position	Diet	Cigarette smoking	Physical activity/ fitness	Blood pressure	Blood cholesterol	Adiposity	Height
Health Survey for England[31]	Aggregated data from three surveys of 18,298 children and young adults in England	1995/97	2-24	Occupational social class Household income	✓	✓	✓	✓		✓	
Ten Towns Study[32]	Mixed longitudinal study. 2,650 primary schoolchildren from 10 towns in England and Wales	1994	8-11	Occupational social class	✓						
National Study of Health and Growth[33]	Mixed longitudinal study. Random sample of 1,662 children in England and Scotland	1992/93	9	Father's occupational social class Mother's educational attainment Number of siblings				✓	✓		
National Diet and Nutrition Survey of Pre-school Children[34]	Nationally representative sample of 2,101 pre-school children in Britain	1992/93	$1\frac{1}{2}$ - $4\frac{1}{2}$	Occupational social class Receipt of state benefits Educational attainment	✓					✓	✓
National Study of Health and Growth[35]	Mixed longitudinal study. Random sample of 581 children in England and Scotland	1992	8-9	Father's occupational social class Father's employment status Mother's educational attainment Number of siblings			✓				
National Fitness Survey[36]	Random sample of 1,308 adults in England	1990	16-34	Occupational social class Educational attainment Housing tenure			✓				

† Study design is cross-sectional unless otherwise stated.

Study name and reference	Description†	Year of risk factor measurement	Age at risk factor measurement (years)	Indicator of socioeconomic position	Diet	Cigarette smoking	Physical activity/ fitness	Blood pressure	Blood cholesterol	Adiposity	Height
Ten Towns Study[37]	Mixed longitudinal study. 3,360 primary schoolchildren from 10 towns in England and Wales	1990	5-7 $^1/_2$	Maternal occupational social class Educational attainment Father's occupational social class				✓			
Ten Towns Study[38]	Mixed cross-sectional study. 3,842 primary schoolchildren from 10 towns in England and Wales	1990	5-7$^1/_2$	Occupational social class of head of household				✓		✓	✓
Conducted in 1981 to 1989											
Young Hearts Project[39]	Longitudinal study. Random sample of 1,015 boys and girls	1989/90 1992/93 (follow-up of 12 year olds)	12 and 15	Occupational social class of head of household	✓	✓	✓	✓	✓	✓	✓
Young People's Leisure and Lifestyles Project[40]	Random sample of 1,171 children from secondary school catchment areas in Scotland	1989	16-22	Occupational social class Parents' educational attainment		✓					
Nine Towns Study[41]	5,006 primary schoolchildren from nine towns in England and Wales	1987/88	5-7$^1/_2$	Occupational social class							✓
Department of Health survey[42]	Longitudinal study. 4,165 children (based on sample in 1988) taken from a random sample of secondary schools in England and Wales	1986/87/88	11-15	Expected school educational level		✓					

† Study design is cross-sectional unless otherwise stated.

Study name and reference	Description†	Year of risk factor measurement	Age at risk factor measurement (years)	Indicator of socioeconomic position	Diet	Cigarette smoking	Physical activity/ fitness	Blood pressure	Blood cholesterol	Adiposity	Height
Department of Health survey on the diets of British schoolchildren[43]	Representative sample of 2,678 schoolchildren in England and Scotland	1983	10-11 and 14-15	Occupational social class	✓						✓
Ministry of Agriculture, Fisheries and Food Dietary Survey[44]	Quasi representative sample of approx. 1,000 young adults from Scotland and Wales	1982	15-25	Occupational social class	✓	✓	✓				✓
National Child Development Study (1958 birth cohort)[45]	Longitudinal study. 6,133 men and 6,141 women born in England, Scotland and Wales in early March 1958	1981	23	Occupational social class						✓	
Conducted in or before 1980											
DHSS survey of British adults[46]	Representative sample of 1,121 adults in England, Scotland and Wales	1980	16-24	Occupational social class of head of household			✓			✓	✓
Child Health and Education Study (1970 birth cohort)[47]	Longitudinal study. Approx. 15,000 children born in England, Scotland and Wales in early April 1970	1980	10	Occupational social class	✓						
National Study of Health and Growth[48]	Mixed longitudinal study. Random sample of 9,815 children in England and Scotland	1972	5-11	Occupational social class Number of siblings Father's employment status Mother's educational attainment						✓	

† Study design is cross-sectional unless otherwise stated.

Study name and reference	Description†	Year of risk factor measurement	Age at risk factor measurement (years)	Indicator of socioeconomic position	Diet	Cigarette smoking	Physical activity/ fitness	Blood pressure	Blood cholesterol	Adiposity	Height
National Study of Health and Growth[49]	Mixed longitudinal study. Random sample of 9,815 children in England and Scotland	1972	5-11 1/2	Occupational social class Father's employment status Number of siblings							✓
Government social survey[50]	5,601 boys from a stratified random sample of secondary schools in England and Wales	1966	11-15	Father's occupational social class Perception of father's occupational social class Headteacher's rating of child's academic ability Child's perception of position in class based on academic performance Vocabulary test		✓					
National Diet and Nutrition Survey of pre-school children[51]	Nationally representative sample of 1,254 pre-school children in Britain	1967/68	1/2-4 1/2	Occupational social class Number of siblings Income Mother's educational attainment	✓						✓
National Child Development Study (1958 birth cohort)[52]	Longitudinal study. 13,127 men and women born in England, Scotland and Wales in early March 1958	1965	7	Occupational social class							✓
National Survey of Health and Development (1946 birth cohort)[53]	Longitudinal study. 1,570 men and 1,456 women born in England, Scotland and Wales in the first week of March 1946	1953/57/61	7, 11, 15	Occupational social class Number of siblings							✓

† Study design is cross-sectional unless otherwise stated.

Study name and reference	Description†	Year of risk factor measurement	Age at risk factor measurement (years)	Indicator of socioeconomic position	Diet	Cigarette smoking	Physical activity/ fitness	Blood pressure	Blood cholesterol	Adiposity	Height
National Survey of Health and Development (1946 birth cohort) and National Child Development Study (1958 birth cohort) combined[54]	Longitudinal study. Men and women born in England, Scotland and Wales in early March of 1946 and of 1958. (Sample size varies according to study and period of follow-up.)	1953/57 (1946 cohort) 1965/69 (1958 cohort)	7, 11	Occupational social class							✓
National Survey of Health and Development (1946 birth cohort) and National Child Development Study (1958 birth cohort) combined[55]	Longitudinal study. Men and women born in England, Scotland and Wales in early March of 1946 and of 1958. (Sample size varies according to study.)	1953/57/62 (1946 cohort) 1965/69/74 (1958 cohort)	7, 11 and 16	Occupational social class						✓	
National Survey of Health and Development (1946 birth cohort) [23]	Longitudinal study. 4,599 men and women born in England, Scotland and Wales in the first week of March 1946	1950	4	Occupational social class	✓						

† Study design is cross-sectional unless otherwise stated.

and five towns characterised by low adult CVD rates. In some of the reviewed studies such as the Scottish Health Survey[25] and the National Fitness Survey,[36] the age range of the participants is wide. Such studies are only included because they present sub-analyses of children and/or young people.

Since 1978 the General Household Survey has collected information biennially on the smoking habits of adults in the UK. The recognition that few comparable data on children were available led to the Department of Health funding biennial surveys of 11-15 year old children from 1982[64] until 1999 when they became annual, alternating between a smoking and drinking focus in even-numbered years[65] and a drugs focus in odd-numbered years.[66] Enquiries regarding socioeconomic position were included for the first time in 1996.[29] Because of the cross-sectional nature of these studies, they were unable to shed light on the time trends in smoking habits in children. To examine this question, the Department of Health also funded a cohort study with the aim of tracking the smoking behaviour of children in 1986, 1987 and 1988[42] during which data on educational aspirations were collected. The former Heath Education Authority (now the Health Development Agency) also commissioned a series of eight studies to complement this work by examining the effectiveness of various teenage anti-smoking campaigns. With the implementation of a new campaign in 1996, a further three studies were conducted and the main report,[30] from the 1996 survey, contains an analysis of social factors in relation to smoking habits.

The widest range of CHD risk factors examined in relation to markers of socioeconomic position is seen in publications from the Scottish Health Survey,[25] the National Diet and Nutrition Survey,[27, 28] the Health Survey for England,[31] and the Young Hearts Project.[39] What is also evident is that for several of the CHD risk indicators – most notably blood pressure and blood cholesterol – there are few sources that provide published information on socioeconomic distribution in childhood. For serum cholesterol this is partially explained by the ethical considerations of drawing blood from children.

In the next section, the associations between individual CHD risk factors and socioeconomic indices will be discussed in turn. Tables 2-9 describe the association of each risk factor with socioeconomic position according to the publications reviewed.

Cigarette smoking

Studies from the 1960s[67-71] (see also the review by Bewley et al[72]) and the 1970s,[73, 74] report an inconsistent association between occupational social class or income and cigarette smoking in schoolchildren. These surveys were, however, of convenience samples and we identified a further eight reports of representative samples of schoolchildren and young adults from the UK that have published data on the social distribution of smoking (see Table 2). The first such survey took place in 1966[50] and because pilot study results indicated a low prevalence of smoking in schoolgirls, comprised teenage boys only. An association between social class and smoking prevalence was seen with the lowest levels evident in the non-manual occupations; this relation broke down in social groups IV and V, possibly due to the low numbers of study participants in these categories. The study investigators also assessed academic performance, as a marker of socioeconomic position, in terms of a vocabulary test,[75] headteacher's perception of pupils' academic ability, and the pupil's self-rating in relation to classroom peers. For all indicators, there was a lower prevalence of smoking among those who achieved academically, or were perceived to either by themselves or by their teachers.

More recently, on aggregating data for children and young adults from the Health Survey for England carried out over three years between 1995 and 1997, Prescott-Clarke and Primatesta[31] found a relation between the occupational social class of the carer and self-reported smoking prevalence, whereby the prevalence of smoking was lowest in both males and females from social class I relative to those in the lower social classes. The same observations have been made elsewhere.[44, 40] By measuring cotinine levels – a biological marker of exposure to tobacco smoke – in 4-24 years olds in the 1996 and 1997 phases of data collection in the Health Survey for England, the investigators were able to objectively assess both direct and passive exposure, with a continine level of 15ng/ml or more used as an indication of a child who smokes regularly and inhales. Cotinine levels were measured in either the saliva or serum of the research participants depending on the age group in question or the survey year. An inverse socioeconomic gradient with cotinine levels in both children (4-15 years) and young people (16-24 years) was seen for social class (see Figure 1 on page 94) and housing tenure (see Figure 2 on page 94). Enquiries about income were only introduced in 1997 when the sample of 16-24 year olds was markedly smaller than in the preceding two years, and thus no data on the income–cotinine relation are available. In the younger age group, however, there were sufficient numbers and a less pronounced income–cotinine association was seen than for the other markers of socioeconomic position.

An insight into why these social gradients in smoking prevalence exist has been provided by De Vries[76] who also reported similar social class patterning in a survey of Dutch adolescents. In this study the understanding of the deleterious health effects of smoking were greatest, and the perception of the peer pressure to smoke were least acute, in children in the higher social strata relative to the lowest.

Table 2 ***Publications of UK studies relating socioeconomic position to cigarette smoking in children and young adults***

Study name and reference	Year of risk factor measurement	Age at risk factor measurement (years)	Findings
Department of Health Ninth National Survey of Smoking in Secondary School Children[29]	1996	11-15	Smoking inversely associated with number of cars (girls only). Children from homes with a computer were less likely to smoke than those without. Higher prevalence of smoking in children whose parents rented their dwelling than in those whose parents were owner-occupiers. Children who expected to stay at school after their GCSEs and children who expected to pass more than five GCSEs were less likely to smoke than those planning to leave school after their GCSEs and those who did not expect to pass five GCSEs, respectively.
Teenage Smoking Attitudes in 1996[30]	1996	11-15	Number of cars *positively* associated with smoking. No association between housing tenure and smoking. Children who expected to stay at school after their GCSEs, children who planned to sit their GCSEs, and children who expected to pass more than five GCSEs were less likely to smoke than those planning to leave school after their GCSEs, those who planned not to sit their GCSEs and those who did not expect to pass five GCSEs, respectively.
Health Survey for England[31]	1995/7	2-24	Occupational social class associated with both cotinine and self-reported levels of cigarette smoking in children and young adults, with the highest levels seen in the lower social groups. Cotinine levels in 4-15 year olds negatively associated with equivalised income and accommodation tenure (i.e. children in social housing had higher cotinine levels than children whose parents owned their accommodation). Too few data on cotinine levels in 16-24 year olds to facilitate analyses.

Study name and reference	Year of risk factor measurement	Age at risk factor measurement (years)	Findings
Young People's Leisure and Lifestyles Project[40]	1989	16-22	In females aged 20-22, occupational social class and parental educational attainment associated with self-reported levels of smoking. In males aged 16-18, parental educational attainment negatively associated with smoking. In other age groups no association seen.
Young Hearts Project[39]	1989/90 1992/93	12 15	Occupational social class of head of household associated with cigarette smoking in 15 year olds, such that the highest levels apparent in the lower social groups. Insufficient data on 12 year olds to facilitate cross-sectional or longitudinal analyses.
Department of Health Survey[42]	1986/87/88	11-15	Expected school educational level negatively associated with smoking.
Ministry of Agriculture, Fisheries and Food Dietary Survey[44]	1982	15-25	Occupational social class associated with self-reported levels of cigarette smoking, with the highest levels apparent in the lower social groups.
Government social survey[50]	1966	11-15	Occupational social class associated with smoking with the lowest levels in the higher social groups, but relation breaks down in lower social groups. Headteacher's rating of child's academic ability, child's perception of position in class based on academic performance, and vocabulary test scores all inversely related to smoking; associations strongest in older groups.

Figure 1 ***Proportion (%) of children and young adults aged 4-24 years with cotinine* levels of 15ng/ml or above by the occupational social class of the head of the household/subject in the Health Survey for England 1995-97***

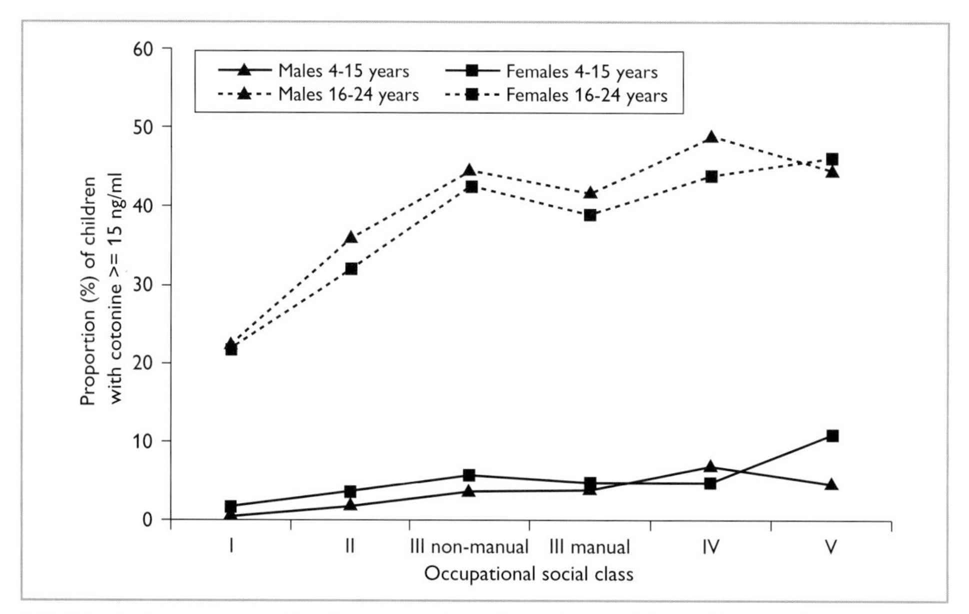

* Cotinine levels were measured in saliva or serum depending on the age of the participants and the survey year. To provide a level for all research participants, serum levels were converted to saliva levels.

Source: See reference 31.

Figure 2 ***Proportion (%) of children and young adults aged 4-24 years with cotinine* levels of 15ng/ml or above by accommodation tenure in the Health Survey for England 1995-97***

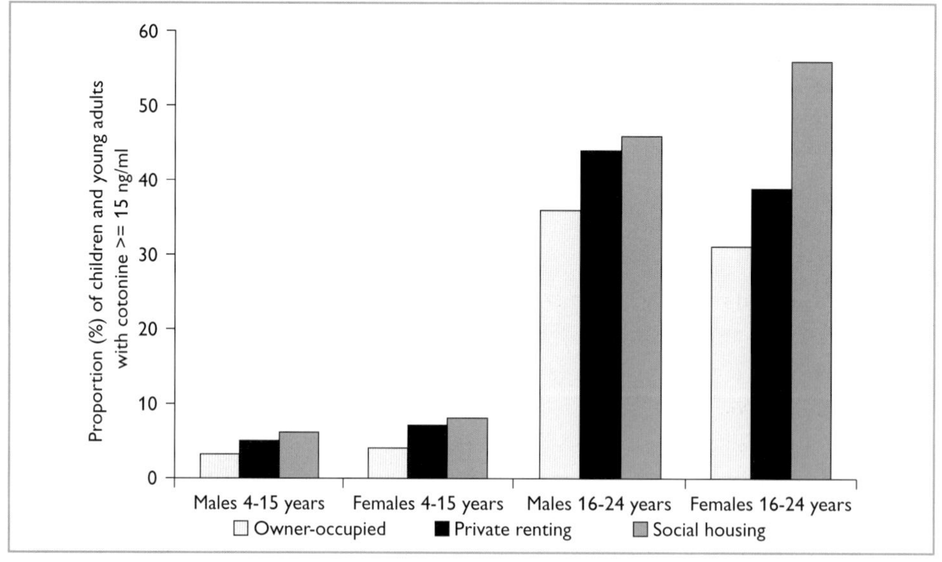

* Cotinine levels were measured in saliva or serum depending on the age of the participants and the survey year. To provide a level for all research participants, serum levels were converted to saliva levels.

Source: See reference 31.

Birthweight

Routinely collected data on over two million live births between 1991 and 1995 in England and Wales[77] show a social class gradient for birthweight, with the distribution moving towards the higher birthweights as one moves from social class V to social class I (see Table 3). This association has been demonstrated repeatedly over the last two decades in the UK[38, 78] and we will therefore not describe individual studies. The role of this socioeconomic gradient in birthweight in generating either past, current, or future socioeconomic gradients in CHD is unknown. What is clear, however, is that a positive socioeconomic–birthweight relation has been observed for as long as records have been available and certainly back to the early part of the 20th century. This consistency in the social patterning of birthweight is in contrast to the evidence that the current negative socioeconomic gradient in coronary heart disease in adults has not always been observed in the past,[79] although this has recently been disputed.[80]

Table 3 ***Proportion (%) of live births inside marriage by occupational social class and birthweight in England and Wales, 1991-95***

	Birthweight							
Social class	*Up to 1,000g*	*1,000-1,499g*	*1,500-1,999g*	*2,000-2,499g*	*2,500-2,999g*	*3,000-3,499g*	*3,500-3,999g*	*Over 4,000g*
I	0.3	0.5	1.1	3.4	13.9	36.1	31.6	13.1
II	0.3	0.5	1.2	3.7	14.3	35.7	31.7	12.6
III non-manual	0.3	0.6	1.3	3.7	15.3	35.8	31.0	12.1
III manual	0.4	0.6	1.4	4.4	16.1	36.1	29.6	11.5
IV	0.4	0.7	1.4	4.9	17.7	35.8	28.4	10.9
V	0.4	0.6	1.7	5.1	18.5	37.0	26.9	9.9

Source: See reference 77.

Height

Childhood height is a product of genetic and environmental factors.[81] In terms of the latter, height may be regarded as an indicator of nutritional status, housing conditions, well-being, and/or psychological stress. The study of the relationship between childhood growth and social background has a long research pedigree,[82] with strong evidence to suggest that the social differentials in height evident in the early part of last century still persist today. For example, in Aberdeen in 1910 all primary schoolchildren aged 5-14 years entering educational institutions underwent a medical examination during which their height was recorded.[83] These data were classified according to the cleanliness of the school which was used as a group level indicator for the socioeconomic position of the parents. For both sexes there was evidence of a graded association with children from the 'poor' schools of consistently shorter stature in comparison with those from schools that were classified as 'well-to-do'. Later surveys which also assessed deprivation at the group level report similar findings.[84-88]

Similarly consistent patterns of association of height with a range of indicators of social position at the level of the individual are also evident, including family size[89-91] and parental occupational social class.[91,92] Notably, in a longitudinal study of children from birth to age five in South Wales,[93] occupational social class differences in height were apparent from as young as two years of age. More recently, a number of representative national surveys of children and young adults have compared height with individual socioeconomic position (see Table 4). One of the most notable of these is the National Study of Health and Growth[59,60] which was established to detect what changes in growth, if any, were evident as a result of the abolition of the free school milk programme in UK schools by the then Conservative government headed by Margaret Thatcher. Using data collected in 1972,[49] Rona et al reported an association between social class and height whereby children of higher stature were from the more affluent households. This observation is consistent with that found in children in the 1946 and 1958 British birth cohort studies[54] and in the Nine[41] and Ten Towns Studies[38] (see Figure 3 on page 99). Statistically significant relationships between height and a range of other markers of socioeconomic position have also been reported (see Table 4).

Gunnell et al,[94] in a re-analysis of data from a cross-sectional study of children examined across Britain in the late 1930s,[95] indicate that of the two components of overall stature – leg length and trunk length – the main source of social variation lies in the former. This finding is in keeping with other observations made in Britain during a similar period[87] and subsequent to it.[92] The authors conclude that leg length may, therefore, be a more sensitive marker of childhood environment than the traditionally used overall height.

To summarise, irrespective of the period of data collection, the unit of analysis (i.e. person or group), and the indicator of socioeconomic position used, a socioeconomic gradient in height has been demonstrated in children of all ages. The reason for these height differences is not well understood but it may be in part attributable to differentials in dietary characteristics across the social groups and this association is examined on page 103.

Table 4 ***Publications of UK studies relating socioeconomic position to height in children and young adults***

Study name and reference	Year of risk factor measurement	Age at risk factor measurement (years)	Findings
National Diet and Nutrition Survey[27]	1997	4-18	Household income (males and females) and occupational social class (females only) associated with height, with the taller children coming from more affluent backgrounds.
National Diet and Nutrition Survey[34]	1992/93	$1\frac{1}{2}$-$4\frac{1}{2}$	Occupational social class associated with height in males, with the taller children coming from more affluent backgrounds; no association in females. Boys from households where head was employed were taller than those where head was unemployed/economically inactive.
Ten Towns Study[38]	1990	5-$7\frac{1}{2}$	Occupational social class associated with height, with the taller children coming from more affluent backgrounds.
Young Hearts Project[39]	1989/90 1992/93	12 15	Occupational social class associated with height in 15 year olds, with the taller children coming from more affluent backgrounds.
Nine Towns Study[41]	1987/88	5-$7\frac{1}{2}$	Occupational social class associated with height, with the taller children coming from more affluent backgrounds.
Department of Health survey of the diets of British schoolchildren[43]	1983	10-11 and 14-15	In both age groups, boys and girls in social class I were taller than those in social class V.
Ministry of Agriculture, Fisheries and Food Dietary Survey[44]	1982	15-25	Occupational social class associated with height in males and females, with the taller children coming from more affluent backgrounds.
DHSS survey of British adults[46]	1980	16-24	Occupational social class positively associated with height in males and females, with the taller children coming from more affluent backgrounds.
National Study of Health and Growth[49]	1972	5-$11\frac{1}{2}$	Height associated with occupational social class with the taller children coming from more affluent backgrounds, and negatively associated with number of siblings.

Study name and reference	Year of risk factor measurement	Age at risk factor measurement (years)	Findings
National Diet and Nutrition Survey of pre-school children[51]	1967/68	$^1/_2$ - $4^1/_2$	Negative association between family size and height in girls but not boys. Evidence in some age groups and sexes that income and educational attainment are negatively associated with height although, when stratified, these analyses are based on small numbers.
National Child Development Study (1958 birth cohort)[52]	1965	7	Height associated with occupational social class with the taller children coming from the more affluent backgrounds, and negatively associated with number of siblings.
National Survey of Health and Development (1946 birth cohort)[53]	1953/57/61	7, 11, 15	Height associated with occupational social class with the taller children coming from more affluent backgrounds, and negatively associated with number of siblings.
National Survey of Health and Development (1946 birth cohort) and National Child Development Study (1958 birth cohort)[54]	1953/7 (1946 cohort) 1965/9 (1958 cohort)	7, 11	Height associated with occupational social class, with the taller children coming from more affluent backgrounds.

Figure 3 ***Mean height of children aged 5-7½ years by parental occupational social class in the Ten Towns Study, 1990***

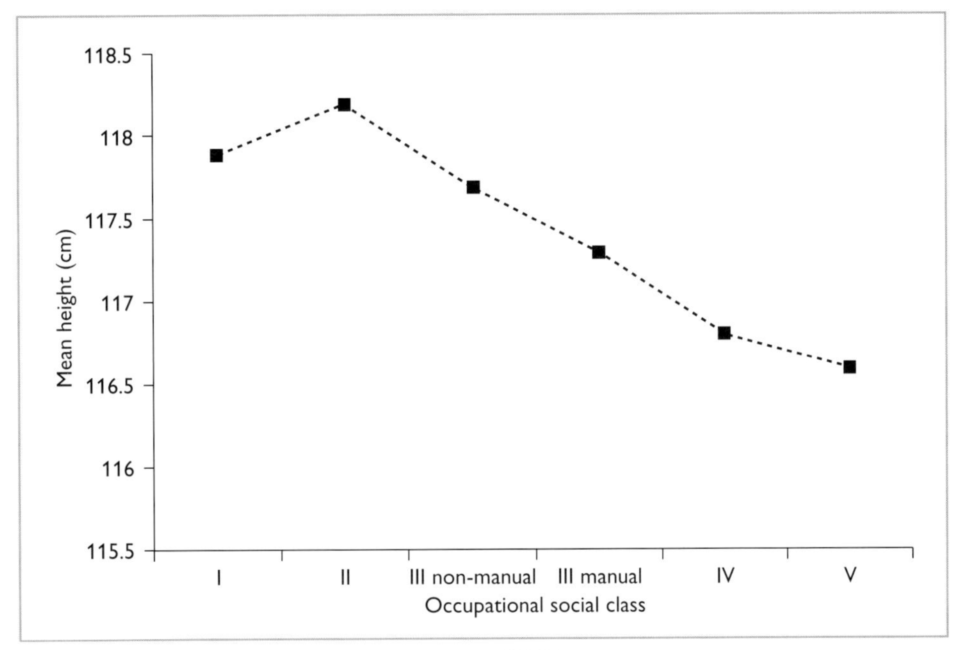

Data are age- and sex-adjusted. P value for heterogeneity <0.0001
Source: See reference 38.

Adiposity

In studies of the anthropometry of children, investigators have typically measured adiposity in terms of body mass index (BMI) or, less commonly, skinfold thickness (see Table 5); waist to hip ratio has been used to assess fat distribution. In several early small-scale studies, skinfold thickness was related to social class with inconsistent results: on aggregating data from five cohorts of children examined between 1950 and 1953 from mixed social backgrounds, Hammond[96] reported no relationship between skinfold thickness and social class. Subsequent surveys of schoolchildren from Glasgow in the 1960s[97] and London during a similar period,[98] yielded discrepant associations between social class and skinfold thickness.

Several studies drawing on nationally representative samples of UK children and young adults were identified (see Table 5). In cross-sectional studies that relate current childhood measures of socioeconomic position – most commonly parental occupational social class – to markers of adiposity, there is little evidence of an association. For example, in 2-15 year olds in the Scottish Health Survey,[25] in 5-11 year olds in the National Study of Health and Growth,[48] in pre-schoolers in the National Diet and Nutrition Survey,[34] in 5-7½ year olds in the Ten Towns Study,[38] in 7 year olds

Table 5 ***Publications of UK studies relating socioeconomic position to adiposity in children and young adults***

Study name and reference	Year of risk factor measurement	Age at risk factor measurement (years)	Findings
Scottish Health Survey[25]	1998	2-15	No association between occupational social class and BMI in boys or girls in any age group.
Health Survey for England[26]	1998	2-15	Occupational social class and household income not related to BMI.
National Diet and Nutrition Survey[27]	1997	4-18	Occupational social class, household income, and receipt of state benefits not associated with BMI or waist to hip ratio.
Health Survey for England[31]	1995/97	2-24	No association between occupational social class and prevalence of obesity (i.e. the proportion of participants in the top BMI quintile) in younger (2-15 year old) males and females. Lowest prevalence of obesity seen in higher social class grouping in 16-24 year olds; stronger association in females than males. No association with income in either sex or age group.
National Diet and Nutrition Survey[34]	1992/93	$1\frac{1}{2}$-$4\frac{1}{2}$	In males, no association between BMI and occupational social class, employment status of head of household, state benefits or mother's educational attainment. In females, obesity more common in lower social groups but positively associated with educational attainment of mother. No association with employment status or benefits.
Ten Towns Study[38]	1990	5-$7\frac{1}{2}$	No association between occupational social class and BMI.
Young Hearts Project[39]	1989/90 1992/93	12 15	Occupational social class not associated with either BMI or sum of skinfold thickness in 12 or 15 year olds.
National Child Development Study (1958 birth cohort)[45]	1981	23	Occupational social class associated with prevalence of obesity with most favourable levels seen in higher social groups.
DHSS survey of British adults[46]	1980	16-24	Weak association between occupational social class and BMI, such that higher BMI apparent in higher social groups.

BMI=body mass index

Study name and reference	Year of risk factor measurement	Age at risk factor measurement (years)	Findings
National Study of Health and Growth[48]	1972	5-11	Occupational social class associated with weight for height (i.e. weight adjusted for height and age) in boys, such that the most favourable levels seen in higher social groups; no association in girls. Number of siblings positively associated with weight for height in girls; no association in boys. Father's employment status and mother's educational attainment not related to weight for height. No association between occupational social class and tricep skinfold thickness. Negative association between number of siblings and tricep skinfold thickness in girls and boys.
National Survey of Health and Development (1946 birth cohort) and National Child Development Study (1958 birth cohort) combined[55]	1953/57/62 (1946 cohort) 1965/69/74 (1958 cohort)	7,11 and 16	In females, association between occupational social class and prevalence of overweight (i.e. weight exceeding standard weight for age, sex and height by 20% or more) in both birth cohorts at various ages whereby the most favourable levels apparent in higher social groups. In males, little evidence of an association.

in the National Child Development Study (1958 birth cohort),[45] and in 2-15 year olds in the 1995/97[31] and the 1998[26] Health Surveys for England (see Figure 4), there were no consistent social class differences in the markers of overweight or obesity used. Despite the increasing secular trends in childhood obesity, particularly in recent years,[99] the observation of little, if any, association between socioeconomic position and obesity in this group seems to persist. However, in contrast, in early adulthood, a social class gradient is apparent in some studies, including 23 year olds in the National Child Development Study (1958 birth cohort)[45] and 16-24 year olds in the Health Survey for England[31] (see Figure 4). There is also growing evidence from UK longitudinal studies[45, 55, 100] that social class in early life is related to subsequent adult adiposity with the lowest risk apparent in the higher social groups. This finding has been supported in a comprehensive review of these and other non-UK studies.[101]

Although being born into the low social classes would not in itself 'cause' obesity, the characteristics of this group in terms of their material circumstances, and the knowledge that informs behaviours such as food intake and physical activity, probably do.[101] The relation of socioeconomic position to each of these behaviours is discussed next.

Dietary characteristics

While detailed but modestly sized dietary studies of schoolchildren from Kent,[102, 103] the West of Scotland,[104] and Edinburgh[105, 106] have been conducted, it is possible to draw on the findings of several large-scale representative surveys of 1½-4½ year olds,[51, 34] schoolchildren,[27, 47] and young people[27] carried out over the last 50 years in the UK (see Table 6).

In 1967/68 a survey of the dietary habits of 1,938 pre-school children aged 6 months to 4½ years was conducted by the Department of Health.[51] This study was repeated 25 years later in 1992/93 in a different cohort of similar size and age range.[34] Despite a lower overall level of fat consumption in the most recent survey in comparison to the 1967/68 cohort, a relation with social class was apparent in both studies with the highest levels of fat consumption seen in children from households where the head was in manual employment. Other indicators of socioeconomic position – receipt of state benefits, employment status of the head of the household, and educational attainment of the mother – as measured in the 1992/93 study showed similar patterns of association.

In an older group of children, Golding et al[47] reported on the dietary habits of 10 year olds in the national Child Health and Education Study (1970 birth cohort study). Although the enquiries were limited to a small number of questions, it was evident that the proportion of children whose carers were in the lowest social groups consumed twice as much confectionery as those in social class I. Similar observations

Figure 4 ***Proportion (%) of children and young adults aged 2-24 years from the highest quintile of body mass index (BMI) by parental/subject's occupational social class in the Health Survey for England 1995-97***

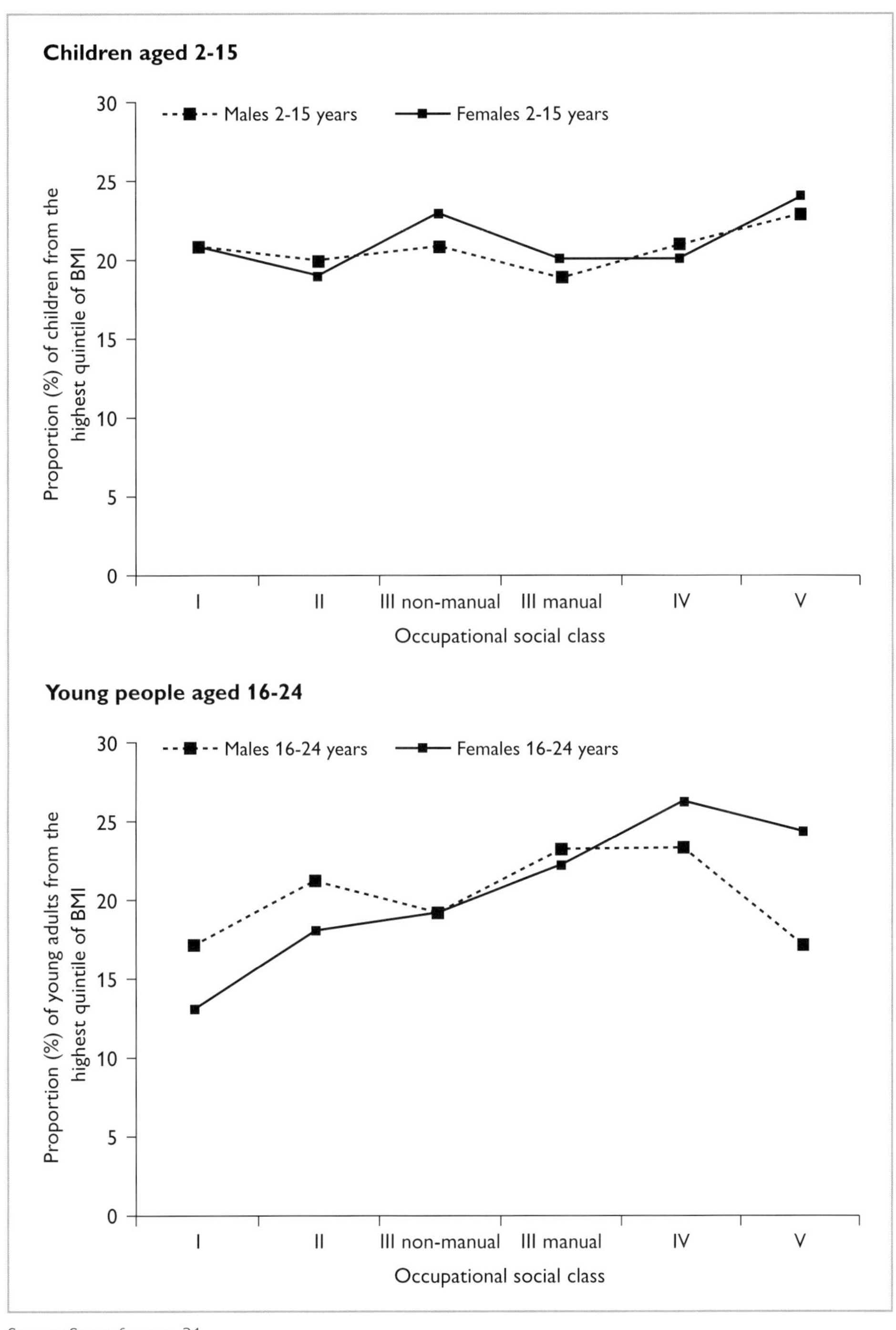

Source: See reference 31.

Table 6 ***Publications of UK studies relating socioeconomic position to dietary characteristics in children and young adults***

Study name and reference	Year of risk factor measurement	Age at risk factor measurement (years)	Findings
Scottish Health Survey[25]	1998	2-15	In boys and girls, occupational social class related to the consumption of wholemeal bread, fruit, and vegetables (green, raw and root) and fried food, with the most favourable levels evident in the higher social groups.
National Diet and Nutrition Survey[27]	1997	4-18	In girls, occupational social class associated with salad, fruit, green beans, and cream and cheese consumption, with the greatest quantities eaten by the most affluent children. In boys, these associations were seen for the consumption of skimmed milk, bread, cream and cheese.
Health Survey for England[31]	1995/97	2-24	Occupational social class and income associated with fruit, vegetable, crisp and chip consumption in 2-15 year old boys and girls, with the most favourable levels evident in the higher social groups. No association seen in older group.
Ten Towns Study[32]	1994	8-11	Occupational social class associated with fruit consumption in girls and boys, with the higher levels seen in the more affluent children.
Young Hearts Project[39]	1989/90 1992/93	12 15	In 12 year olds: occupational social class associated with polyunsaturates:saturates ratio (boys only) and total energy intake. In 15 year olds: occupational social class associated with fat and fruit intake. In all cases the most favourable levels seen in the higher social groups.
National Diet and Nutrition Survey[34]	1992/93	$1\frac{1}{2}$-$4\frac{1}{2}$	Occupational social class and income associated with absolute fat consumption with higher levels reported in the poorer groups. Fat consumption also higher in the children of parents who received state benefits (i.e. family credit and income support) in comparison with those who did not.

Study name and reference	Year of risk factor measurement	Age at risk factor measurement (years)	Findings
Department of Health survey of the diets of British schoolchildren[43]	1983	10-11 and 14-15	Occupational social class associated with fat consumption with higher levels reported in the poorer groups.
Ministry of Agriculture, Fisheries and Food Dietary Survey[44]	1982	15-25	Association between occupational social class and fat consumption in same direction as above but stronger in females than males.
Child Health and Education Study (1970 birth cohort)[47]	1980	10	Occupational social class associated with chocolate, cheese and brown bread consumption, with highest levels seen in the lower social groups.
National Diet and Nutrition Survey of pre-school children[51]	1967/68	$^1/_2$-$4^1/_2$	Fat consumption higher in children from households where head is in manual compared with non-manual employment. Positive association of income of head of the household, but not educational attainment of the mother, with fat consumption.
National Survey of Health and Development (1946 birth cohort)[23]	1950	4	Occupational social class associated with fruit, vegetable, and cake consumption with highest levels seen in the highest social groups. Chip consumption levels most favourable in more affluent children.

Figure 5 *Proportion (%) of daily fresh fruit consumption in children aged 8-11 years according to parental occupational social class in the Ten Towns Study, 1994*

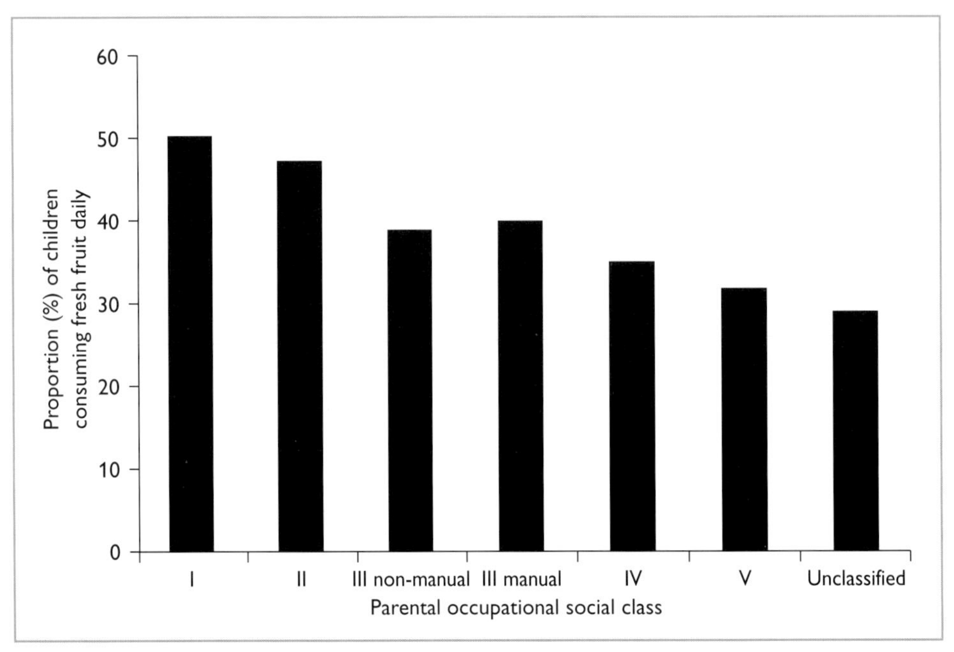

Source: Figures supplied by Peter Whincup based on further analyses[32] of data from a report of the Ten Towns Study

were made in the Health Survey for England[31] where, in 2-15 year olds, there was an increase from social classes I and II (combined) to IV and V (combined) in the prevalence of children consuming sweet foods, soft drinks and crisps. In keeping with this observation, Whincup,[107] in reporting on further analyses of data from the Ten Towns Study,[32] found that children from the lower social groups in England and Wales are less likely to favour fruit and vegetables (see Figure 5).

Physical activity and cardiorespiratory fitness

Like food consumption, physical activity is a multi-dimensional behaviour, the accurate assessment of which is problematic in all age groups, particularly children.[108] It has become increasingly common, therefore, for investigators to use previously validated physical activity questionnaires – of which there are several[109] – when surveying the physical activity levels of child populations. However, in the eight studies identified herein (see Table 7), a validated questionnaire was not used, so the findings should be treated with some caution.

Table 7 ***Publications of UK studies relating socioeconomic position to physical activity and/or cardiorespiratory fitness in children and young adults***

Study name and reference	Year of risk factor measurement	Age at risk factor measurement (years)	Findings
Scottish Health Survey[25]	1998	2-15	Occupational social class not consistently associated with physical activity in boys or girls.
National Diet and Nutrition Survey[27]	1997	4-18	Occupational social class and household income not associated with physical activity.
Health Survey for England[31]	1995/97	2-24	No clear pattern of association between physical activity, occupational social class and household income.
National Study of Health and Growth[35]	1992	8-9	No association of cardiorespiratory fitness with any of the indicators of socioeconomic position with the exception of number of siblings (in girls only).
National Fitness Survey[36]	1990	16-34	Occupational social class and educational attainment associated with physical activity, such that higher levels reported in men who were more affluent or better educated. Council house tenants less likely to be active than owner-occupiers or those in privately rented accommodation.
Young Hearts Project[39]	1989/90 1992/93	12 15	Occupational social class associated with physical activity in girls but unrelated to cardiorespiratory fitness in either sex.
Ministry of Agriculture, Fisheries and Food Dietary Survey[44]	1982	15-25	Prevalence of no exercise greatest in lower occupational groups.
Department of Health survey of British adults[46]	1980	16-34	Quantity of recreational exercise greatest in higher social groups.

No consistent pattern of association between socioeconomic position and indices of physical activity was apparent.[31, 39, 44, 36, 25, 27] The direction of these relationships does not seem to depend on age at measurement. In young adults (16-24 years) in the Health Survey for England,[31] for example, there was no evidence of a relationship between social class and physical activity, whereas in the National Fitness Survey[36] an association was observed in a similar age group.

The issue of inaccuracy of self-reported physical activity data has been addressed by Kikuchi et al[35] in the National Study of Health and Growth (NSHG) and Van Lenthe et al in the Young Hearts Project[39] where cardiorespiratory fitness – a physiological outcome of frequent physical activity and therefore an objective marker of this behaviour – was assessed in primary and secondary schoolchildren, respectively. No association with father's occupation nor mother's educational attainment (NSHG only) was evident.

Blood pressure

While both blood pressure and parental occupational social class were recorded in a survey of adolescents drawn from Nottinghamshire and Derbyshire general practice registries[110] (one of the first UK studies, along with the Brompton Longitudinal Study[111] to measure CHD risk factors in children) their relationship was not explored. Despite a recent review[112] of the socioeconomic position–blood pressure relation reporting an absence of any data from the UK for children, we were able to identify six relevant studies[31, 25, 27, 39, 33, 37] which draw on nationally representative UK samples (see Table 8) and a further three[113-115] which were based on convenience samples.

In children, height is strongly correlated with blood pressure such that tall children have higher blood pressure in comparison with those of shorter stature. Because height is also associated with occupational social class in this group with the taller children coming from more affluent backgrounds (see page 95), one would expect higher levels of blood pressure in the higher social class groups.[112] In most,[25, 27, 39, 37] but not all studies,[33] however, there was little evidence of any association between the given marker of socioeconomic position (i.e. occupational social class, household income, receipt of benefits, or parental educational attainment) and the measure of blood pressure employed (i.e. systolic, diastolic or mean). This was supported in some[113] but not all[114, 115] of the studies using non-representative samples of schoolchildren. The balance of evidence at the current time, therefore, suggests little evidence of an association between socioeconomic position indices and blood pressure levels in children and young people.

Table 8 ***Publications of UK studies relating socioeconomic position to blood pressure in children and young adults***

Study name and reference	Year of risk factor measurement	Age at risk factor measurement (years)	Findings
Scottish Health Survey[25]	1998	2-15	No association between occupational social class and systolic or diastolic blood pressure in boys or girls.
National Diet and Nutrition Survey[27]	1997	4-18	Occupational social class, household income and household benefit status not associated with mean blood pressure.
Health Survey for England[31]	1995/97	2-24	No association between occupational social class and height-adjusted systolic blood pressure in children or young adults. Income negatively associated with height-adjusted systolic blood pressure in 5-15 year old females but not males. No association in young adults.
National Study of Health and Growth[33]	1992/93	9	Occupational social class associated with diastolic blood pressure, whereby lowest levels seen in children from affluent backgrounds.
Ten Towns Study[37]	1990	5-7½	No association of mother's or father's occupational social class or educational attainment with systolic blood pressure.
Young Hearts Project[39]	1989/90 1992/93	12 15	No association between occupational social class and systolic or diastolic blood pressure in boys or girls.

Table 9 ***Publications of UK studies relating socioeconomic position to blood cholesterol in children and young adults***

Study name and reference	Year of risk factor measurement	Age at risk factor measurement (years)	Findings
National Diet and Nutrition Survey[27]	1997	4-18	Occupational social class, household income, and receipt of state benefit not associated with plasma total cholesterol or plasma HDL cholesterol.
National Study of Health and Growth[33]	1992/93	9	Number of siblings inversely associated with blood cholesterol. No association with father's occupational social class and mother's educational attainment.
Young Hearts Project[39]	1989/90 1992/93	12 15	Inconsistent associations between occupational social class, total and HDL cholesterol.

Blood cholesterol

Only three[27, 39, 33] published studies relating occupational social class to blood cholesterol in a representative sample of UK children were located (see Table 9). These studies generally reported no relationship[27, 33] and this observation was also made in preliminary analyses of data from the Ten Towns study (Peter Whincup – personal communication). The inconsistent pattern of association of occupational social class with total and HDL cholesterol seen in some age groups in the Young Hearts Project[39] may be explained by the small sample size therein.

Emerging CHD risk factors

Although high levels of some physiological variables such as C-reactive protein,[116] homocysteine,[117] and fibrinogen[118] when measured in adults appear to be predictive of subsequent CHD, their association with CHD when assessed in childhood is unknown. This notwithstanding, some studies have explored the relation of these emerging risk factors with parental occupational social class in children. In the Ten Towns study, Cook et al found that both C-reactive protein[119] and fibrinogen[120] were unrelated to the occupational social class of the head of the household. Although no UK study exploring the socioeconomic position–homocysteine association was identified, a survey of Norwegian schoolchildren reported no relationship.[121]

Conclusions

The aim of this chapter was to review the relation of socioeconomic position to CHD risk factors in children and young adults.

The main finding was that, of the 11 variables associated with CHD risk that were examined in this review, associations with markers of socioeconomic position were evident for:

- cigarette smoking
- birthweight
- indices of adiposity (in young adults)
- height, and
- some aspects of diet, specifically fat and fibre consumption.

The same relationships have been demonstrated in UK adults.

No clear association was seen for the other variables, that is:

- physical activity/cardiorespiratory fitness
- indices of adiposity (in children)
- blood pressure
- blood cholesterol, and
- some emerging risk factors.

Notably, obesity does not appear to show a relation with socioeconomic position in children under approximately 15 years of age, although a negative obesity–socioeconomic gradient seems to emerge in studies of young adults. The reasons for this are not clear. It should be a priority for further work to understand why associations emerge so relatively late in childhood and whether this indicates the existence of a particular window of opportunity in adolescence for interventions.

At present, there is an interest in addressing inequalities in health by focusing on 'poor' or 'socially excluded' children and young people. However, the findings of our review indicate that, for several modifiable CHD risk factors, there is an incremental gradient across the socioeconomic spectrum. To this extent, policies aimed at reducing inequalities may need to have a broader reach.

Overall, what is notable from this review is that there is a relative paucity of published data on which to make a comprehensive assessment of socioeconomic gradients in several CHD risk factors in childhood and early adulthood. There is, however, considerable scope to undertake analyses of existing databases (e.g. General Household Survey,[122] for young adults, and the Avon Longitudinal Study of Pregnancy and Childhood[123]) which would go beyond what is already in the public domain. Although the practice of investigators on the national health surveys to include samples of children in their studies is increasing, the recently published report *Health in England: Investigating the Links between Social Inequalities and Health*[124] was notable in not collecting information on individuals under the age of 16 years.

Acknowledgements

The authors are grateful to Peter Whincup for providing the graph featured in Figure 5; to Martin Jarvis and Eileen Goddard for drawing our attention to the various Health Education Authority and Department of Health-sponsored surveys on teenage smoking; and to Jan Gregory (National Diet and Nutrition Survey[27]) and Anne McMunn (Health Survey for England[31] and the Scottish Health Survey[25]) for discussing their work. Our thanks also go to Peter Whincup, George Davey Smith, David Gunnell, Martin Jarvis, and Eileen Goddard for providing detailed feedback on an earlier version of this chapter. We would welcome any corrections or suggested additions to this review.

Dr David Batty
Research Fellow in Epidemiology
Epidemiology Unit
Department of Epidemiology and Population Health
London School of Hygiene and Tropical Medicine
Keppel Street
London WC1E 7HT

References

1 Office for National Statistics. 1997. *Mortality Statistics Cause: Review of the Registrar General on Deaths by Cause, Sex and Age, in England and Wales, 1995. Series DH2: 22.* London: The Stationery Office.

2 Dawber TR, Meadors GF, Moore FE. 1951. Epidemiological approaches to heart disease: the Framingham study. *American Journal of Public Health*; 41: 279-86.

3 Labarthe DR. 1998. *Epidemiology and Prevention of Cardiovascular Diseases.* Gaithersburg, Maryland: Aspen Publishers Inc.

4 Wannamethee SG, Shaper AG, Whincup PH, Walker M. 1998. Adult height, stroke, and coronary heart disease. *American Journal of Epidemiology*; 148: 1069-76.

5 McKee M, Shkolnikov V, Leon DA. 2001. Alcohol is implicated in the fluctuations in cardiovascular disease in Russia since the 1980s. *Annals of Epidemiology*; 11: 1-6.

6 Navas-Nacher EL, Colangelo L, Beam C, Greenland P. 2001. Risk factors for coronary heart disease in men 18 to 39 years of age. *Annals of Internal Medicine*; 134: 433-39.

7 McCarron P, Davey Smith G, Okasha M, McEwen J. 2000. Blood pressure in young adulthood and mortality from cardiovascular disease. *Lancet*; 355: 1430-31.

8 Klag MJ, Ford DE, Mead LA, He J, Whelton PK, Liang KY et al. 1993. Serum cholesterol in young men and subsequent cardiovascular disease. *New England Journal of Medicine*; 328: 313-18.

9 Must A, Jacques PF, Dallal GE, Bajema CJ, Dietz WH. 1992. Long-term morbidity and mortality of overweight adolescents. A follow-up of the Harvard Growth Study of 1922 to 1935. *New England Journal of Medicine*; 327: 1350-55.

10 Gunnell DJ, Frankel SJ, Nanchahal K, Peters TJ, Davey Smith G. 1998. Childhood obesity and adult cardiovascular mortality: a 57-year follow-up study based on the Boyd Orr cohort. *American Journal of Clinical Nutrition*; 67: 1111-18.

11 Gunnell DJ, Davey Smith G, Frankel S, Nanchahal K, Braddon FE, Pemberton J et al. 1998. Childhood leg length and adult mortality: follow up of the Carnegie (Boyd Orr) Survey of Diet and Health in Pre-war Britain. *Journal of Epidemiology and Community Health*; 52: 142-52.

12 Barker DJP. 1998. *Mothers, Babies and Health in Later Life*. Edinburgh: Churchill Livingstone.

13 McCarron P, Davey Smith G, Okasha M, McEwen J. 2001. Smoking in adolescence and young adulthood and mortality in later life – prospective observational study. *Journal of Epidemiology and Community Health*; 55: 334-35.

14 Paffenbarger RS, Wing AL. 1969. Chronic disease in former college students. X. The effects of single and multiple characteristics on risk of fatal coronary heart disease. *American Journal of Epidemiology*; 90: 527-35.

15 Katzmarzyk PT, Perusse L, Malina RM, Bergeron J, Despres J, Bouchard C. 2001. Stability of indicators of the metabolic syndrome from childhood and adolescence to young adulthood. The Quebec Family Study. *Journal of Clinical Epidemiology*; 54: 190-95.

16 McGill HC, McMahan CA, Herderick EE, Malcom GT, Tracy RE, Strong JP. 2000. Origin of atherosclerosis in childhood and adolescence. *American Journal of Clinical Nutrition*; 72: 1307S-15S.

17 McGill HC Jr, McMahan CA, Zieske AW, Malcom GT, Tracy RE, Strong JP. 2001. Effects of nonlipid risk factors on atherosclerosis in youth with a favorable lipoprotein profile. *Circulation*; 103: 1546-50.

18 Napoli C, Glass CK, Witztum JL. 1999. Influence of maternal hypercholesterolemia during pregnancy on progression of early atherosclerotic lesions in childhood: Fate of Early Lesions in Children (FELIC) study. *Lancet*; 354: 1234-41.

19 Davey Smith G, Shipley MJ, Rose G. 1990. Magnitude and causes of socioeconomic differentials in mortality: further evidence from the Whitehall Study. *Journal of Epidemiology and Community Health*; 44: 265-70.

20 Pocock SJ, Shaper AG, Cook DG, Phillips AN, Walker M. 1987. Social class differences in ischaemic heart disease in British men. *Lancet*; 2: 197-201.

21 Davey Smith G, Hart C, Blane D, Gillis C, Hawthorne V. 1997. Lifetime socioeconomic position and mortality: prospective observational study. *British Medical Journal*; 314: 547-52.

22 Marmot MG, Davey Smith D, Stansfeld S, Patel C, North F, Head J et al. 1991. Health inequalities among British civil servants: the Whitehall II study. *Lancet*; 337: 1387-93.

23 Prynne CJ, Paul AA, Price GM, Wadsworth MEJ. 2000. Social class differences in foods eaten by a national sample of four-year old children in 1950 (abstract). *Proceedings of the Nutrition Society*.

24 World Health Organization Study Group. 1990. *Prevention in Childhood and Youth of Adult Cardiovascular Diseases: Time for Action.* Technical report series 792. Geneva: World Health Organization.

25 Shaw A, McMunn A, Field J. 2000. *The Scottish Health Survey 1998.* Edinburgh: The Scottish Executive Health Department.

26 Health Survey for England: children's reference tables '98. (http://www.doh.gov.uk/stats/crtables.htm – accessed 22 April 2001).

27 Gregory J, Lowe S. 2000. *National Diet and Nutrition Survey: Young People Aged 4 to 18 Years. Volume 1: Report of the Diet and Nutrition Survey.* London: The Stationery Office.

28 Smithers G, Gregory JR, Bates CJ, Prentice A, Jackson LV, Wenlock R. 2000. The National Diet and Nutrition Survey: Young People Aged 4-18 Years. *Nutrition Bulletin*; 25: 105-11.

29 Jarvis L. 1997. *Smoking Among Secondary School Children in 1996: England.* London: The Stationery Office.

30 Jarvis L. 1997. *Teenage Smoking Attitudes in 1996*. London: The Stationery Office.

31 Prescott-Clarke P, Primatesta P. 1999. *Health Survey for England. The Health of Young People '95-'97.* London: HMSO.

32 Cook DG, Carey IM, Whincup PH. 1997. Effect of fresh fruit consumption on lung function and wheeze in children. *Thorax*; 52: 628-33.

33 Rona RJ, Qureshi S, Chinn S. 1996. Factors related to total cholesterol and blood pressure in British 9 year olds. *Journal of Epidemiology and Community Health*; 50: 512-18.

34 Gregory JR. 1995. *National Diet and Nutrition Survey: Children Aged 1½ to 4½ years. Volume 1: Report of the Diet and Nutrition Survey*. London: HMSO.

35 Kikuchi S, Rona RJ, Chinn S. 1995. Physical fitness of nine year olds in England: related factors. *Journal of Epidemiology and Community Health*; 49: 180-85.

36 Allied Dunbar, Health Education Authority and Sports Council. 1992. *Allied Dunbar National Fitness Survey.* London: Sports Council.

37 Whincup PH, Cook DG, Papacosta O. 1992. Do maternal and intrauterine factors influence blood pressure in childhood? *Archives of Disease in Childhood*; 67: 1423-29.

38 Whincup PH, Cook DG, Papacosta O, Walker M. 1992. Childhood blood pressure, body build, and birthweight: geographical associations with cardiovascular mortality. *Journal of Epidemiology and Community Health*; 46: 396-402.

39 Van Lenthe FJ, Boreham CA, Twisk JW, Strain JJ, Savage JM, Davey Smith G. 2001. Socio-economic position and coronary heart disease risk factors in youth. Findings from the Young Hearts Project in Northern Ireland. *European Journal of Public Health*; 11: 43-50.

40 Glendinning A, Shucksmith J, Hendry L. 1994. Social class and adolescent smoking behaviour. *Social Science and Medicine*; 38: 1449-60.

41 Whincup PH, Cook DG, Shaper AG. 1988. Social class and height. *British Medical Journal*; 297: 980-81.

42 Goddard, E. 1990. *Why Children Start Smoking*. London: HMSO.

43 Committee on Medical Aspects of Food Policy. 1989. *The Diets of British Schoolchildren. Report on Health and Social Subjects Number 36.* London: HMSO.

44 Bull NL. 1985. Dietary habits of 15-25 year olds. *Human Nutrition: Applied Nutrition*; suppl 1; 39A: 1-68.

45 Power C, Moynihan C. 1988. Social class and changes in weight-for-height between childhood and early adulthood. *International Journal of Obesity*; 12: 445-53.

46 Knight I, Eldridge J. 1984. *The Heights and Weights of Adults in Britain.* London: HMSO.

47 Golding J, Haslum M, Morris AC. 1984. What do our ten year old children eat? *Health Visitor*; 57: 178-79.

48 Rona RJ, Chinn S. 1982. National Study of Health and Growth: social and family factors and obesity in primary school children. *Annals of Human Biology*; 9: 131-45.

49 Rona RJ, Swan AV, Altman DG. 1978. Social factors and height of primary schoolchildren in England and Scotland. *Journal of Epidemiology and Community Health*; 32: 147-54.

50 Bynner JM. 1969. *The Young Smoker*. London: HMSO.

51 Department of Health and Social Security. 1975. *A Nutrition Survey of Pre-school Children in 1967-68. Report on Health and Social Subjects: 10.* London: HMSO.

52 Goldstein H. 1971. Factors influencing the height of seven year old children – results from the National Child Development Study. *Human Biology*; 43: 92-111.

53 Douglas JWB, Simpson HR. 1964. Height in relation to puberty, family size and social class. A longitudinal study. *Milbank Memorial Fund Quarterly*; 42: 20-35.

54 Kuh DL, Power C, Rodgers B. 1991. Secular trends in social class and sex differences in adult height. *International Journal of Epidemiology*; 20: 1001-09.

55 Peckham CS, Stark O, Simonite V, Wolff OH. 1983. Prevalence of obesity in British children born in 1946 and 1958. *British Medical Journal (Clinical Research Edition)*; 286: 1237-42.

56 Wadsworth ME, Kuh DJ. 1997. Childhood influences on adult health: a review of recent work from the British 1946 national birth cohort study, the MRC National Survey of Health and Development. *Paediatric and Perinatal Epidemiology*; 11: 2-20.

57 Power C. 1992. A review of child health in the 1958 birth cohort: National Child Development Study. *Paediatric and Perinatal Epidemiology*; 6: 81-110.

58 Butler NR, Golding J, Howlett B. 1986. *From Birth to Five. A Study of the Health and Behaviour of Britain's 5-year-olds.* Oxford: Pergamon.

59 Rona RJ. 1995. The National Study of Health and Growth (NSHG): 23 years on the road. *International Journal of Epidemiology*; 24; suppl. 1: S69-S74.

60 Rona RJ, Chinn S. 1999. *The National Study of Health and Growth.* Oxford: Oxford University Press.

61 Erens B, Primatesta P. 1999. *Health Survey for England. Cardiovascular Disease '98.* London: HMSO.

62 Whincup PH, Cook DG, Shaper AG, Macfarlane DJ, Walker M. 1988. Blood pressure in British children: associations with adult blood pressure and cardiovascular mortality. *Lancet*; 2: 890-93.

63 Shaper AG, Pocock SJ, Walker M, Cohen NM, Wale CJ, Thomson AG. 1981. British Regional Heart Study: cardiovascular risk factors in middle-aged men in 24 towns. *British Medical Journal*; 283: 179-86.

64 Dobbs J, Marsh A. 1983. *Smoking Among Secondary School Children.* London: HMSO.

65 Goddard E, Higgins V. 1999. *Smoking, Drinking and Drug Use Among Young Teenagers in 1998.* London: The Stationery Office.

66 Goddard E, Higgins V. 2000. *Drug Use, Smoking and Drinking Among Young Teenagers in 1999.* London: The Stationery Office.

67 O'Rourke A, O'Sullivan N, Wilson-Davis K. 1968. A Dublin schools' smoking survey. I. *Irish Journal of Medical Science;* 7: 123-30.

68 Bynner JM. 1971. The dilemma facing health educators. Second World Conference on Smoking and Health, 1971.

69 Flynn M. 1961. Smoking habits of school children in County Westmeath. *Journal of the Irish Medical Association*; XLVIII: 87-97.

70 Holland W, Halil T et al. 1969. Indications for measures to be taken in childhood to prevent chronic respiratory disease. *Milbank Memorial Fund Quarterly*; 47: 215-27.

71 McKennell AC, Thomas RK. Adults' and adolescents' smoking habits and attitudes. 1967. London: British Ministry of Health.

72 Bewley BR, Day I, Ide L. 1973. *Smoking by Children in Great Britain – A Review of the Literature.* London: Social Science Research Council.

73 Bewley BR, Bland JM. 1977. Academic performance and social factors related to cigarette smoking by schoolchildren. *British Journal of Preventive and Social Medicine*; 31: 18-24.

74 Rawbone RG, Keeling CA, Jenkins A, Guz A. 1978. Cigarette smoking among secondary schoolchildren in 1975. Prevalence of respiratory symptoms, knowledge of health hazards, and attitudes to smoking and health. *Journal of Epidemiology and Community Health*; 32: 53-58.

75 Raven JC. 1965. *Mill Hill Vocabulary Scale Manual.* London: Lewis.

76 De Vries H. 1995. Socio-economic differences in smoking: Dutch adolescents' beliefs and behaviour. *Social Science and Medicine*; 41: 419-24.

77 Macfarlane A. 2000. *Birth Counts. Statistics of Pregnancy and Childbirth.* London: The Stationery Office.

78 Bartley M, Power C, Blane D, Davey Smith D, Shipley M. 1994. Birth weight and later socioeconomic disadvantage: evidence from the 1958 British cohort study. *British Medical Journal*; 309: 1475-78.

79 Marmot MG, Adelstein AM, Robinson N, Rose GA. 1978. Changing social-class distribution of heart disease. *British Medical Journal*; 2: 1109-12.

80 Davey Smith G. Socioeconomic differentials. In: Kuh D, Ben-Shlomo Y (eds.) 1997. *A Life Course Approach to Chronic Disease Epidemiology*. Oxford: Oxford University Press: 242-73.

81 Mascie-Taylor CG. 1991. Biosocial influences on stature: a review. *Journal of Biosocial Science*; 23: 113-28.

82 Floud R, Wachter K, Gregory A. 1990. *Height, Health and History. Nutritional Status in the United Kingdom, 1750-1980.* Cambridge: Cambridge University Press.

83 Rose G. 1910. *First Annual Report by the Medical Officer on the Medical Inspection of the Schools under his Supervision.* Aberdeen: Aberdeen School Board.

84 White E, Wilson A, Greene SA, Berry W, McCowan C, Cairns A et al. 1995. Growth screening and urban deprivation. *Journal of Medical Screening*; 2: 140-44.

85 Reading R, Raybould S, Jarvis S. 1993. Deprivation, low birth weight, and children's height: a comparison between rural and urban areas. *British Medical Journal*; 307: 1458-62.

86 Wright CM, Aynsley-Green A, Tomlinson P, Ahmed L, MacFarlane JA. 1992. A comparison of height, weight and head circumference of primary school children living in deprived and non-deprived circumstances. *Early Human Development*; 31: 157-62.

87 Norman HB. 1939. Public-school and secondary-school boys. A comparison of their physique. *Lancet*; 2: 442-45.

88 Menzies F. 1940. *Report by the School Medical Officer on the Average Heights and Weights of Elementary School Children in the County of London in 1938.* London: London County Council.

89 Bransby ER, Burn JL, Magee HE. 1946. Effects of certain social conditions on the health of school children. *British Medical Journal*; 2: 767.

90 Grant MW. 1964. Rate of growth in relation to birth rank and family size. *British Journal of Preventive and Social Medicine*; 18: 35-42.

91 Topp SG, Cook J, Holland WW, Elliott A. 1970. Influence of environmental factors on height and weight of schoolchildren. *British Journal of Preventive and Social Medicine*; 24: 154-62.

92 Billewicz WZ, Thomson AM, Fellowes HM. 1983. A longitudinal study of growth in Newcastle upon Tyne adolescents. *Annals of Human Biology*; 10: 125-33.

93 Elwood PC, Sweetnam PM, Gray OP, Davies DP, Wood PD. 1987. Growth of children from 0-5 years: with special reference to mother's smoking in pregnancy. *Annals of Human Biology*; 14: 543-57.

94 Gunnell DJ, Davey Smith D, Frankel SJ, Kemp M, Peters TJ. 1998. Socio-economic and dietary influences on leg length and trunk length in childhood: a reanalysis of the Carnegie (Boyd Orr) survey of diet and health in pre-war Britain (1937-39). *Paediatric and Perinatal Epidemiology*; 12; suppl 1: 96-113.

95 Rowett Research Institute. 1953. *Family Diet and Health in Pre-war Britain*. Dunfermline: Carnegie United Kingdom Trust.

96 Hammond WH. 1955. Measurement and interpretation of subcutaneous fat, with norms for children and young adult males. *British Journal of Preventive and Social Medicine*; 9: 201-11.

97 Durnin JVA, Lonergan ME, Good J, Ewan A. 1974. A cross-sectional and nutritional and anthropometric study, with an interval of 7 years, on 611 young adolescent school children. *British Journal of Nutrition*; 32: 169-79.

98 Whitelaw AGL. 1971. The association of social class and sibling number with skinfold thickness in London schoolboys. *Human Biology*; 43: 414-20.

99 Chinn S, Rona RJ. 2001. Prevalence and trends in overweight and obesity in three cross sectional studies of British children, 1974-94. *British Medical Journal*; 322: 24-26.

100 Hardy R, Wadsworth M, Kuh D. 1998. Association between childhood obesity and social class and adult obesity across the life course in a British national cohort (abstract). *Journal of Epidemiology and Community Health*; 52: 693.

101 Parsons TJ, Power C, Logan S, Summerbell CD. 1999. Childhood predictors of adult obesity: a systematic review. *International Journal of Obesity*; 23; suppl. 8: S1-S107.

102 Holland WW, Halil T. 1969. Factors influencing the onset of chronic respiratory disease. *British Medical Journal*; 2: 205-08.

103 Cook J, Altman DG, Moore DMC. 1973. A survey of the nutritional status of schoolchildren. Relation between nutrient intake and socio-economic factors. *British Journal of Preventive and Social Medicine*; 27: 91-99.

104 Anderson AS, MacIntyre S, West P. 1994. Dietary patterns among adolescents in the west of Scotland. *British Journal of Nutrition*; 71: 111-22.

105 Ruxton CH, Kirk TR, Belton NR, Holmes MA. 1996. Relationships between social class, nutrient intake and dietary patterns in Edinburgh school children. *International Journal of Food Sciences and Nutrition*; 47: 341-49.

106 Ruxton CH, O'Sullivan KR, Kirk TR, Belton NR, Holmes MA. 1996. The contribution of breakfast to the diets of a sample of 136 primary-schoolchildren in Edinburgh. *British Journal of Nutrition*; 75: 419-31.

107 Whincup P. 2000. *Cardiovascular Risk Factors in Childhood and Adolescence. Diet and Physical Activity in Children: Preventing Adult Obesity and Heart Disease* (Conference report). London: The Coronary Prevention Group.

108 Batty GD. 1998. Physical activity measurement in children. *Australian and New Zealand Journal of Public Health*; 22: 165.

109 Pereira MA. 1997. A collection of physical activity questionnaires for health-related research. *Medicine and Science in Sports and Exercise*; 29: S1-S205.

110 Orchard TJ, Rodgers M, Hedley AJ, Mitchell JRA. 1980. Changes in blood lipids and blood pressure during adolescence. *British Medical Journal*; 280: 1563-67.

111 de Swiet M, Fayers P, Shinebourne EA. 1976. Blood pressure survey in a population of newborn infants. *British Medical Journal*; 2: 9-11.

112 Colhoun HM, Hemingway H, Poulter NR. 1998. Socio-economic status and blood pressure: an overview analysis. *Journal of Human Hypertension*; 12: 91-110.

113 MacIntyre S, West P. 1991. Lack of class variation in health in adolescence: an artefact of an occupational measure of social class? *Social Science and Medicine*; 32: 395-402.

114 Beresford SAA, Holland WW. 1973. Epidemiology and treatment of raised blood pressure. *Proceedings of the Royal Society of Medicine*; 66: 1009-11.

115 Law CM, Barker DJP, Bull AR, Osmond C. 1991. Maternal and fetal influences on blood pressure. *Archives of Disease in Childhood*; 66: 1291-95.

116 Kuller LH, Tracy RP, Shaten J, Meilahn EN. 1996. Relation of C-reactive protein and coronary heart disease in the MRFIT nested case-control study. Multiple Risk Factor Intervention Trial. *American Journal of Epidemiology*; 144: 537-47.

117 Stampfer MJ, Malinow MR, Willett WC, Newcomer LM, Upson B, Ullmann D et al. 1992. A prospective study of plasma homocyst(e)ine and risk of myocardial infarction in US physicians. *Journal of the American Medical Association*; 268: 877-81.

118 Meade TW. 1994. Haemostatic function and arterial disease. *British Medical Bulletin*; 50: 755-75.

119 Cook DG, Mendall MA, Whincup PH, Carey IM, Ballam L, Morris JE et al. 2000. C-reactive protein concentration in children: relationship to adiposity and other cardiovascular risk factors. *Atherosclerosis*; 149: 139-50.

120 Cook DG, Whincup PH, Miller G, Carey IM, Adshead FJ, Papacosta O et al. 1999. Fibrinogen and factor VII levels are related to adiposity but not to fetal growth or social class in children aged 10-11 years. *American Journal of Epidemiology*; 150: 727-36.

121 Tonstad S, Refsum H, Sivertsen M, Christophersen B, Ose L, Ueland PM. 1996. Relation of total homocysteine and lipid levels in children to premature cardiovascular death in male relatives. *Pediatric Research*; 40: 47-52.

122 Bridgwood A. 2000. *Living in Britain: Results from the 1998 General Household Survey. Series GHS. Office for National Statistics. Social Survey Division 28.* London: The Stationery Office.

123 Golding J, Pembrey M, Jones R. 2001. ALSPAC – the Avon Longitudinal Study of Parents and Children. I. Study methodology. ALSPAC Study Team. *Paediatric and Perinatal Epidemiology*; 15: 74-87.

124 Mason V. 2000. *Health in England 1998: Investigating the Links between Social Inequalities and Health.* London: The Stationery Office.

Chapter 5

Ethnic minority young people and health

Dr Marie-Claude Gervais

Department of Social Psychology, London School of Economics

Hamid Rehman

Ethnos Research and Consultancy

This chapter:

- provides a demographic, sociocultural and psychological profile of the ethnic minority populations in the UK
- summarises research findings in relation to coronary heart disease, stroke and hypertension, and diabetes
- discusses explanations proposed for variations in disease patterns found among ethnic minority populations, and
- argues for the need for targeted programmes if the health of ethnic minorities is to improve.

Key themes

- There are important differences in disease patterns between certain ethnic minority groups compared with the general population. Rates of coronary heart disease and non-insulin dependent diabetes are considerably higher among the South Asian population. Hypertension and stroke are high among the African-Caribbean and Bangladeshi populations. Many ethnic minority groups are at risk of haemoglobin disorders.
- The reasons for such inequalities are not clear-cut. Biological, socioeconomic, cultural, and environmental explanations have been advanced, in conjunction with individual differences in lifestyles and matters of access to health services.
- To make sense of the evidence, and to devise more effective interventions, it is useful to think of the main groups as comprising three generations, each with their own distinctive sociocultural experiences and identities.
- Programmes and interventions aimed at the general population often fail to reach the ethnic minority groups. Specifically targeted initiatives are required if the burden of ill health experienced by many ethnic minority groups is to be alleviated.

Introduction

The aim of this chapter is to summarise research on the health status and health needs of young members of black and minority ethnic groups in the UK. However, in conducting the review we have found very little information on the specific needs of young people from ethnic minority groups. Young ethnic minority people are much neglected both in terms of health research and service provision. Very little is known about the specific needs and views of these groups, and not enough specialist services or health campaigns are aimed at them. We will therefore summarise what is currently known about the health of ethnic minority groups in general, and highlight areas where information is available for young people.

The paucity of research about the health of ethnic minority youth is particularly troubling in three ways. First, the ethnic minority population is known to suffer from disproportionately poor health. In the context of a government policy which seeks to reduce inequalities in health, it seems especially urgent to address the needs of ethnic minority groups. Second, the early years of life are a time when many lifestyle choices are established. Some of these lifestyles may increase the vulnerability of people to health problems such as coronary heart disease or hypertension. Thirdly, many young people engage in particularly high-risk behaviours (for example, the misuse of illegal drugs and alcohol, or the practice of unsafe sex). It is therefore important to assess the extent to which these – or other more culturally-specific – practices are found among ethnic youth.

There are important differences in disease patterns between certain ethnic minorities and the general population. The reasons for such inequalities are not clear-cut. Biological, socioeconomic, cultural, and environmental explanations are advanced, in conjunction with individual differences in lifestyles and matters of access to health services. The research shows that the health and information needs of ethnic minorities in the UK are not being met. The situation portrayed by the accumulated evidence leaves little doubt: black and ethnic minority groups in the UK need more support, more resources, and greater sensitivity to their life experiences. Services aimed at the general population often fail to meet the needs of ethnic minority communities. The current disparity that exists between the health status of the black and minority ethnic groups and that of the white population cannot be justified.

This chapter provides a brief demographic profile of the ethnic minorities in the UK. It summarises the research findings in relation to three key health conditions: coronary heart disease; stroke and hypertension; and diabetes. It also discusses some of the explanations for the variations in the health of black and minority ethnic groups and considers lifestyle factors in detail.

A profile of the black and ethnic minority population

Demographic profile

The 1991 Census identified just over 3 million people, or 5.5% of the population of the UK, as belonging to one of the ethnic minority groups. More recent estimates from the 1997 Labour Force Survey[1] show that this figure has grown to 6.4%. Table 1 shows the size of the different populations.

Table 1 ***The ethnic composition of the UK population, 1997***

	Number (000s)	Percentage of total
White	52,936	93.6%
All ethnic minority groups	3,599	6.4%
African-Caribbean	526	0.9%
Black African	352	0.6%
Black – Other	307	0.5%
Indian	925	1.6%
Pakistani	587	1.0%
Bangladeshi	209	0.4%
Chinese	157	0.3%
Other Asian	192	0.3%
Other	344	0.6%

Source: See reference 1.

The largest groups are Indians, African-Caribbeans, Pakistanis, black Africans, Bangladeshis and Chinese. South Asians (Indians, Pakistanis and Bangladeshis) form about half of the ethnic minority population and the black groups make up a further quarter of the population. All ethnic minority populations have a younger age profile than the white population, with about a third (31%) aged under 14 compared to about a fifth (18%) of the white population. Just under a half of the ethnic minority population were born in the UK. This figure increases to 90% for those aged below 30.

The ethnic minority population is largely concentrated in a few geographical areas, with the exception of the Chinese who are widely dispersed. Greater London is where the concentration of ethnic minority groups is the highest. Nearly half (44.8%) of all ethnic minority groups live there, compared with one in ten of the white population. A further quarter of the population lives in the West Midlands, West Yorkshire and the Greater Manchester area.

There are also significant variations in the concentration of individual ethnic groups. The black population is heavily concentrated in the Greater London area, with 85% of the black African and 60% of the African-Caribbean population residing there. Among the South Asian groups, about half of the Indian and Bangladeshi populations and a fifth of the Pakistani population live in the Greater London area. In contrast, 60% of Pakistani, 20% of the African Caribbean and only 5% of the black African population live in the Greater Manchester, West Yorkshire and West Midlands areas.

Sociocultural and psychological profile by generation

Beyond the demographic profile given above, it is useful to think of the main ethnic minority groups in the UK as comprising three generations, each with their own distinctive sociocultural experiences and identities.

Across all communities, the older age group (which includes those aged roughly 50 and above) mainly comprises the original migrants who left their respective countries to settle in the UK in search of greater economic prosperity. It also includes the parents of later migrants who arranged for their relatives to come and join them. In most communities, the elders tend to be poorly educated and, with the exception of people of African-Caribbean descent, they also tend to speak, read and write little or no English. Their way of life and sense of identity are rooted in a different country. Ethnic minority elders very often live under extremely harsh material and social conditions. Their level of participation in mainstream British society is severely impaired both by difficulties in communication and by discrimination.

The middle generation (which comprises those aged roughly between 30 and 50) is more diverse. It includes two main sub-groups: the now grown-up children of the older settlers, as well as migrants who arrived here in mid-life. The first sub-group is not characterised predominantly by its adherence to the culture of their parents. In most cases, they are cultural 'hybrids', raised according to their parents' original culture but in the wider context of British society. They have been to school, they often speak both English and their traditional language, and they can draw on two sets of cultural resources, but they also experience the tensions between these diverse ways of life and their attendant expectations. Full participation in mainstream British society is still limited by a sense of exclusion and the experience of racism despite the erosion of linguistic barriers. The second sub-group tends to be much more traditional since they keep very close ties with the country they have recently left. They experience many of the same difficulties originally faced by the older migrants, although the overt racism they face has somewhat reduced since British society has become more open and has developed infrastructures to facilitate integration.

The younger generation (aged roughly below 30) is more heterogeneous still. This group comprises the growing number of youth who are born and raised in the UK. As stated above, more than 90% of the ethnic minority population aged below 30 were born in the UK. Not only do they master English, but they often speak no other language, despite their parents' best efforts to keep their traditional culture alive. The experiences of the UK-born youth are highly diverse. For some, full participation is achieved and simply taken for granted. For others, discrimination continues to make it difficult for them to feel that they truly belong here. Skin colour serves as a reminder that they are 'different'. Yet these young people know their parents' culture only indirectly through their family and the occasional visit to their parents' country of origin. Others still seek to retrieve a strong identification with their parents' culture. The maintenance and resurrection of very traditional lifestyles among the younger segments of some communities must be understood as an attempt to restore a positive sense of identity in the face of widespread exclusion. At the opposite end of the spectrum, we also find a growing number of young people of mixed ethnic, racial or religious parentage. In this case, the dominant approach seems to be one of internationalism and an active quest for diversity, but very little is known about this group of youth.

Of course, this portrayal oversimplifies a complex situation. It does not account for the specificity of each community, for the range of religious, regional or linguistic differences between them, and the individual experiences within them. Yet, we must go beyond statistics to understand key aspects of community life among the youth and how this might impact on their health.

This kind of profile provides an essential framework to make sense of the evidence concerning the health of ethnic minority youth. It is also necessary for devising more realistic intervention programmes.

Inequalities in health of black and minority ethnic groups

Limitations of data

When discussing the health of black and minority ethnic groups in the UK it is important to note that much of what is known about the health of these populations is based on country of birth as recorded on death certificates. This presents serious problems, especially in the case of young people, most of whom are born in the UK. Further, country of birth does not always reflect ethnicity. For example, an Indian born in Jamaica would be classified as African-Caribbean but would have very little in common with that ethnic group. Finally, mortality data merely describe variations in mortality rates but suggest no explanation for the inequalities in health recorded between ethnic minority groups.

The situation is improving. Three national health and lifestyles surveys have generated much needed evidence on the health status and knowledge, attitudes and behaviours towards a variety of health-related topics among the largest ethnic minority groups.[2-4] Some of the results are discussed below. In addition, a recent national survey of ethnic minorities has yielded crucial data on employment patterns and income levels, and family and household structures as well as health.[5] The routine recording of information on ethnicity for people admitted into hospital was introduced in April 1996. The 1999 Health Survey for England has a specific ethnic focus and provides data on disease and illness.[6] These help to overcome some of the gaps existing in ethnic research and allow for better explanations for the variations in health. Still, health issues among ethnic youth must too often be extrapolated rather than demonstrated.

Variations in health

There are important differences in disease patterns between certain ethnic minority groups compared with the general population. Rates of coronary heart disease and non-insulin dependent diabetes are considerably higher among the South Asian population. Hypertension and stroke are high among the African-Caribbean and Bangladeshi populations. African-Caribbeans, especially young men, are over-represented in mental health services. Many ethnic minority groups are at risk of haemoglobin disorders.

Some of the key findings from the research in relation to coronary heart disease, stroke and hypertension, and diabetes are summarised below. The data do not refer specifically to ethnic youth. Inferences drawn from the entire ethnic group to the young segment of each group will largely depend on the kind of explanations offered to account for the discrepancies recorded. For instance, if biological/genetic explanations are favoured, then one may legitimately generalise from the adult population to the youth. However, if lifestyle factors and socioeconomic conditions are deemed more important, then empirical research will have to determine the extent to which lifestyles and socioeconomic conditions have changed between each generation within any one community.

Coronary heart disease

- For the period 1988-92, among South Asians the mortality rate from coronary heart disease was 38% higher among men and 43% higher among women when compared to the population of England and Wales.[7]

- The pattern shows some variations between the groups, with the highest rates being among Bangladeshi men (47% higher than the population of England and Wales), followed by Pakistani men (42% higher), and Indian men (37% higher).[7]

- The Caribbean population has lower rates than the general population[7] as do the Chinese.[8]

- For the period 1979-83, the relative risks of coronary heart disease in young South Asian men aged 20-29 and 30-39, compared with the population of England and Wales, were 3.1 and 2.1, respectively. These figures are much higher than the relative risk associated with men of South Asian origin in the age group 20-69 which is 1.36.[9]

- These findings are of particular concern when the relatively young age profile of the South Asian population in the UK is considered. This suggests that, unless the relative burden of ill health is addressed, it will have a dramatic effect on both South Asian communities and healthcare providers.

- Mortality rates from coronary heart disease among South Asians have not declined as fast as they have in the general population.[10]

Stroke and hypertension

- Significantly higher rates of mortality from stroke are found across all ethnic minority groups, compared with the general population. The highest rates are found among Bangladeshis (2.5 times the national average), followed by African-Caribbeans (1.8), Pakistanis (1.7), and Indians (1.3).[7]

- Between 1988 and 1992, mortality from hypertension among African-Caribbeans was 3.5 times greater than among the white population of England and Wales. Among South Asians the rate was 1.5 times the national average.[11]

- Estimates suggest that between 25% and 35% of African-Caribbeans are hypertensive, compared with 10%-20% of the white population.[12]

Diabetes

- Mortality rates from diabetes are higher among all ethnic minority groups when compared with the general population.

- Bangladeshis have a 6.5-fold excess; Pakistanis a four-fold excess; and Indians a three-fold excess. African-Caribbean men exceed the national average by 3.6-fold, while among African-Caribbean women the excess is six-fold.[13]

- Twenty per cent of South Asians aged 40-69 have type 2 diabetes, compared with 5% of whites.[14] The condition remains undiagnosed for 40% of Asians.[15]

Explanations for variations in the health of black and minority ethnic groups

The aetiology of disease is complex. Environmental, social, economic, biological and cultural issues as well as individual lifestyle and behaviours have a bearing on people's health. The following explanations have been put forward for the variations in disease patterns found among ethnic minority populations. We will briefly discuss the genetic/biological and socioeconomic explanations. Greater emphasis is placed on lifestyle factors and inequalities in access to health services.

Genetic/biological factors

A number of researchers have argued that the higher prevalence of certain conditions among ethnic minorities can be explained by genetic factors. For example, McKeigue et al[16] suggest that South Asians may face an additional risk of heart disease compared with other ethnic groups because of the relatively high prevalence of the metabolic disorder insulin resistance syndrome, which is genetically determined. The strengths of this approach are well known, but it may be worth pointing out some of its limitations. Firstly, it relies on mortality data, which is problematic as 'ethnicity' is recorded on death certificates as country of birth. Secondly, this approach assumes that all members forming the group 'South Asians' are genetically and culturally identical. In reality they consist of very different groups with different cultures, religions, migration patterns, and socioeconomic positions.[17]

Social and economic factors

The material and social conditions in which many ethnic minority groups find themselves are particularly harsh. Most ethnic minority groups live in deprived inner city areas. Unemployment levels are generally higher in these groups and people tend to be unemployed for longer. Income levels are lower and many members of ethnic groups live in poorer housing.[18, 5, 19] There is a growing body of evidence to suggest that such factors are more immediate and powerful predictors of poor health than are strictly biological/genetic factors.[20] Indeed, it is first and foremost as members of socially and economically disadvantaged groups that members of black and minority ethnic populations suffer from poor health, and not as Chinese, African-Caribbeans, or Bangladeshis *per se*.

Specific social and psychological experiences

Psychological stress has an important impact on health. There are a number of social and psychologically stressful experiences that are confined to ethnic minorities, most notably racism. The experience of racism – both direct and indirect – is pervasive. It contributes to disengagement from mainstream society, limits improvements in socioeconomic conditions, and creates fear and frustration. The consequence of direct racism, frequently experienced in the form of racial harassment, goes beyond the actual events themselves. The impact affects not only the individual concerned, but their family, friends and the community at large.

In one survey, 13% of ethnic minority respondents reported having been subjected to some form of racial harassment in the 12 months prior to the survey and about a quarter of respondents worried about being racially harassed.[21] Six to eight per cent of the ethnic minority groups feel that the racism in their area has a bad effect on their health.[2]

High levels of unemployment among ethnic minorities are another source of stress. The Health Education Authority survey[2] found that 17% of African-Caribbean, 10% of Indians, 11% of Pakistanis and 14% of Bangladeshis worry enough about being unemployed to feel that this has a bad effect on their health. This compares with 6% of the general population.

About one in six of all ethnic minorities feel that the amount of violent crime in their area affects their health. This reflects the concentration of the ethnic minority groups in urban, inner city areas with associated higher levels of crime.

Lifestyle factors

It is now accepted that changes in certain lifestyle factors – such as smoking, diet and physical activity – can reduce the prevalence of conditions such as coronary heart disease and stroke. Health education aimed at altering such behaviours is an important way of reducing the prevalence of these conditions among ethnic minority populations.

The extent to which individuals engage in health-promoting behaviours and are prepared to modify risky behaviours such as smoking and unhealthy eating will depend, to some extent, on how they assess their own health, on their health behaviours, on their awareness of what healthy behaviour is, and on their awareness of the relationship between their behaviour and health or illness.

Recent survey results show that, within black and minority ethnic groups, knowledge about the risk factors associated with health is very limited. Knowledge about diseases associated with smoking, lack of physical activity, and diet is generally poor. This is particularly worrying as these are the main risk factors associated with conditions such as coronary heart disease, hypertension and stroke – conditions which are found to be disproportionately higher among many of the ethnic minority communities. This evidence suggests that current health promotion programmes are not reaching these communities.

Ethnic minority youth and health

The Health Survey for England 1999[6] was the first national survey to assess the health and lifestyles of the ethnic minority children aged 2 to 15 years. Key findings from the survey are given below. For each section, issues for discussion and potential explanations (in italics) are suggested to make sense of the otherwise purely descriptive data.

Self-reported health

Longstanding and limiting longstanding illness

Overall, for both boys and girls, Indian, Pakistani, Bangladeshi and Chinese children were significantly less likely to report any longstanding illness than children in the general population. For limiting longstanding illness, this remained the case only for Bangladeshi boys and Chinese girls.

It could be that the threshold at which some children from ethnic minority backgrounds report a longstanding illness is higher than in the general population, but that this difference is smaller when people consider the case of 'limiting' longstanding illness.

Self-assessed general health

The proportion of boys reporting 'good' or 'very good' health in the general population was 91%. All ethnic minority boys except the Chinese were less likely to report 'good' or 'very good' health than boys in the general population. Among girls no significant differences were found.

Psychological health

Psychological health was only tested in the 13-15 age groups. No significant differences were found but the sample sizes were very small.

Methodological difficulties must be invoked here. Much qualitative evidence suggests that there are differences in psychological health between ethnic groups, and between them and the general population. Low self-esteem and poor mental health are commonly reported among African-Caribbean boys, for instance. Suicide rates are disproportionately high among South Asian young women. The experience of racism and discrimination – common across all groups but particularly frequent in the Chinese community – is also known to have a debilitating effect on health.

Smoking

Questions about smoking were asked of those aged between 8 and 15. The rates reported for 'ever having smoked a cigarette' are very similar in the general population and the African-Caribbean group: 19% of white boys and 21% of white girls aged 8-15 report ever having smoked a cigarette, compared with 21% of African-Caribbean children (boys and girls). Much lower figures are found across all the other ethnic groups. Among boys, 10% of Indian, 10% of Pakistani, 8% of Bangladeshi and 6% of Chinese report ever having smoked. Among girls, the figures drop to 7% for Indian, 5% for Pakistani, 1% for Bangladeshi and 3% for Chinese.

Smoking is a highly normative behaviour and one which is subject to peer pressure. In South Asian and Chinese communities – where smoking is culturally frowned upon for both children and women – smoking rates among children are very low. Children do not smoke in front of their parents as this causes serious offence. And, because smoking is culturally frowned upon in these cultures, it is likely that under-reporting is very common among South Asian and Chinese children. By contrast, in the white and African-Caribbean groups, and despite health messages to the contrary, smoking is valued as part of a 'cool' and 'rebellious' teenage identity.

Alcohol consumption

Questions about alcohol consumption were asked of those aged between 8 and 15. Again, the rates reported for ever having drunk a whole alcoholic drink (rather than merely tasted one) are much lower among the South Asian and Chinese children than among African-Caribbean and white children. Moreover, whenever drinking is at all common, the rates are higher for boys than for girls. Among the boys, 40% of white, 31% of African-Caribbean, 18% of Chinese, 12% of Indian and 1% of both Pakistani and Bangladeshi boys report ever having had a whole alcoholic drink. Among girls,

32% of white, 25% of African-Caribbean, 11% of Chinese, 8% of Indian, 2% of Pakistani and 1% of Bangladeshi girls report ever having had a whole alcoholic drink.

Again, cultural and religious differences must be invoked. In the Muslim Pakistani and Bangladeshi communities – where alcohol consumption is prohibited on religious grounds – the children respect these proscriptions and do not drink until well into young adulthood (if at all).

Physical activity
With the exception of African-Caribbean children, generally lower rates of participation in sports and exercise are found among ethnic minority children than in the general population. In the general population, 63% of boys participate in regular sport and exercise. Among ethnic minority boys the figures are 68% of African-Caribbean, 59% of Indian, 46% of Pakistani, 48% of Bangladeshi and 51% of Chinese. The figures for girls are 56% for the general population, 55% for African-Caribbean, 34% for Indian, 31% for Pakistani, 27% for Bangladeshi and 53% for Chinese.

It is likely that South Asian and Chinese parents put a stronger emphasis on educational achievements than do white or African-Caribbean parents. The presence of sporty role models in these two groups and their virtual absence from the South Asian and Chinese communities are also possible explanatory factors.

Body mass index
Compared with the general population, mean body mass index (BMI) was higher among African-Caribbean and Indian boys, while for Bangladeshi boys mean BMI was lower than for boys in the general population. Among girls, BMI was higher for African-Caribbean and lower for Bangladeshi and Chinese compared with the general population.

Differences in genetic make-up and differences in diet are the two most likely causes of the reported differences in BMI.

Discussion and speculations

African-Caribbean boys and girls have much in common with the general population on a range of indicators. South Asian (Indian, Pakistani and Bangladeshi) and Chinese children are also quite similar on a number of indicators.

On the whole, it is extremely difficulty to identify in this data set developing 'trends' that could explain the very significant inequalities in health noted among the adult population. The degree to which ethnic minority children take on the behaviours of their elders remains unclear. Research is needed to establish the extent to which ethnic minority children follow the cultural lifestyles espoused by their parents.

Below, we speculate on the reasons for the apparent differences (and, more often, lack of differences) between children from the ethnic minority groups, and between the latter and children from the majority white population.

Cultural and religious differences

South Asian and Chinese children are much more obedient and respectful of authority (parental or otherwise) than are both white and African-Caribbean children. Deference to authority, respect for hierarchy, an emphasis on self-discipline and hard work, and a collectivist ethos more generally, still prevail among South Asian and Chinese children. This value system is gradually eroding, but children from these ethnic minority backgrounds do not tend to challenge parental authority or to engage in socially unacceptable behaviours until later in life (if at all).

Socioeconomic factors

Although poor socioeconomic conditions disproportionately affect ethnic minority groups, and although these conditions are known to have a detrimental effect on health, it takes a long period for these effects to manifest themselves. It is not surprising therefore that differences should not yet be large among young children.

One exception has to do with respiratory problems. Asthma is the most common chronic childhood disease in the UK. For both boys and girls, respiratory problems were more common in the African-Caribbean and white groups than among South Asian and Chinese groups (whose rates were significantly lower than those found in the general population).

The causes of asthma and other respiratory problems are unclear, but explanatory factors include outdoor and indoor pollution, exposure to allergens, smoking, and diet. It seems plausible that ethnic minority families – who tend to live in polluted inner cities – should be more affected by outdoor pollution. In addition, it is likely that ethnic minority children are differentially affected by passive smoking – the main source of indoor pollution – on the basis of their parents' smoking habits. Although South Asian and Chinese *men* smoke very heavily, women do not, which means that the households as a whole are likely to be less polluted. By contrast, in African-Caribbean and white households, both parents are likely to be smokers. This could suggest that the children are more likely to develop health problems as a result of passive smoking.

Age groups

In many cases, very young children (from the age of 2) are aggregated together with young teenagers (up to the age of 15). Thus, although there may be highly significant differences among teenagers from different ethnic minority groups, these differences are somewhat minimised or obscured by the conflation of all the children under one age group.

Conditions which do not affect children
Some of the conditions assessed in the survey,[6] such as high blood pressure, do not affect children in any significant way. It is therefore not surprising that differences should not be noted in this population.

The need for targeted programmes

The situation of black and minority ethnic groups can be significantly improved. Initiatives aimed at improving the social and economic circumstances of the more deprived communities of this country will impact on the lives of ethnic minority communities.

However, unless ethnic minority needs are specifically targeted, such programmes and initiatives will fail to alleviate the burden of ill health experienced by ethnic minorities. This point is made forcibly by Acheson:[20]

"… failure to make specific consideration of minority ethnic issues risks increasing ethnic inequalities by unintentionally favouring policies that benefit the ethnic majority. Thus policies to consider inequalities in health should include consideration of the application of these policies to minority ethnic groups as a matter of course."

In particular, these policies should attempt to reach those members of ethnic minority groups who:

- cannot speak English
- have limited knowledge of the health service
- have restricted access to the health service
- find the information presented to them inappropriate or irrelevant (largely because it embodies the norms of the dominant white culture)
- are systematically dissatisfied by their experiences of health services (often because they experience institutional or direct discrimination).

Below we list some issues that need to be considered when promoting health among ethnic minority young people.

- Specifically targeted programmes need to be developed on those conditions known to disproportionately affect members of black and minority ethnic groups. This is particularly important in the case of coronary heart disease among South Asians.

- All health promotion materials should reflect the fact that the UK is a multi-cultural society. At minimum, this means the routine use of images depicting not only black, Asian or Chinese faces, but also aspects of various ethnic ways of life. This is important as it shows ethnic minority groups that they 'belong'. This recognition is central to integration and psychological well-being.

- Much crucial information fails to reach black and minority ethnic youth, either because it is in a format that does not make sense to them, or because it is not disseminated effectively.

- Health messages and health promotion activities need to be developed for each community (in line with its own health needs and culture) and be disseminated through appropriate channels. Grassroots community groups have a key role to play here. In addition, the family and religion play an important role in the identity and socialisation of many young ethnic minority people. They may be potent resources for reaching out to young people.

- Health service professionals need to be trained to develop a 'multi-cultural awareness', i.e. to develop and to communicate a sensitivity and positive attitude towards ethnic, cultural or religious differences. Such training should not perpetuate static stereotypes. Rather, it should involve teaching health professionals to develop listening and communication skills, and it should affirm the patient's right to be different.

- Similar training is also necessary for staff in schools. Furthermore, any policies to promote healthy eating in schools must take into consideration the religious and cultural aspects of ethnic minority diets.

- Interaction between local and national bodies needs to be strengthened. Local emphases are crucial to take account of differences in the life circumstances and identities of different groups of people; national emphases are crucial to provide the 'big picture', to coordinate local projects, and to ensure learning gains across projects and organisations.

- There are many examples of good practice at the local level with ethnic minority people that need to be recorded, and shared with other local projects throughout the country. There is a definite tendency to 'reinvent the wheel' rather than to build on best practice and experience.

- The practice of short-term funding of community-based health projects needs to change. It has a detrimental effect on ethnic minorities. Often, just as people begin to get used to a project, the funding is withdrawn and the project ends. Such experiences contribute to the widespread sense of marginalisation and mistrust in public bodies found across ethnic minority groups (especially among youth), and often result in disengagement from future health projects.

Acknowledgements

We are grateful to Dr Catherine Campbell for use of her paper Report of the Expert Working Group on the Health of Young Black and Minority Ethnic People in Britain *(unpublished).*

References

1 Schuman J. 1999. The ethnic minority populations of Great Britain: Latest estimates. *Population Trends: 96*; 33-43.

2 Health Education Authority. 1994. *Black and Minority Ethnic Groups in England: Health and Lifestyles Survey*. London: Health Education Authority.

3 Health Education Authority. 1999. *The Health and Lifestyles of the Chinese Population in England*. London: Health Education Authority.

4 Health Education Authority. 2000. *Black and Minority Ethnic Groups in England: The Second Health and Lifestyles Survey*. London: Health Education Authority.

5 Modood T, Berthoud R, Lakey J, Nazroo J, Smith P, Virdee S, Beishon S. 1997. *Ethnic Minorities in Britain: Diversity and Disadvantage*. London: Policy Studies Institute.

6 Erens B, Primatesta P, Prior G. 2001. *Health Survey for England: The Health of Minority Ethnic Groups 1999*. London: The Stationery Office.

7 Balarajan R. 1995. Ethnicity and variations in the nation's health. *Health Trends*; 27: 114-19.

8 Harland JO, Unwin N, Bhopal RS, White M, Watson W, Laker M et al. 1997. Low levels of cardiovascular risk factors and coronary heart disease in a UK Chinese population. *Journal of Epidemiology and Community Health*; 51: 636-42.

9 Balarajan R. 1991. Ethnic differences in mortality from ischaemic heart disease and cerebrovascular disease in England and Wales. *British Medical Journal*; 302: 560-64.

10 Wild S, McKeigue P. 1997. Cross sectional analysis of mortality by country of birth in England and Wales, 1970-92. *British Medical Journal*; 314: 705-10.

11 Raleigh VS, Kiri V, Balarajan R. 1997. Variations in mortality from diabetes mellitus, hypertension and renal disease in England and Wales by country of birth. *Health Trends*; 28: 122-27.

12 Beevers G, Beevers M. Hypertension: Impact upon black and ethnic minority people. In: Hopkins A, Bahl V (eds.) 1993. *Access to Health Care for People from Black and Ethnic Minorities*. London: Royal College of Physicians.

13 Raleigh V. 1997. Diabetes and hypertension in Britain's ethnic minorities: Implications for the future of renal services. *British Medical Journal*; 314: 209-13.

14 McKeigue P, Sevak L. 1994. *Coronary Heart Disease in South Asian Communities: A Manual for Health Promotion*. London: Health Education Authority.

15 Simmons D, Williams DRR, Powell MJ. 1989. Prevalence of diabetes in a predominantly Asian community: Preliminary findings of the Coventry diabetes study. *British Medical Journal*; 298: 18-21.

16 McKeigue P, Shah B, Marmot M. 1991. Relation of central obesity and insulin resistance with high diabetes prevalence and cardiovascular risk in South Asians. *Lancet*; 337: 382-86.

17 Nazroo JY. 1998. *Genetic, Cultural or Socio-economic Vulnerability? Explaining Ethnic Inequalities in Health*. London: Blackwell Publishers Ltd.

18 Balarajan R. 1997. *Ethnic Diversity in England and Wales*. London: National Institute for Ethnic Studies in Health and Social Policy.

19 Berthoud R. 1998. *The Incomes of Ethnic Minorities*. ISER Report 98-1. Colchester: University of Essex, Institute of Social and Economic Research.

20 Acheson D. 1998. *Independent Inquiry into Inequalities in Health*. London: The Stationery Office.

21 Virdee S. 1997. Racial harassment. In: Modood T, Berthoud R, Lakey J, Nazroo J, Smith P, Virdee S, Beishon S. 1997. *Ethnic Minorities in Britain: Diversity and Disadvantage*. London: Policy Studies Institute.

Chapter 6

Health-related behaviour in low-income families

Dr Paul Harker

South and East Dorset Primary Care Trust

Dr Ann Hemingway

Institute of Health and Community Studies, Bournemouth University

This chapter:

- discusses findings from qualitative studies of coronary heart disease risk-related behaviour among low-income women and their children
- looks at adverse influences outside the family on such behaviour, and
- makes recommendations for action to reduce the problems of low-income families at risk from coronary heart disease.

Key themes

- Adverse socioeconomic conditions affect the health-related behaviour of women and therefore their children.
- A theoretical model for coronary heart disease risk behaviour in the workplace appears to be applicable to the home environment of mothers and children, particularly but not exclusively to low-income families.
- A perception of high workload demand, characterised by lack of control and absence of social support, has to be addressed if children and adults are to be receptive to lifestyle education.
- Multi-strand interventions are required which should include the provision of: high quality, low-cost childcare; parent access to training opportunities; and the development of community forums (including young people) with agency support to develop their own health promotion programmes.

Introduction

Social issues such as low family income and poor housing in childhood have been linked with adult risk of coronary heart disease (CHD). This chapter looks in detail at the behavioural influences and responses which operate under adverse circumstances. It focuses on the findings of a recent research study to examine those factors and relevant related theory.

The demand-control-support model[1] was developed in relation to occupational psychosocial factors which increase the risk of CHD. There appears to be a strong association between measures of poor psychosocial work environment and risk of CHD.[2] The Whitehall study showed that those who described low decision latitude had a greater relative risk of developing CHD and the relationship was significant after adjusting for negative affectivity, social class and biomedical risk factors.[3]

Home can act as a place of work for mothers on low income (often combined with an external work contract) and the demand-control-support model can then be applied to the home as a 'workplace'. Childhood behaviour is most influenced by the relationship with the parents within the home, particularly in the pre-school years, and thus the effect of the home as workplace can bring to bear on the child as well as the parent.

The characteristics of the model are:

- high workload demand from self, partner and children
- lack of control and low decision latitude in relation to conditions inside and outside the home
- absence of social support, both emotional and instrumental, from partner, family and friends.

The role a mother has as a carer within a family can be viewed as particularly relevant in terms of its impact on the health and lifestyle of the family members overall[4] and invariably the lifestyle of parents and young children are intertwined. Almost one-third (2.7 million) of children in the UK live with lone parents (90% lone mothers), and 60% of these live on a low income.[5] An understanding of the knowledge, attitudes and behaviour relevant to CHD risk for these parents and their children can be gained by considering the social influences on such low-income, often isolated mothers who are relying on benefits. One study which has looked at this group is the Boscombe Public Health Action Area Study.

The Boscombe Public Health Action Area Study

The first stage of this case study, which is currently being undertaken within Boscombe, one of the Dorset urban Public Health Action Areas, has considered the CHD risk factors in the lifestyles of low-income women aged 18-46 and their children (where low income is defined as below half average income [EU definition cited in Acheson 1998[6]]). This study has taken a qualitative approach using a grounded theory method to analyse and guide the interviews with the participants. The study is being undertaken in an area of high density, multiple occupation housing with a rapid turnover of population (in excess of 25% per year). The women within the study were theoretically sampled mapping the characteristics of the local population (n=19).

The interviews were in-depth discussions including reflections on the women's own lifestyles and those of their children. A quarter of the women interviewed were in paid work, although none of the women were earning enough to escape benefits. The high workload demand, low control and lack of social support influences which were revealed related both to the unpaid and paid work the women did, inside and outside of the home.

High workload demand

The burden of caring for a child or children alone on a low income exposes a parent to high or continuous work demands. A typical quote from a participant underlines this:

"She needs watching all the time ... it's not as easy as if someone else was here and I could just get on with it ... I could improve (our diet) if the circumstances were different."

This woman was living with her 10-month old daughter in a bed-sit, in sub-standard conditions; the shared kitchen had no door and outside there were open stairs. The demands on the women were seen as relentless and all consuming:

"Yes, I can (make changes) but my whole way of life centres around them really so is dependent on their well being" (Lone mother with two daughters aged 1 and 5.)

These demands were highlighted as the root cause of their stress, which in some cases led to illness. The stress of caring for children, possibly on their own and in difficult circumstances, was overwhelming, and the frustrations experienced from managing on a low income were apparent in many aspects of their lifestyles.

Parents' coping mechanisms for life stresses, such as smoking,[7] drinking, or over-eating, sometimes leading to weight problems, may affect children directly, and may also lead to children learning negative coping mechanisms early in life which can be maintained into adulthood and which may, within their family circumstances, go unchallenged. Parental alcohol abuse can be both a cause of and a response to stress, and affect child and subsequent adult behaviour. An estimated 920,000 children are currently living in a home where one or both parents drink alcohol excessively.[8] The psychological impact on children can be immense, often leading to the development of alcohol problems for themselves and difficulties with combating other negative coping mechanisms such as smoking and an unhealthy diet.

Individuals who use smoking to cope with stress and who are negatively controlled by a smoking partner and friends are least likely to take assistance to quit the habit. This becomes particularly worrying with pregnant mothers, who will neglect future physical health matters in favour of alleviation of current stresses. Living on a low income not only restricts purchasing choices, such as of healthy food, but also engenders individual and group behaviours such as smoking which can be regarded as valuable by those with few pleasures.[7,9] Postnatal depression, while of course not confined to low-income families, can both cause and/or exacerbate dysfunction if not recognised and treated.[10]

Lack of control and low decision latitude

When asked about their dietary intake, the women in Boscombe made it clear that their decisions were influenced and controlled by their children and those they lived with. The majority of the women interviewed considered themselves to be overweight at the time of interview, and all had tried different methods to lose weight, many of which had involved a cost, and their efforts had been ineffective. The women were aware of what constitutes a healthy diet, namely eating fruit and vegetables each day and having less fatty food, as has been shown in other studies.[11] However, the women's own dietary intake was dictated by practical issues of income and 'what the children would eat'. For example, a lone parent of two children, one aged 3 years and one aged 3 months said:

"I will cook something she likes, which is probably very unhealthy, like sausages, eggs ... you know something childy."

The women viewed chips, burgers and sausages as child-friendly food, and said that their children were not keen on, nor satisfied with fruit, vegetables or salads. They said that the problem with their own dietary intake was that for practical reasons they ate with the children and the kind of things the children liked to eat were not healthy:

"I couldn't buy different for me, him and for them ... I couldn't afford it ... I did try."

Good intentions were not realised:

"I kept finding salad going off in the fridge." (Mother of two, aged 2 and 4, with a partner)

The diet which the women thought their partners and children preferred, and which they thus provided, was high in fats and markedly lacking in fruit and vegetables.

From investigations of dietary patterns of families and extended families on a low income in Boscombe,[12] the following points emerged:

- Mothers are mainly concerned that their children eat what they are given; and are less concerned that what they are given is a balanced diet.
- As the chaotic lifestyle of some dysfunctional families leads children to assert their independence earlier, they are able to help themselves to snacks and drinks throughout the day as and when they choose, without parental guidance, effectively controlling their own diets.
- Where there was the traditional 'generation gap' between parents and grandparents, and these grandparents took an active role in the extended family scenario, visiting grandchildren experienced more traditional, balanced meal patterns.
- Grandparents appeared to have a greater appreciation of the valuable contribution fruit and vegetables make to children's diets. Some children said it was more common to eat fruit when visiting grandparents than when at home.

The practical problems relating to preparing food while caring for young children, in potentially unsafe surroundings, was apparent. The majority of the women interviewed lived in private rented accommodation in an inner urban area and expressed concerns over the standard of cooking equipment and food storage available. The women stated that often grills or cookers did not work or were not present, thereby preventing or limiting food preparation. Refrigerators and freezers were faulty or absent, and their contents vulnerable to theft:

"When I was living in a B & B (we were homeless) and I had to give my children take-away – the guilt because I was not feeding them properly was awful. I had nowhere to prepare anything." (Lone mother of two, aged 7 and 11)

In cases where all food had to be stored, prepared and consumed in the same room, there were concerns over accidents during preparation and disposal of waste.

A chaotic lifestyle within a family may lead to children snacking inappropriately. The comments and observed behaviour within this study showed that food may be used in difficult circumstances as a distraction or a pacifier, or indeed as a reward. If one is caring for children on a low income, the only achievable treats may be in terms of snacks and drinks, since trips out, toys, games or clothes may be well beyond the family budget.

Receiving benefits or working at a low pay, low status job may expose one to a low level of decision latitude or deflated sense of control.[9] Having no influence over when or how one receives one's benefits, or being unable to influence how or when one works, heightens this.

All of the women had plans for their own study or work-related development, but these were generally inhibited by caring responsibilities and financial constraints, with lack of realistically priced and reliable childcare being the main drawback. This inhibition of ambition caused frustration and reduced the perception of control in the short term. Karasek and Theorell[1] discuss "feeling like your feet are stuck to the floor" in high demand, low control situations, and how this can cause psychological strain.

The educational attainment of parents, and their interest in and value of education, affect the achievement of their children. European research[13] has indicated a direct relationship between the educational achievement of mothers and the degree of consideration given to healthy family food. Mothers with higher educational attainment considered health more frequently than cost. They applied more food restrictions and were generally less permissive in indulging a child's preferences than mothers with low educational attainment. Diet in infancy is mainly influenced by the mother's culture, employment and coping skills, which inform the choice of breast or bottle-feeding and timing of the introduction of solids.

Some women had downsized their work ambitions if they were alone caring for children, even though they had educational qualifications which would allow access to a variety of occupations. The reasons stated for this related to the need to have little or no responsibility at work, so that if there were problems with illness or childcare they were not failing their employer. Casual work seemed to be appealing as they could leave or not attend if caring responsibilities needed to take precedence:

"Something where I can just clock in and clock out – I don't really care how mundane – if the children are sick I can phone up and say they are and I am not letting anyone down." (Lone parent and trained operating department assistant, parent of two children, aged 1 and 5)

Karasek and Theorell[1] have pointed out that low pay, low status jobs are often demanding and lacking in decision latitude. Most notable is the large number of these occupations populated primarily by women. The women in the study who worked primarily undertook jobs such as waitressing, sewing, childcare or shop work. Interestingly, of the women who worked, none had only one job, multiple casual jobs being the norm, and there was a preference for 'low levels of responsibility' which fitted in with their caring responsibilities.

Choices for exercise were severely limited by finance, mobility, safety of local areas to exercise in (especially in the winter months), and childcare responsibilities. If the women had to pay for childcare as well as having to pay to attend a class, they were discouraged from attending. If in addition they had to pay to travel to a class, then regular attendance would be outside their budget. Once again, influencing factors include the high level of demand of caring for children that was placed on the women, as well as in some cases caring for sick partners or ageing relatives. Their low budget and lack of access to transport (most not having use of a car) also inhibited their control over whether they attended exercise groups or classes. Lack of support from friends and family to relieve caring responsibilities meant limited choices.

Many of the women expressed anxieties over the level of traffic and the resulting dangers inherent in allowing their children out to play in the local area. In addition anxieties were expressed over the safety of the limited play areas provided locally, as they had found syringes and needles in the gardens of their own homes (normally houses of multiple occupation) and in the council play areas. Anxieties were also expressed regarding paedophiles, and in some cases the women felt that ex-partners might put their children at risk, either due to the risk of violence or abduction. Thus the children were kept in to play at home, often in a home which contained dangers such as unscreened fires and unsafe cooking facilities and stairs. These caring strategies are pragmatic within the realities of the families' circumstances, but the end result may be sedentary children and adults, and a rise in accidents in the home. Diets may also suffer in such circumstances as parents' ability to distract or amuse children can be limited by the surroundings, so the cheapest solution may be to offer food or drinks.

Absence of social support

The women interviewed gained little social support. Few of the women originated from the area, and those who did had often lost contact with family members. The main source of support was from other women in the area in similar circumstances to themselves, from church groups, and from local health professionals such as health visitors. Lack of social support may be of even greater importance when changes in accommodation and/or employment take place on the birth of another child into a family.

Changes which occurred to the women in the study and their children were commonly related to the breakdown of a relationship; a reduction in income and a change in accommodation would often result. Birth cohort studies carried out in the UK have shown over several decades that there are both short-term and long-term disadvantages to children after parental separation. Early effects include lower self-esteem and increased health, educational and social difficulties, while longer term effects include earlier age of school leaving, lower vocational achievement, earlier serious relationships, departure from the family home, pregnancy, marriage and divorce. The causal relationship between these outcomes and parental divorce is, however, hotly disputed.[14]

Interestingly, none of the women interviewed had internet access in their own home for themselves or their children. In rented accommodation the likelihood of having an extra phone point, as well as the expense of purchasing a computer was considered by the women to be an unattainable goal. In the US this issue has been termed 'the digital divide' as it has been recognised that educationally children may be disadvantaged by having no internet access throughout their education. Lack of computer access seriously disadvantages mothers and children for information access and development of basic IT skills.

Discussion

We have concentrated on families on a low income, but it is apparent that coronary heart disease risk behaviour can operate within less socially excluded families. Junk eating and drug-taking, for example, can be a problem in affluent families. One or both parents may have an emphasis on striving and control, a so-called 'Type A' personality. It is believed that such behaviour can be learned in the home through transference of parental values to children.[15] Type A behaviour is said to be associated with high blood pressure and consequent risk of CHD. Such families do exhibit high workload demand, and lack-of-control features, but these should be more amenable to self-help correction when they have a high educational attainment, are not on a low income and have greater social support. Culture may also affect parental response to low income. Black British or Afro-Caribbean lone parent families in one study were able to provide more nutritious meals than white counterparts.[16]

Parental example is not the only social influence which affects risk of coronary heart disease. Children who are separated from parents are more influenced by peers, as are young people beginning to break away from the family. Smoking in 11-16 year olds may have more to do with personality than with external influences such as parental attitude and peer group reinforcement.[17] This view is in contrast with studies which rate parental example as an important influence on adolescent smoking.[18, 19] Others emphasise the influences of 'style' in younger smokers and later the group socialisation of smoking and its use to relieve stress in teenagers.[20] After the age of 16, young people who have started smoking may be more likely to continue if they face limited opportunities and a low income.

Advertising targets families with low decision latitude. Ninety-nine per cent of foods and drinks advertised to children during Saturday morning children's TV contain either high fat, high sugar or high salt.[21] A recent review of the effects of television on child health in the US points out that in a typical portrayal, television characters eat vast quantities of unhealthy food and yet remain thin. Content analysis of US television has found that alcohol, tobacco or illicit drugs are present in 70% of prime-time dramatic programmes and half of all music videos.[22] A study of cigarette advertising and the onset of smoking in 11-12 year old children in the North and South of England found that cigarette advertising increased children's awareness of smoking at a more generic level. It also encouraged them to take up the habit, beginning with any cigarettes which were available and affordable.[23]

School settings can be used for preventive action but effects have been limited to small supplementation of diet (poor uptake of school meals and few breakfast clubs) and delaying onset of smoking.[24] Action often requires using timetable time and scarce school resources. Constraints of the National Curriculum and school targets also have an inhibiting effect which can, for example, lead to the decline in exercise opportunities at school. Children and young people may be given the knowledge of how to be healthy but the effect on behaviour is transitory if they are growing up in a dysfunctional family.

A theory of family stress or non-coping was formulated after the Great Depression of the 1930s in the US by Reuben Hill, based on those families who survived the Depression contrasted with those who did not. They were families who had lost their jobs and were in extreme poverty. From qualitative material, Hill theorised that there are two complex variables which act to buffer the family from acute 'stressors' and reduce the direct correlation between multiple stressors and family crisis. The 'B' variable refers to a complex of internal and external family resources and social support available to the family, including internal and external social connectedness. Hill theorised that social isolation significantly increased the impact of the multiple stressors on family functioning. The second 'C' factor was the extent to which the family perceived their circumstances as a disaster or an opportunity. Approaches to substance misuse in the US, such as the Families and Schools Together (FAST) programme are based on measures to address the B variable, while taking into account the C factor.[25]

A UK programme to address the problems of low-income families with risk of coronary heart disease should include the following:

Reduce high workload demand

- Make it easier for mothers to combine parenting and part-time work through a supportive benefits system.

- Provide more high quality, low-cost childcare services to relieve parents. The National Childcare Strategy, which has announced a three-fold increase in the annual investment in childcare from £66m in 2000 to over £200m by 2003-04, is good news.

- Joint agency identification of health problems related to housing deficiencies and provision of special funds to correct them, along the lines of a scheme in Cornwall to reduce asthma risk.[26]

- Provision of greater local council powers over neglectful landlords and scrutiny of houses in multiple occupation featured in the consultation paper *Licensing of houses in multiple occupation*.[27]

Increase decision latitude

- Coordinate the support given to mothers through statutory and voluntary services to ensure time to talk, and give the right support and provide a wider net to detect and 'treat' postnatal depression.

- Help parents access attractive training opportunities.

- Develop exercise opportunities tailored to mothers.

- Provide support for shopping and cooking of food through measures which ensure low-cost, healthy food supplies and cookery groups.

- Develop community approaches to smoking cessation which include mentoring and buddy support.

Build social capital

- Develop community forums, with charitable status and agency support, to develop their own health promoting programmes.

- Support community newsletters which help to build social networks.

- Open community cafés with cyber and childcare facilities.

- Give direct help to parents to avoid a non-coping dysfunctional future. Extending the Sure Start (0-4s and parents) and New Start (outreach to 16-17 year olds) programmes to cover more of the country, and particularly rural areas, and extending the new Children's Fund (targeted at 5-13 year olds), should help.

- Integrate community, school and youth club/young people's advisory centre action which helps young people consider making changes for improvement.

Support should be available for all parents, including those who are apparently coping with adversity. They can help others by their example and they themselves can receive support to prevent being tipped over the edge into dysfunction.

Developments such as Health Action Zones, Public Health Action Areas, Healthy Living Centres, Sure Start and New Start programmes offer excellent opportunities for the prevention of heart disease through addressing underlying behavioural responses to social adversity.

We select three interventions as the most cost-effective. These are:

- high quality, low-cost childcare

- parent access to attractive training opportunities, and

- development of community forums (including young people), with charitable status and agency support, to develop their own health promotion programmes.

This selection is based on the reality that these three developments will underpin the other recommendations. The three priorities are inter-linked because in particular, the building of local community influence on local lives is most likely to ensure creation of training opportunities, some of which will provide more qualified childcarers. It is also most likely to generate acceptability and sustainability of local health promotion initiatives.

There is some objective evidence of the effectiveness of building social capital in reducing coronary heart disease in adults,[28] and of Sure Start-type pre-school social capital interventions[29] in reducing adult dysfunctional behaviour. We calculate the cost of community development, paid by health and local authority funding, at £80,000 per annum, per community of up to 5,000 persons, over three years. Thereafter each community should be capable of raising and sustaining grant funding and drawing on its own resources. This calculation is based on the Building Social Capital programme in West Howe, Bournemouth, which employs a full-time community development worker. The returns on such an investment – as Health Action Zone experience is revealing – are not immediate in terms of a decline in cardiovascular morbidity, nor indeed other examples of physical and mental morbidity, for which such a programme can be expected to pay dividends. The gains for children will be over a lifetime and we should be optimistic, although current knowledge is limited by the existing evidence, that this type of endowment policy can be expected to pay dividends in the long term, for heart and other health gain.

References

1 Karasek R, Theorell T. 1990. *Healthy Work: Stress Productivity and the Reconstruction of Working Life.* New York: Basic Books.

2 Theorell T, Karasek RA. 1996. Current issues relating to psychosocial job strain and cardiovascular disease research. *Journal of Occupational Health Psychology;* 1: 9-26.

3 Bosma H, Marmot MG, Hemingway H, Nicholson AC, Brunner E, Stansfield SA. 1997. Low job control and risks of CHD in Whitehall II (Prospective cohort study). *British Medical Journal;* 314: 558-65.

4 Spencer N. 1996. *Poverty and Child Health.* Oxford: Radcliffe Medical Press.

5 Child Poverty Action Group. 1998. *Real Choices for Lone Parents and Their Children.* London: Child Poverty Action Group.

6 Acheson D. 1998. *Independent Inquiry into Inequalities in Health.* London: The Stationery Office: 17.

7 Graham H. 1988. Women and smoking in the UK: the implications for health promotion. *Health Promotion;* 4: 371-82.

8 Alcohol Concern. 2000. Britain's ruin? Alcohol's role in social exclusion. *Alcohol Concern Magazine;* 15: 2.

9 Blackburn C. 1991. *Poverty and Health.* Oxford: Oxford University Press.

10 Murray L, Cooper PJ. 1997. Effects of postnatal depression on infant development. *Archives of Disease in Childhood;* 77: 99-101.

11 Health Education Authority. 1989. *Diet, Nutrition and Healthy Eating in Low Income Groups.* London: Health Education Authority.

12 Luckett N. 2000. *Bournemouth Food Initiative Needs Assessment Report.* Bournemouth: Dorset Health Care NHS Trust.

13 Hupkens CLH, Knibbe RA, Drop MJ. 2000. Social class differences in food consumption: the explanatory value of permissiveness and health and cost considerations. *European Journal of Public Health;* 10: 108-13.

14 Tripp JH, Cockett M. 1999. Parents, parenting and family breakdown. *Archives of Disease in Childhood.* Annotations 104-07.

15 Thorenson C. 1991. Type A and teenagers. In: Lerner R et al (eds.) *Encyclopedia of Adolescence, Volume 2.* New York: Garland Press.

16 Dowler E, Calvert C. 1995. *Nutrition and Diet in Lone Parent Families in London.* London: Family Policy Studies Centre.

17 Lynch P. 1995. Adolescent smoking – an alternative perspective using personal construct theory. *Health Education Research;* 10; 1: 95-106.

18 Smith C, Roberts C, Moore L. 1995. Parents and adolescent smoking. *Journal of the Institute of Health Education;* 33: 4: 104-09.

19 Green G, Macintyre S, West P, Ecob R. 1991. Like parent, like child? Association between drinking and smoking behaviour of parents and their children. *British Journal of Addiction;* 86: 745-58.

20 Allbutt H, Amos A, Cunningham-Bailey S. 1995. The social image of smoking among young people in Scotland. *Health Education Research;* 10; 4: 443-54.

21 Co-op. 2000. *Blackmail.* Manchester: CWS Ltd.

22 Bar-on M. 2000. The effects of television on child health: implications and recommendations. *Archives of Disease in Childhood;* 83: 289-92.

23 While D, Kelly S, Wenyong H, Charlton A. 1996. Cigarette advertising and onset of smoking in children: questionnaire. *British Medical Journal;* 313: 398-99.

24 Dennehy A, Smith L, Harker P. 1997. *Not to be Ignored – Young People, Poverty and Health.* London: Child Poverty Action Group.

25 McDonald L. 1996. Families and Schools Together (FAST): a substance abuse prevention program which clusters families under stress for social support. Paper for the conference on family systems approaches to substance abuse prevention, Maryland USA, January 25-26.

26 Somerville M, Mackenzie I, Owen P, Miles D. 2000. Housing and health: does installing heating in their homes improve the health of children with asthma? *Public Health;* 114: 434-39.

27 Accessed from: www.housing.odpm.gov.uk/information/consult/lhmoe/index.htm

28 Kalawachi I et al. 1996. A prospective study of social networks in relation to total mortality and cardiovascular disease in men, in the USA. *Journal of Epidemiology and Community Health;* 50 (3): 245-51.

29 Hertzman C, Wiens M. 1996. Child development and long term outcomes: a population health perspective and summary of successful interventions. *Social Science and Medicine;* 43: 1083.

Chapter 7

The diets of children and young people: implications for coronary heart disease prevention

Karen McColl

Independent consultant in nutrition and public health

This chapter:

- describes recent evidence on what children and adolescents in Great Britain are eating and drinking
- provides an overview of the findings of the 2000 report on the National Diet and Nutrition Survey on young people aged 4 to 18 years[1] in relation to coronary heart disease, and
- describes recent policy initiatives designed to help improve the diets of young people and reviews the policy implications of the recent dietary survey findings.

Key themes

- The results of recent surveys, particularly the National Diet and Nutrition Survey on young people aged 4 to 18 years,[1] suggest that young people's diets are too high in saturated fat, sugars and salt. It is also startlingly clear that very few young people are eating enough fruit and vegetables. Furthermore, young people appear to be relatively inactive.

- There is particular cause for concern about the diets of children and adolescents living in poorer households.

- There is a need for continued, and coherent, efforts to:
  - reduce the proportion of food energy from total fat, saturated fat and non-milk extrinsic sugars
  - reduce salt intakes and the prevalence of sodium intakes above the RNI (Reference Nutrient Intake)
  - increase the consumption of fruit and vegetables, especially in those groups where consumption is particularly low
  - ensure that children growing up in disadvantaged households have access to an adequate and high quality diet, and
  - promote physical activity in young people in ways which are likely to be carried on into adulthood.

- Policy initiatives to achieve these goals should include a whole school approach to improving nutrition, action to address the commercial messages about food which children are exposed to, and ensuring provision of clear, honest and meaningful nutrition information to enable young people to choose a healthy diet. In addition, government should work with the food industry to improve the foods which make up the diets of young people.

- Efforts to promote access to affordable, good quality, nutritious food for low-income families should be a priority.

Introduction

Diet is one of the major risk factors contributing to the development of cardiovascular disease, the biggest single cause of death in the UK. Coronary heart disease has been selected by the government as one of four key health priorities.

A diet high in fat, particularly saturated fat, and low in complex carbohydrates, fruit and vegetables is known to increase the risk of chronic diseases. It is estimated that consumption of at least five portions of fruit and vegetables a day (around 400g) could prevent up to one-fifth of the deaths from chronic diseases in the UK.[2]

The relationships between heart disease risk factors in childhood and health in later life are complex. The diets of children can, however, have a direct impact on the development of risk factors relevant to heart disease, such as overweight and obesity, blood cholesterol levels and blood pressure. Furthermore, there is evidence that dietary habits in childhood and adolescence also influence eating patterns in later life.[3] The diets of children and young people, therefore, are of fundamental importance to the future health of the nation.

There has been increasing recognition of the importance of children's diets in recent years and there has also been growing concern about the eating and physical activity patterns of children and teenagers. Poor nutrition in young women and pregnant women contributes to low birthweight in babies. There is now growing evidence that this, in turn, contributes to the development of chronic diseases, such as coronary heart disease, in later life (see Chapter 1).

There are many important aspects of the nutritional health of young people. These include oral health, bone health and vitamin and mineral status. In addition, there are many components of young people's diets which may contribute to the development of cancer, hypertension and other non-communicable diseases.

This review, however, concentrates on the nutritional factors involved in the development of coronary heart disease. The key factors considered are, therefore, energy intake, fat intakes and the pattern of fatty acid consumption, total carbohydrate, non-milk extrinsic sugars, and the consumption of fruit and vegetables. Physical activity is also considered.

National Diet and Nutrition Survey: Young People Aged 4 to 18 Years

In June 2000, the government published the most significant piece of research into children's and young people's eating patterns and nutritional status to emerge in recent decades. The *National Diet and Nutrition Survey: Young People Aged 4 to 18 Years* is the most detailed survey of children's diets ever undertaken.[1] This survey forms part of the National Diet and Nutrition Survey programme which also includes surveys of adults, older people and pre-school children.[4-6] The main aims of the survey were to provide detailed information on the dietary behaviour, nutritional status and oral health of young people.

The previous government survey on young people's nutrition, *The Diets of British Schoolchildren*, was carried out in 1983.[7] This survey was carried out to examine the impact of the abolition of nutritional standards for school meals in the 1980 Education Act. The 1983 survey studied two age groups: children aged 10-11 years, and young people aged 14-15 years. The 1983 survey found that the diets of schoolchildren generally provided more than the recommended amount of energy from fat and that the diets of some children, particularly girls, provided intakes below the then recommended levels of riboflavin, iron and calcium.

This chapter concentrates on the findings of the National Diet and Nutrition Survey report on the survey of young people aged 4-18[1] and the policy implications of these findings.

Survey methodology

The survey was carried out on a nationally representative sample of 2,672 young people aged 4-18 years who were living in private households in Great Britain. Of these, 2,127 were interviewed about their sociodemographic circumstances, medication and eating and drinking habits. A weighed dietary record of all food and drink consumed over seven days was obtained for 1,701 young people (80% of those completing the interview). The survey also included a record of bowel movements for the same seven days, physical measurements of the young person, blood pressure measurements, a request for a sample of blood and urine and an assessment of dental health. Young people aged between 7 and 18 kept a seven-day physical activity diary. The field work took place over a period of 12 months, to take account of possible seasonal differences in eating habits.

Methodological issues

The energy intakes reported in the survey, based on the seven-day weighed dietary intakes, were below the Estimated Average Requirements (EAR) for each age/sex group in the survey. For girls aged between 15 and 18, the mean reported energy intake was as low as 77% of the EAR.

Young people in this survey, however, were taller and heavier than those studied in earlier surveys of the same age group. This suggests that energy intakes are, therefore, unlikely to be inadequate and that there is significant under-reporting of energy intake (and therefore food intake) in the survey population.

The survey design did include specific measures to address the issue of under-reporting. Interviewers checked the completeness of diaries, paying particular attention to the oldest group of girls and to the completeness of 'eating out' diaries which have been identified as a specific source of under-reporting. Despite these measures to try and reduce the impact of under-reporting, it remains likely that there was significant under-reporting and that this was a particular problem in specific age groups, most notably the oldest age group of girls.

A separate analysis was undertaken to identify and exclude respondents who were classified as 'under-reporters' because their energy intake appeared to be below the minimum energy requirements for their age and sex. The proportion of under-reporters ranged from 17% and 13% respectively of boys and girls aged between 4 and 6 years, to 64% of boys and 74% of girls aged between 15 and 18. There were relatively few over-reporters in all age groups except for the 4 to 6 year olds (12% for boys and 10% for girls).

The effect of excluding under-reporters on the average intakes was substantial. Mean energy intake, for example, was 21% higher in boys aged 15-18 years when under-reporters were excluded. At 28%, the differential was even higher for 15-18 year old females. Similarly, intakes of macronutrients increased by as much as 33% when under-reporters were excluded. The percentage differences were greatest for sugars (non-milk extrinsic sugars) and smallest for protein. In general, the percentages of food energy derived from macronutrients, however, remained similar to the overall results when under-reporters were excluded. The two exceptions were sugars and saturated fatty acids (see Tables 5 and 6). For boys aged 11-18 and girls aged 15-18, the proportion of food energy from non-milk extrinsic sugars (NMES) increased significantly when under-reporters were excluded.

Caution is advised in interpreting these results because of the limitations of the methodology to define 'under-reporters', which may overestimate the proportion of under-reporters. Nevertheless, this analysis reinforces the findings of the feasibility study for this survey that there is a high incidence of under-reporting in young people, particularly those aged between 11 and 18. Furthermore, it appears that the young people in the survey, in addition to under-reporting daily energy intakes, selectively under-reported foods high in sugars and saturated fats. This bias should be borne in mind when considering the survey findings.

Survey results

Energy intake and expenditure, and body mass index

As outlined above, average energy intakes were below the Estimated Average Requirement (EAR) for all groups (see Table 1). The young people in the survey, however, were taller and heavier than those in other surveys of the same age group. This suggests, therefore, that the actual energy intakes of the population are not inadequate and may be explained, at least partially, by under-reporting of food consumption. The survey report also suggests that the energy needs of young people are lower than in previous surveys.

Heights and weights were recorded and body mass index (BMI) calculated for 1,946 young people. The mid upper-arm circumference was measured for 1,943 young people and waist and hip circumferences were recorded for 987 young people aged between 11 and 18 years. This enabled calculation of the waist to hip ratio which is an indicator of the distribution of body fat. Table 2 shows the results for mean BMI, mid-upper arm circumference and waist to hip ratio.

The results were compared with the results of the *Health Survey for England: The Health of Young People*[8] carried out in 1995-97, and the National Study of Health and Growth[9] carried out in 1994. These comparisons suggest that results for this survey are broadly similar to the findings of the previous studies, confirming the general perception than children are getting fatter.

When assessing childhood overweight and obesity, it is necessary to consider age-specific BMI. Further analysis of this data set would be required to assess the real extent of overweight and obesity in the young people surveyed. The survey suggests that the growing concern about childhood obesity is not misplaced.[10, 11]

The data were analysed to identify the characteristics independently associated with BMI for all those aged 4-18 years. For both boys and girls, systolic blood pressure, average daily energy intake, and whether or not they were currently dieting to lose weight, were positively associated with BMI.

For boys, but not girls, several other characteristics were associated with BMI. These included the proportion of energy from total fat, and the proportion of energy from total sugars. In addition, boys living in London and the South East had a lower than average BMI, and those living in Scotland a higher BMI than the overall average. Household income was also significant: boys living in households with a gross weekly income of less than £160 had, on average, a lower BMI.

BMI in girls was associated with puberty (higher in girls for whom menarche had occurred), and was inversely related with father's reported height and a manual social class background.

Linked to obesity and overweight is the issue of slimming. Overall, 2% of boys and girls reported dieting to lose weight. This increased to 16% for girls aged 15-18 years. It is clear that body weight and body image is an important issue for many young women and policy interventions to tackle the childhood obesity epidemic must be sensitive to this issue.

Food consumption

The survey contains considerable detail on the amount and frequency of foods consumed by young people as well as the nutritional analysis of their diets. There is also a wealth of information on what young people eat and when. Much of this

Table 1 ***Energy intakes as a percentage of Estimated Average Requirement (EAR), 4-18 year olds, Great Britain, 1997, by sex and age group***

Age in years	Mean energy intake (MJ)	Estimated Average Requirement (EAR) for energy (MJ)	Intake as % of EAR
Males			
4-6	6.39	7.16	89%
7-10	7.47	8.24	91%
11-14	8.28	9.27	89%
15-18	9.60	11.51	83%
Females			
4-6	5.87	6.46	91%
7-10	6.72	7.28	92%
11-14	7.03	7.92	89%
15-18	6.82	8.83	77%

Source: See reference 1.

Table 2 ***Body mass index (BMI), mid-upper arm circumference and waist to hip ratio, Great Britain, 1997, by sex and age group***

Age in years	Mean BMI	Mean mid-upper arm circumference (cm)	Waist to hip ratio
Males			
4-6	16	18	N/a
7-10	17	20	N/a
11-14	19	24	0.83
15-18	22	28	0.81
All males	19	23	0.82
Females			
4-6	16	18	N/a
7-10	18	21	N/a
11-14	20	24	0.77
15-18	23	27	0.75
All females	19	23	0.76

Source: See reference 1.

information is extremely valuable for the development of relevant, appropriate and effective food-based dietary guidelines. The ability to analyse this information and find out which foods contribute most fat, saturated fat and sugars in children's diet should enable the formulation of effective strategies to improve children's nutrition.

The foods most commonly consumed by young people were white bread, savoury snacks, chips and other potatoes, savoury sauces and condiments, biscuits and chocolate confectionery. All of these foods were consumed by over 80% of the young people during the seven-day survey period. Three-quarters of the young people consumed carbonated soft drinks (non low-calorie) and 45% consumed low-calorie versions. About two-thirds ate sugar confectionery.

Dietary guidelines for both adults and young people have tended to focus on nutrient intakes of the diet as a whole rather than particular foods. There have been two important exceptions to this rule: fruit and vegetables. As outlined on page 153, current UK advice is to eat at least five portions of a variety of fruit and vegetables each day. This survey is important in helping to develop understanding of current fruit and vegetable consumption patterns in young people.

On average the young people ate less than half of the recommended 400g (the equivalent of 'five portions') of fruit and vegetables per day. Table 3 shows the average consumption of vegetables and fruit in boys and Table 4 shows the results for girls.

It is clear that vegetables are less commonly eaten than many other foods. Only 47% of boys and 59% of girls ate raw and salad vegetables (excluding tomatoes), 40% ate cooked leafy green vegetables and 60% ate other cooked vegetables. This is a stark contrast with the 84% who ate chocolate confectionery and 75% who drank carbonated soft drinks.

The main difference between boys and girls in relation to vegetable consumption is that girls were more likely to eat raw and salad vegetables and raw tomatoes than boys. This is true for all age groups except 11-14 year olds.

There were strong regional variations in consumption of vegetables. Only one-fifth of boys in Scotland, for example, ate leafy green vegetables, one third ate 'other' raw or salad vegetables, and 30% ate cooked carrots. In London and the South East, by comparison, over half of the boys ate all of these categories of vegetable.

Children in households with a gross weekly income of less than £160 per week were less likely to eat raw and salad vegetables than those in households with an income of £600 per week or more. Girls in the lower income households were also less likely to eat green beans and 'other' vegetables. Girls in households in receipt of benefits were less likely to eat raw and salad vegetables or green beans, and boys in this group were less likely to eat raw carrots than children in households not in receipt of benefits.

Table 3 shows the consumption of fruit and fruit juice by boys in the survey and Table 4 describes fruit consumption by females. Only around a quarter of young people (24% of boys and 28% of girls) ate citrus fruit during the recording period. Less than two-thirds ate apples and pears (53% for boys, 57% for girls). Fruit juice was consumed by 46% of boys and 51% of girls.

There are no statistically significant differences between all boys and all girls for fruit consumption. When non-consumers are excluded, however, girls eat significantly more (i.e. larger quantities) of apples, pears and other fruit.

The proportion of young people who ate fruit decreased with age – more young children ate fruit than older boys and girls. For most foods, the quantities consumed tended to increase with age, particularly for boys. The mean amounts of fruit consumed by boys, however, increased very little with age. The mean amount of fruit consumed by girls did increase with age. There was little variation in the consumption of fruit by region.

Boys in households where the head of household was a manual worker were less likely to consume fruit (apples, pears, bananas, other fruit and fruit juice) than boys in non-manual households. Children in homes where the gross weekly household income is less than £160 per week are less likely to drink fruit juice and, for girls, eat other fruit, compared with children in homes with a weekly income of £600 or over. Children in households receiving benefit were less likely to drink fruit juice and, for girls, eat citrus or other (mainly soft) fruit than children in households not in receipt of benefits.

Boys were more likely to eat breakfast cereals (not high fibre or wholegrain) and sausages, and to drink beer and lager. Girls of all ages were more likely to eat raw tomatoes and other raw and salad vegetables.

There are more variations in the amounts of different types of foods eaten by boys and girls in older age groups than in the younger groups. In children aged between 4 and 6 years, for example, boys ate significantly larger amounts of cereal-based milk puddings and sausages than girls of the same age. Girls aged 4-6 ate more raw and salad vegetables. In the 15-18 year old age group, boys ate significantly more pizza, white bread, breakfast cereals, biscuits, semi-skimmed milk, several types of red meat and meat products such as burgers, kebabs and sausages, baked beans and potatoes (including chips) and drank more beer. Apart from raw and salad vegetables, as described above, there were no other foods that 15-18 year old girls were more likely to consume than their male counterparts.

It is difficult to generalise about the other food consumption differences between socioeconomic groups. Boys in households in receipt of benefits were less likely to eat chocolate confectionery than those in households which did not receive benefit. Girls in benefit-receiving households, however, were more likely to consume sugar confectionery than those not receiving benefits. Boys in the less advantaged group according to all three of the indicators (social class, income and receipt of benefits) were less likely to consume cream or semi-skimmed milk and were more likely to consume whole milk. Boys and girls in the households in receipt of benefits, and girls in the lower-income households, were less likely to consume alcoholic drinks.

Table 3 *Consumption of fruit and vegetables, males aged 4-18, Great Britain, 1997, by age group*

	Males aged 4-6 years			Males aged 7-10 years			Males aged 11-14 years			Males aged 15-18 years		
	Mean consumption for all (consumers and non-consumers) *(g in 7 days)*	Percentage of consumers	Mean consumption – consumers only *(g in 7 days)*	Mean consumption for all (consumers and non-consumers) *(g in 7 days)*	Percentage of consumers	Mean consumption – consumers only *(g in 7 days)*	Mean consumption for all (consumers and non-consumers) *(g in 7 days)*	Percentage of consumers	Mean consumption – consumers only *(g in 7 days)*	Mean consumption for all (consumers and non-consumers) *(g in 7 days)*	Percentage of consumers	Mean consumption – consumers only *(g in 7 days)*
Vegetables												
Raw carrots	17	16	101	12	16	79	6	10	59	14	11	131
Other raw and salad vegetables	26	37	71	35	44	80	53	53	100	64	51	124
Raw tomatoes	15	26	57	23	27	85	25	33	76	44	42	104
Peas	45	59	75	37	49	76	51	48	105	60	44	137
Green beans	7	16	44	7	13	56	10	12	78	19	17	112
Baked beans	134	64	208	124	63	197	156	60	261	203	62	325
Leafy green vegetables	134	46	75	34	41	82	30	32	91	45	38	117
Carrots – not raw	44	59	74	41	54	75	49	51	95	54	47	115
Tomatoes – not raw	3	8	45	7	8	87	8	11	76	16	15	106
Vegetable dishes	42	20	203	26	16	164	44	17	252	54	20	262
Other vegetables	56	55	103	62	58	107	77	61	126	82	57	144
Fruit												
Apples and pears	191	70	271	180	59	307	123	48	255	115	39	293
Citrus fruits	52	26	196	56	29	192	42	21	197	56	19	294
Bananas	109	47	232	97	42	232	71	32	221	83	33	254
Canned fruit in juice	8	8	103	10	7	151	6	5	129	3	4	70
Canned fruit in syrup	14	11	127	10	8	120	7	5	123	11	5	219
Other fruit	66	42	159	82	38	214	45	23	191	39	21	185
Fruit juice	311	48	646	380	50	766	382	50	851	433	43	1015

Source: See reference 1.

Table 4 Consumption of fruit and vegetables, females aged 4-18, Great Britain, 1997, by age group

	Females aged 4-6 years			Females aged 7-10 years			Females aged 11-14 years			Females aged 15-18 years		
	Mean consumption for all (consumers and non-consumers) *(g in 7 days)*	Percentage of consumers	Mean consumption – consumers only *(g in 7 days)*	Mean consumption for all (consumers and non-consumers) *(g in 7 days)*	Percentage of consumers	Mean consumption – consumers only *(g in 7 days)*	Mean consumption for all (consumers and non-consumers) *(g in 7 days)*	Percentage of consumers	Mean consumption – consumers only *(g in 7 days)*	Mean consumption for all (consumers and non-consumers) *(g in 7 days)*	Percentage of consumers	Mean consumption – consumers only *(g in 7 days)*
Vegetables												
Raw carrots	10	19	52	11	16	65	7	13	51	21	19	103
Other raw and salad vegetables	50	52	91	56	49	107	56	56	94	104	66	149
Raw tomatoes	26	30	81	33	35	90	31	67	79	67	54	116
Peas	35	52	64	49	50	93	41	46	84	39	39	96
Green beans	6	15	38	7	12	52	9	12	77	12	12	97
Baked beans	98	62	152	121	60	191	106	50	201	127	44	272
Leafy green vegetables	36	44	77	37	42	84	50	40	117	54	40	127
Carrots – not raw	42	58	69	43	53	76	40	44	86	47	50	89
Tomatoes – not raw	3	5	52	9	8	105	7	8	83	7	9	79
Vegetable dishes	36	15	222	41	16	235	56	21	254	110	28	369
Other vegetables	61	60	97	73	60	116	85	52	154	118	63	179
Fruit												
Apples and pears	190	66	275	179	61	277	148	47	299	155	44	336
Citrus fruits	62	29	204	80	33	226	56	23	225	60	20	286
Bananas	99	50	189	87	38	217	52	28	175	65	30	210
Canned fruit in juice	7	6	126	15	9	156	8	4	173	5	3	157
Canned fruit in syrup	15	13	117	14	10	134	10	6	157	1	1	100
Other fruit	84	42	191	102	42	231	60	28	204	89	24	349
Fruit juice	344	53	617	373	48	737	373	47	741	428	45	899

Source: See reference 1.

Nutritional patterns

The energy intake and expenditure patterns of young people have been described on page 155. The survey also identified the nutrient composition of the young people's diets. The main results of this nutritional analysis are presented in this section, and the findings compared with current nutritional guidelines.

Recommendations published in the report of the Committee on Medical Aspects of Food Policy (COMA)[12] are referred to as the current UK recommendations. In addition, because the science has moved on since that report was published, recommendations from some dietary guidelines recently published by international bodies such as the World Health Organization and the European Commission are also included.

Table 5 shows the contribution of nutrients to the overall diet of 4-18 year olds, by showing the contribution of each macronutrient as a percentage of food energy. Table 6 shows the same figures, but excluding the results for young people classified as 'under-reporters'.

Protein

The average daily protein intake was 61.6g for boys and 51.2g for girls. This protein contributed 13.1% of food energy for both boys and girls. These mean intakes were higher than the Reference Nutrient Intake (RNI). The main sources of protein were meat and meat products which contributed around a third, cereal and cereal products (just over a quarter), and milk and milk products (18%).

Fat and fatty acids

The average proportion of food energy coming from fat intake (total fat) was 35% for boys and 36% for girls. Although the absolute amounts of fat consumed increased with age, there was no increase in the mean proportion of food energy derived from fat with age. The current UK recommendation (dietary reference value) for adults is for 35% energy from total fat[12] and the intakes for boys and girls were close to this level. It is widely recognised that an even lower population average fat intake is desirable. The World Health Organization has recommended that fat intake should be less than 30%.[2]

It is not only the total amount of dietary fat, and its contribution to energy intake, that are important for heart health. The relative proportions of different fatty acids are also important.

In the National Diet and Nutrition Survey of 4-18 year olds, the average proportion of energy from saturated fat was 14.2% for boys and 14.3% for girls. For both sexes the proportion of food energy from saturated fatty acids decreased with age. The diets of both boys and girls were above the UK recommendation for adults that no more than

Table 5 ***Energy intakes and percentage of food energy from macronutrients, 4-18 year olds, Great Britain, 1997, by sex and age group***

	Males Age in years					Females Age in years				
	4-6	*7-10*	*11-14*	*15-18*	*All*	*4-6*	*7-10*	*11-14*	*15-18*	*All*
Total energy (MJ)	6.39	7.47	8.28	9.60	8.01	5.87	6.72	7.03	6.82	6.65
Food energy (MJ)	6.39	7.47	8.27	9.37	7.95	5.87	6.72	7.02	6.69	6.61
% food energy from:										
Protein	12.9	12.4	13.1	13.9	13.1	12.7	12.8	12.7	13.9	13.1
Carbohydrate	51.6	52.4	51.7	50.5	51.6	51.4	51.3	51.2	50.6	51.1
Total fat	35.5	35.2	35.2	35.9	35.4	35.9	35.9	36.1	35.9	35.9
Saturated fatty acids	14.8	14.3	13.8	13.9	14.2	15.3	14.5	14.0	13.8	14.3
NMES	16.2	17.5	16.9	15.8	16.7	17.6	16.7	16.2	15.3	16.4

Source: See reference 1.

Table 6 ***Energy intakes and percentage of food energy from macronutrients, excluding 'under-reporters', 4-18 year olds, Great Britain, 1997, by sex and age group***

	Males Age in years				Females Age in years			
	4-6	*7-10*	*11-14*	*15-18*	*4-6*	*7-10*	*11-14*	*15-18*
Total energy (MJ)	6.71	8.02	9.46	11.59	6.10	7.13	8.14	8.75
% food energy from:								
Protein	13.0	12.5	12.7	13.0	12.8	12.7	12.5	13.1
Carbohydrate	52.3	52.8	52.9	52.4	52.1	52.0	51.8	51.3
Total fat	34.7	34.8	34.4	34.6	35.2	35.3	35.6	35.7
Saturated fatty acids	14.5	14.1	13.6	13.9	15.1	14.4	14.2	14.0
NMES	16.8	18.0	19.1	18.8	18.1	17.8	17.5	18.0

Source: See reference 1.

11% of food energy should be from saturated fatty acids.[12] The EU-funded Eurodiet project proposed that saturated fats should provide less than 10% of food energy.[13]

Intakes of *trans* fatty acids contributed an average of 1.4% of food energy for boys and 1.3% for girls. The COMA dietary reference value (DRV) is for a population average of not more than 2% of food energy from trans fatty acids.[12]

Average daily intakes of *cis* monounsaturated fatty acids were 24.6g for boys and 20.6g for girls. This is equal to 11.7% and 11.8% of food energy respectively. The DRV recommendation is that *cis* monounsaturates should provide 13% of food energy as a population average.

Intakes of total *cis* polyunsaturated fatty acids, which include the n-3 and n-6 groups of fatty acids, contributed 5.9% of food energy for boys and 6.1% for girls. These intakes are close to the DRV recommended by COMA for 6.5% of food energy intake. The survey did not include information on individual fatty acids, so it is not possible to say whether young people were meeting COMA's specific recommendations on linoleic (one of the n-6 group) and α-linolenic acid.

The four main sources of total fat, saturated fat, *trans* and *cis* monounsaturated fatty acids in the diets were cereals and cereal products, milk and milk products, meat and meat products, and vegetables, potatoes and savoury snacks.

Foods in the cereals and cereal products group – mainly biscuits, buns, cakes and pastries – contributed just over a fifth of total fat and similar proportions of saturated fat and *cis* monounsaturated fatty acids. This food group made a substantial contribution to *trans* fatty acid consumption, providing about a third of the intake.

Milk and milk products contributed 20% of the total fat and 30% of the saturated fat of 4-6 year old boys, but this declined to 13% and 20%, respectively, among the 15-18 year olds. A similar reduction is seen for girls and reflects declining milk consumption with age, particularly of whole milk.

Meat and meat products contributed 21% to the total fat intake and 19% to the saturated fat intake for boys. For girls the figures were 18% and 16% respectively. The main sources of fat in this group were sausages, meat pies and pastries which provided 8% of total fat intake for boys and 6% for girls. In older boys, burgers and kebabs were a significant source of saturated fat, providing 4% of the saturated fatty acid intake in the 15-18 year old age group.

Vegetables, potatoes and savoury snacks contributed 18% and 20% of the total fat for boys and girls, respectively. Foods in this group contributed 13% of saturated fat intake for boys and 15% for girls and they also contributed 21% and 23% of the *cis* monounsaturated fatty acids. The main sources of total fat, saturated fat and *cis* monounsaturated fat were roast and fried potatoes, chips, and savoury snacks.

Another important source of total fat, saturated and *cis* monounsaturated fat in the diets of the young people was the 'fat spreads' group, which contributed 9% to the total fat intake and 8% to both the saturated and *cis* monounsaturated fatty acid intake. Fat spreads contributed a higher proportion of *trans* fatty acids – 13% for boys and girls.

For boys and girls, chocolate confectionery contributed 6% of total fat and of *cis* monounsaturated fatty acids intake, 9% of the saturated fat intake and a similar proportion for *trans* fatty acids.

The main sources of *cis* n-3 polyunsaturated fatty acids were vegetables, potatoes and savoury snacks, cereals and cereal products, and meat and meat products. A third of the intake came from vegetables, potatoes and savoury snacks, mainly from chips and roast or fried potatoes. The main sources of n-6 polyunsaturated fatty acids were vegetables, potatoes and savoury snacks (27% for boys and 29% for girls), cereals and cereal products (23% and 21%), fat spreads (16% for both boys and girls) and meat and meat products (18% for boys and 16% for girls).

There were no significant regional differences in fat intake or in the proportion of food energy derived from total fat, saturated fat, trans or polyunsaturated fatty acids. Girls in Scotland and the North, however, obtained more food energy from *cis* monounsaturated fatty acids than girls in the Central and South West regions.

Analysis of fat intake as a proportion of food energy by socioeconomic characteristics revealed no statistically significant differences. There were some differences, however, in intakes of the different types of fatty acids. Boys from homes where the head of household was a manual worker had diets richer in *cis* monounsaturated fatty acids and polyunsaturated fatty acids. Boys in homes in the second highest income bracket had a significantly lower proportion of food energy from *cis* polyunsaturated fatty acids than boys in the lower income households. Girls in the highest income household group had a lower proportion of food energy from *cis* monounsaturated fatty acids than girls in the lowest income group.

Tables 7 and 8 compare the results with the findings of earlier surveys. Comparison of the 4-6 year olds with the 1992/3 National Diet and Nutrition Survey of pre-school children[6] suggests a reduction in the proportion of food energy derived from saturated fat in the diets of young children, particularly boys. The diets also appear to have become less rich in *trans* fatty acids although they are becoming more rich in *cis* monounsaturated fatty acids and in *cis* n-6 polyunsaturated fats.

Comparison of the 10-11 year olds and the 14-15 year olds with the results from the 1983 Diets of British Schoolchildren survey[7] suggests that average fat intakes have fallen by around 14% in the 10-11 year olds and 20% for the older age group. The proportion of food energy from fat also appears to have fallen, but not by as much. There has been a reduction of around 4% in the younger age group and 6% for the older group.

Results for the 15-18 year old age group can be compared with the results for 16-24 year olds in the Dietary and Nutritional Survey of British Adults carried out in 1986/87[4]. These results suggest that the overall percentage of food energy from fat has fallen, possibly by as much as 10% since the earlier survey. There also appears to have been a decrease in the proportion of food energy from saturated and *trans* fatty acids and from *cis* monounsaturated fats. At the same time there has been an increase in the proportion of energy derived from *cis* n-3 polyunsaturated fatty acids.

Carbohydrate and sugars

The average daily intake of total carbohydrate (excluding non-starch polysaccharides) in the National Diet and Nutrition Survey of 4-18 year olds was 260g for boys and 214g for girls. This corresponded to 51% of the food energy for both boys and girls (see Table 5). The Eurodiet project has recommended that carbohydrates should provide an average of more than 55% of total energy.[13]

For sugars, the average daily intakes were 117g for boys and 97g for girls. When intrinsic and milk sugars are excluded from the analysis, the remaining sugars – non-milk extrinsic sugars (NMES) – provided on average 16.7% of food energy for boys and 16.4% for girls (see Table 5). In both cases, this is considerably higher than the recommended COMA limit of not more than 11%.[12] The main contributors of non-

Table 7 ***Macronutrient contribution to food energy among children and young people in Great Britain: comparison of national surveys***

	Survey year	Average daily energy intake (MJ)	Average fat intake (g/day)	Percentage of food energy from:			Base (Number of subjects)
				Protein	*Carbohydrate*	*Fat*	
Males							
3½ to 4½ years*	1992/93	5.36	50.1	12.4	52.3	35.3	250
4-6 years †	1997	6.39	60.1	12.9	51.6	35.5	184
10-11 years**	1983	8.67	87.6	12.0	50.5	37.4	902
10-11 years †	1997	7.98	75.8	12.8	51.5	35.7	140
14-15 years**	1983	10.40	106.3	12.3	49.8	37.9	513
14-15 years †	1997	9.13	86.5	13.5	50.6	35.9	110
16-24 years***	1986/87	10.29	103.5	13.7	42.9	40.2	214
15-18 years †	1997	9.6	89.0	13.6	49.3	35.9	179
Females							
3½ to 4½ years*	1992/93	4.98	47.2	12.7	51.7	35.5	243
4-6 years †	1997	5.87	55.9	12.7	51.4	35.9	171
10-11 years**	1983	7.69	78.9	11.8	50.2	37.9	821
10-11 years †	1997	7.04	67.2	12.7	51.2	36.6	118
14-15 years**	1983	7.85	82.2	12.4	48.8	38.7	461
14-15 years †	1997	6.90	65.9	13.2	50.8	36.1	113
16-24 years***	1986/87	7.11	73.6	14.0	44.9	39.8	189
15-18 years †	1997	6.82	64.0	13.6	49.7	35.9	210

† = National Diet and Nutrition Survey: Young People Aged 4 to 18 Years[1]

* = National Diet and Nutrition Survey: Children Aged 1½ to 4½ Years[6]

** = The Diets of British Schoolchildren[7]

*** = The Dietary and Nutritional Survey of British Adults[4]

Table 8 ***Energy intake and contribution of macronutrients: comparison with other surveys of children and young people in Great Britain***

Year of survey and reference details	Sex	Age	Average daily energy intake (MJ)	Percentage of food energy from: Protein	Carbohydrate	Fat	Base (Number of subjects)
1991/2	M	7-8	7.78	11.8	50.8	37.4	65
Ruxton et al, 1996[14]	F	7-8	7.16	11.9	50.3	37.8	71
1988	M	7-10	7.59	N/a	N/a	36.6	25
Nelson et al, 1990[15]	F	7-10	6.92	N/a	N/a	35.0	26
1988, 1990	M	8-11	7.61	N/a	51	37	111
Hunt et al, 1995[16]	F	8-11	6.53	N/a	50	39	148
1988	M	11-12	7.74	N/a	N/a	37.5	76
Nelson et al, 1990[15]	F	11-12	7.45	N/a	N/a	38.4	67
1988/9	M	12	8.96	N/a	N/a	N/a	18
McNeill et al, 1991[17]	F	12	8.14	N/a	N/a	N/a	43
1990/1	M	12	11.0	11	50	39	251
Strain et al, 1994[18]	F	12	9.2	11	50	38	258
1990/1	M	15	13.1	11	50	39	252
Strain et al, 1994[18]	F	15	9.1	11	49	39	254
1982	M	15-18	10.1	13	43	42	198
Bull, 1985[19]	F	15-18	7.8	13	43	43	184
1986/7	M	16-17	11.4	12.5	44.2	41.4	2,006
Crawley, 1993[20]	F	16-17	8.8	12.5	43.9	41.6	2,754
1986/7	M	16-29	10.7	13.0	43.5	39.2	105
Barker et al, 1988[21]	F	16-29	7.6	12.9	44.5	39.7	110

milk extrinsic sugars were drinks (mainly soft drinks), sugars, preserves and confectionery.

High consumers of sugars (young people in the upper 2.5 percentile) were obtaining more than a quarter of their food energy from NMES, mainly soft drinks and foods in the sugar, preserves and confectionery category.

It is probable that the survey results underestimate the actual intakes of sugars. A separate analysis of findings which specifically excluded 'under-reporters' showed a significant increase in the proportion of food energy derived from non-milk extrinsic sugars (see Table 6).

Salt intake

Intakes of sodium, *excluding* salt added during cooking or at the table, were on average 2,630mg per day for boys and 2,156mg for girls. This represents at least twice the RNI value for children under 10 years old and also exceeds the RNI for older children.[12]

Vitamins and minerals

Most of the young people in the survey had adequate vitamin intakes and the vitamin content of the diet appears to have improved over time.[22] Average intakes of vitamins were above the RNIs with the exception of vitamin A. In older children, a fifth of girls and 12% of boys had vitamin A intakes below the lower reference nutrient intake (LRNI) and a fifth of girls had riboflavin intakes below the LRNI.

In the younger children, average intakes of most minerals were above the RNIs, with the exception of zinc. In older children, however, average intakes were below the RNI for zinc, potassium, magnesium and calcium in older boys and girls, and iron in older girls. Furthermore, significant proportions had intakes below the LRNI levels. For zinc, a quarter of the youngest girls, over a third of 11-14 year old girls and 10% of boys and older girls had intakes below the LRNI. Intakes of potassium were below the LRNI for a fifth of 11-14 year old girls, over a third of the 15-18 year old girls, and for 15% of the older boys. Up to 50% of older girls had iron intakes below the LRNI.

Physical and biochemical measurements

Mean systolic blood pressure was 110mmHg for boys and 108mmHg for girls, respectively, and diastolic blood pressure was 56mmHg for both boys and girls. Increased systolic pressure was associated with the use of salt at the table for boys and girls, and with use of salt in cooking for girls.

Mean plasma total cholesterol concentration was 4.03mmol/l for boys and 4.24mmol/l for girls. Around 8% of boys and 11% of girls had a concentration at or above the target level of 5.2mmol/l.

There were no significant differences between blood cholesterol levels and haematological analytes for 4-10 year olds according to the type of school lunchtime meal.

Analysis of blood and plasma for nutritional status showed that there was generally good nutritional status for vitamin A and vitamin B_{12} and there was no evidence of a high risk group for magnesium, selenium, copper and vitamin E. There was, however, evidence that some children or young people had poor nutritional status for iron, vitamin D, vitamin C, folate, riboflavin and thiamin.

In the 4-6 year old age group, 3% of boys and 8% of girls had blood haemoglobin levels below the WHO limit for anaemia. In older boys and girls, 13% of boys and 27% of girls had low serum ferritin levels, which suggests that they might have low iron stores. Thirteen per cent of 11-18 year olds had poor vitamin D status.

School meals

Two separate analyses of the contribution of school meals to schoolchildren's diets were undertaken as part of the survey.

The first analysis included all of those in the 4-10 year old age group who had consumed at least one school meal during the survey (340 children). In this case, meals which comprised only of savoury snacks, confectionery, biscuits, cakes, or drinks were excluded from the definition of meals.

The results from this group were compared with the *Balance of Good Health* food guide,[23] which forms the basis of the new school meals regulations. School meals provided a greater proportion of starchy foods and protein-rich foods than the overall daily diet, and a lower proportion of milk and dairy foods and fatty/sugary foods. The *Balance of Good Health* recommends, however, that at least 30% of foods should comprise fruit or vegetables. Only 9% of the school meals in this study comprised fruit and vegetables (13% if drinks are excluded from the analysis). The *Balance of Good Health* also requires that no more than 10% of food should comprise fatty/sugary foods. For the 4-10 year olds in this survey, 19% of their school meals comprised fatty/sugary foods.

A comparison of the nutritional content of the diets of those children consuming free school meals, paid school meals or no school meals was conducted. Children who did not take a school meal during the survey had significantly lower fat, fibre and protein intakes and higher sugar and vitamin C intakes than those who ate free school meals. When compared with those paying for school meals, those who did not take a school meal had significantly lower energy, fat, fibre, protein, calcium and vitamin A intakes.

The second analysis included all young people aged 4-10 and 11-18 who took a school meal on at least three days of the seven-day survey period. A school meal was taken to include any food obtained on the school premises and eaten between noon and 2pm.

Analysis of the contribution of school meals to nutrient intakes revealed that, for both 4-10 year olds and 11-18 year olds, children who had a free school meal tended to obtain more energy and nutrients from their school meal than children who paid for the meal.

Further analysis of the foods consumed showed that buns, cakes and pastries contributed 30% of sugars (NMES) and between 13% and 15% of energy, fat and saturated fat intakes. Chips provided 20% of vitamin C intakes, and between 11% and 15% of energy, fatty acids, carbohydrate, fibre and folate intakes. A further 7% of saturated fat intakes were provided by meat pies and pastries.

Physical activity
The physical activity of young children (4-6 years old) was assessed by questioning their parents. Ninety-five per cent of parents of the young children in the survey reported that their child was fairly or very active.

Young people aged 7-18 in the survey recorded physical activity information in a diary. Their activity levels were then estimated using a number of measures.

The Health Education Authority (HEA) recommends that young people should participate in at least one hour's activity of at least moderate intensity each day.[24] In the 7-18 age group, around 40% of boys and 60% of girls spent on average less than one hour per day in such activities, thus failing to meet the HEA recommendation.

In the 7-18 group, girls were less active than boys and physical activity levels decreased with age. In the oldest age group 56% of boys and 69% of girls failed to meet the HEA one-hour a day recommendation described above.

Around half of the sample walked to school, one-third went by car, and about one-fifth took the bus. Between 1% and 6% cycled to school.

Regional and socioeconomic variations
As outlined above there were differences in the foods consumed between the different regions and socioeconomic groups. Although there were few significant differences in energy and macronutrient intakes between regions, the intakes of most vitamins and minerals tended to be lower in Scotland and in Northern England. Many of these differences persisted when differences in energy intake were taken into account – suggesting a lower density of vitamins and minerals in the diet. Boys and girls in Scotland and the North also tended to have lower levels of vitamin C and folate in their blood.

Young people, particularly boys, in households of lower socioeconomic status had lower intakes of energy, fat, some other macronutrients and most vitamins and minerals. Some of these intakes were still lower after the differences in energy intake were taken into account: vitamin C, calcium, phosphorus, magnesium and iodine for boys and girls, pantothenic acid for boys and riboflavin, niacin, carotene and manganese for girls. Biochemical analyses for folate, riboflavin, vitamin D and iron were also lower in the disadvantaged socioeconomic groups.

Policy implications of the survey findings

The children and young people in the National Diet and Nutrition Survey of 4-18 year olds derived, on average, around 35% of their energy intake from fat, and saturated fat provided over 14% in both boys and girls. Carbohydrates provided just over half of food energy and, within this, non-milk extrinsic sugars accounted for around 16% of food energy. Intakes of sodium were twice the recommended level, even though salt added during cooking or at the table was excluded.

Given the methodological issues outlined on page 154, the results of the survey should be treated with caution. The survey does suggest, however, that young people are eating diets with a lower fat content than the equivalent group of young people in 1983. Despite this improvement, fat intakes, although not above the current COMA recommendation,[12] are considerably higher than the 30% goal recently published by the World Health Organization.[2]

The survey also suggests that young people's diets are still too high in saturated fat, sugars and salt. It is also startlingly clear that very few young people are eating enough fruit and vegetables and that a worrying number of children and adolescents are not eating any fruit and vegetables at all.

The measures of physical activity in the survey, coupled with the findings on energy intake and body weight, also suggest that most young people are relatively inactive.

The survey also gives considerable cause for concern about the diets of young people living in poorer households. The findings relating to children and adolescents, particularly males, in households receiving benefits point to inadequate and poorer quality diets.

At the time of publication of the report, the Food Standards Agency highlighted some bold contrasts emerging from the survey. These were:

"• *whereas 33 per cent of 15-18 year old girls smoke, only 20 per cent eat citrus fruit;*

- *they drink two-thirds more fizzy drinks than milk (1500g v 900g)*

- *boys eat, by weight, nearly four times as many biscuits than leafy green vegetables*

- *girls eat, by weight, more than four times as much sweets and chocolate than leafy green vegetables."*[25]

The range of factors which influence what young people eat and how active they are is very broad. It follows, therefore, that there is also broad scope for potential policy options to influence these factors.

The policy context

When the survey was published, the Food Standards Agency undertook to work with industry and government to improve the diet of young people, and a cross-government alliance was announced to coordinate relevant initiatives, ensure that the priority areas are tackled and to set targets.[25] Other measures under consideration were a review of food labelling and a code of practice on the promotion of food to children.[25]

In recent years, there have been a number of relevant initiatives designed to improve the health, and in particular, the diet of children and younger people. Many of these initiatives have centred around the school. (For more details of these initiatives, see Chapter 12.)

School meals

Local education authorities and governing bodies were not obliged to provide a school meal service until 1 April 2001, when it became their duty to offer a paid school meals service where parents request it. The new regulations also require that local education authorities delegate funding for school meals to all secondary schools. This means that a school's governing body has responsibility for all aspects of school meal provision.

Nutritional standards for school meals had been abolished in 1980 but these were reintroduced on 1 April 2001. These standards are food-based rather than the nutrient-based standards that many public health groups advocated for and which were also backed by the Education and Employment Select Committee. At the time of publication of this report, the Department for Education and Skills is looking at how it should monitor and evaluate the effect of these nutritional standards on the diets of children and young people.

School meals are free for: children whose parents receive income support or jobseekers allowance benefits; older children who receive these benefits themselves; and the children of asylum-seekers. Current estimates are that nationally about 3% of primary school children and 5% of secondary school pupils are eligible for free school meals but do not take them. In some areas the figures are considerably higher. The Department for Education and Skills is funding the Child Poverty Action Group to look at ways of maximising the uptake of free school meals. The results of the survey of 4-18 year olds[1] underline the importance of free school meals as a source of nutrients for children from lower income homes.

Healthy Schools Programme

The government's Healthy Schools Programme was launched in 1998 and was followed by the introduction of the National Healthy School Standard in 1999. The programme promotes a whole-school approach to health which ensures that what is taught in classrooms is matched by what pupils find in the school environment.

Healthy eating is one of the themes for the programme along with physical activity, sex and relationships, drugs, alcohol and tobacco, and citizenship. It is up to the individual school, in conjunction with their local health and education partnership, to decide which themes to prioritise. Healthy eating may not always rank highest in a school's priorities.

The Healthy Schools Programme is an opportunity for schools to implement a whole-school approach to improving nutrition by promoting consistent healthy eating messages in the classroom, the dining room, in tuckshops and in vending machines.

National School Fruit Scheme

The *NHS Plan*,[26] published in 2000, announced a National School Fruit Scheme where every child in nursery and 4-6 year olds in infant schools will be entitled to a free piece of fruit each school day. The scheme will be fully operational by 2004.

Reducing inequalities

In addition to the policy initiatives mentioned above, there have been a number of more far-reaching initiatives which may well have an impact on the diets of children and young people.

5 A DAY initiatives

Following publication of the *NHS Plan*, five local 5 A DAY pilot initiatives were set up by the Department of Health in 2001 to test the feasibility and practicalities of evidence-based community approaches to improving access to and increasing consumption of fruit and vegetables in low-income areas. The lessons learnt from the first five pilots are set out in a series of Department of Health publications which offer practical advice on the planning, setting up and running of an effective local 5 A DAY initiative.

Treasury spending review

The 2002 Treasury spending review[27] identified the need for a long-term government-wide strategy to ensure that health inequalities objectives are reflected in departments' mainstream programmes. As part of the strategy, the review identified the need for targeted services for disadvantaged communities to help families improve their children's nutrition and establish healthy eating patterns early in life.

Health poverty index

It is likely that access to affordable nutritious food will be included in the new health poverty index which is currently being devised.[28] This should make it easier to identify areas where access to such food is difficult and to track the situation if it deteriorates or improves.

Other measures

A number of other relevant measures were announced under the *NHS Plan*, including reform of the Welfare Foods Scheme to ensure that children in poverty have access to a healthy diet (see page 265), and collaboration with the food industry to improve the balance of salt, fat and sugar in foods.

European Union and international issues

In addition to the national policy context, there are clearly influences from outside the UK which affect the diets of children and adolescents. The Common Agricultural Policy, for example, through its effects on price, distribution and promotion of produce, is a major influence on food consumption. This includes the availability of fruit and vegetables to young people. Food labelling rules are decided at EU level and it is likely that there will be further harmonisation of the framework for advertising and promoting foods across Europe.

It has been argued, therefore, that EU member state governments can take only limited action to improve the diets of their populations without corresponding change in these EU policies.[29, 30] There has been growing awareness of the influence of EU policies on dietary patterns in member states. This has led, in turn, to a recognition of the proper role of the EU in improving nutrition. The Commission's *White Paper on Food Safety*, for example, signalled a new commitment to nutrition and the possibility of *'a comprehensive and cohesive nutrition policy'*.[31] Further evidence of increasing EU activity in this area is witnessed by the recent EU-funded Eurodiet project, organised by the University of Crete, which produced a framework for European dietary guidelines,[13] and the promotion of nutrition was a key priority of the French presidency of the EU in 2000.[32] The European Commission is currently preparing a status report on the European Commission's work in the field of nutrition which should provide the basis for the development of an EU Action Plan on Nutrition.

A further influence to consider in the policy context is the Codex Alimentarius and the rules of the World Trade Agreement which can also influence the price, availability, compositional standards and labelling of foodstuffs.

The UK government has also wholeheartedly supported WHO Europe's proposal for a Food and Nutrition Policy and Action Plan which includes a nutrition strategy "geared to ensure optimal health, especially in low-income groups and during critical periods throughout life, such as infancy, childhood, pregnancy, and lactation, and older age".[33]

Conclusions

The National Diet and Nutrition Survey of 4-18 year olds[1] confirms that continued efforts are needed to improve the diets of children and young people in order to improve health in the adults of tomorrow. These efforts should seek to:

- reduce the proportion of food energy from total fat, saturated fat and non-milk extrinsic sugars
- reduce salt intakes and the prevalence of sodium intakes above the RNI
- increase the consumption of fruit and vegetables, particularly in those groups where consumption is particularly low, and
- ensure that children growing up in disadvantaged households have access to an adequate and high quality diet.

This should be coupled with policies to promote physical activity in young people in ways which are likely to be carried on into adulthood.

It is encouraging that a wide range of initiatives are already underway to address these issues. Many of these initiatives are centred around the school. It is hoped that interventions such as the introduction of the National School Fruit Scheme will make a real difference. It will be important to monitor carefully the impact of the scheme and of the introduction of legislation on school meals.

There remains a need, however, to look at the whole-school approach to improving nutrition. Further initiatives to improve food and nutrition education in the school curriculum and to develop practical food skills in young people are required. Healthy eating should be a key part of the Healthy Schools Programme and schools should receive all the necessary support and encouragement to promote healthy eating in a positive and imaginative way throughout the school.

Although schools are a very important part of children's lives, they are not the only influence on young people. Efforts to improve children's diets need to look beyond the school gate. Commercial messages which children receive about foods are often in direct contradiction to the nutritional messages they receive. Food advertising and promotional campaigns, for example, are frequently targeted at children. Sponsorship programmes in schools are another source of commercial information. It is clear that these commercial messages may have an important influence over young people's choices.

Young people who do want to choose a healthy diet need to have access to the information to enable them to do so. This means that food labels must be clear and meaningful in relation to healthy eating messages. The current system of nutrition labelling does not meet these criteria. Control of health claims is also important so that both young people and adults are able to trust and rely on the messages on food labels to enable them to choose healthy foods. In addition, the increasing importance of food eaten outside the home means that clear nutrition information about food from cafés, restaurants, snack bars and fast food restaurants is also essential.

Furthermore, efforts to improve children's diets should seek to improve the foods which make up these diets. The results of the survey of 4-18 year olds[1] provide information on those foods which contribute significant amounts of fat, saturated fat, salt and sugars. There is a very important role for the government to work with manufacturers to ensure an improvement in the nutritional quality of their foods.

Finally, the survey provides a reminder that there are social inequalities in the health of children. Policies to promote access to affordable, good quality, nutritious food for low-income families must be a priority. All efforts to reduce social inequalities and tackle social exclusion may have an impact on child nutrition. A healthy diet in childhood is one important foundation for a long and healthy adult life. Healthy diets for *all* young people should be the goal.

References

1 Gregory J, Lowe S, Bates CJ, Prentice A, Jackson LV, Smithers G, Wenlock R, Farron M. 2000. *National Diet and Nutrition Survey. Young People Aged 4 to 18 Years. Volume 1: Report of the Diet and Nutrition Survey.* London: The Stationery Office.

2 World Health Organization. 1990. *Diet, Nutrition and the Prevention of Chronic Disease: Report of a World Health Organization Study Group. Technical Report Series: 797.* Geneva: World Health Organization.

3 Chiva M, Mischlich D. Du bon usage des sens dans l'alimentation. In: Baudier F, Barthelemy L, Michaud C, Legrand L (eds). 1995. *Education Nutritionelle: Equilibres à la Carte.* Paris: Comité Français d'Education pour la Santé.

4 Gregory J, Foster K, Tyler H, Wiseman M. 1990. *The Dietary and Nutritional Survey of British Adults.* London: HMSO.

5 Finch S, Doyle W, Lowe C, Bates CJ, Prentice A, Smithers G, Clarke PC. 1998. *National Diet and Nutrition Survey: People Aged 65 Years and Over. Volume 1: Report of the Diet and Nutrition Survey.* London: The Stationery Office.

6 Gregory JR, Collins DL, Davies PSW, Hughes JM, Clarke PC. 1995. *National Diet and Nutrition Survey: Children Aged 1½ to 4½ Years. Volume 1: Report of the Diet and Nutrition Survey.* London: HMSO.

7 Department of Health. 1989. *The Diets of British Schoolchildren. Report on Health and Social Subjects No 36.* London: HMSO.

8 Prescott-Clarke P, Primatesta P. 1999. *Health Survey for England. The Health of Young People '95-'97.* London: HMSO.

9 Chinn S, Price CE, Rona RJ. 1989. The need for new reference curves for height. *Archives of Disease in Childhood*; 64: 1545-53.

10 Fruhbeck G. 2000. Childhood obesity: time for action, not complacency. *British Medical Journal*; 320: 328-29.

11 Sokol RJ. 2000. The chronic disease of childhood obesity: the sleeping giant has awakened. *Journal of Pediatrics*; 136: 711-13.

12 Department of Health. 1991. *Dietary Reference Values for Food Energy and Nutrients for the United Kingdom. Report on Health and Social Subjects No 41.* London: HMSO.

13 Kafatos G, Codrington CA (eds.) 2001. Eurodiet Core Report. *Public Health Nutrition;* 4, 2 (A).

14 Ruxton CHS, Kirk TR, Belton NR. 1996. Energy and nutrient intakes in a sample of Edinburgh 7-8 year olds: a comparison with United Kingdom dietary reference values. *British Journal of Nutrition;* 75: 151-60.

15 Nelson M, Naismith DJ, Burley V et al. 1990. Nutrient intakes, vitamin-mineral supplementation, and intelligence in British schoolchildren. *British Journal of Nutrition*; 64: 13-22.

16 Hunt C, Rigley L. 1995. A study of the dietary habits, heights and weights of primary schoolchildren. *Nutrition and Food Science;* 4: 5-7.

17 McNeill G, Davidson L, Morrison DC et al. 1991. Nutrient intake in schoolchildren: some practical considerations. *Proceedings of the Nutrition Society*; 50: 37-43.

18 Strain JJ, Robson PJ, Livingstone MBE et al. 1994. Estimates of food and macronutrient intake in a random sample of Northern Ireland adolescents. *British Journal of Nutrition*; 72: 343-52.

19 Bull N. 1985. Dietary habits of 15-25 year olds. *Human Nutrition. Applied Nutrition;* 39A; Suppl. 1, 1-68.

20 Crawley HF. 1993. The energy, nutrient and food intakes of teenagers aged 16-17 years in Britain. *British Journal of Nutrition*; 70: 15-26.

21 Barker ME, McClean SI, McKenna PG et al. 1988. *Diet, Lifestyle and Health in Northern Ireland.* Coleraine: Centre for Applied Health Studies.

22 Buttriss J. 2000. Diet and nutritional status of 4-18 year olds: Public health implications. *Nutrition Bulletin*; 25: 209-17.

23 Health Education Authority. 1994. *National Food Guide: The Balance of Good Health.* London: Health Education Authority.

24 Biddle S, Sallis J, Cavill N (eds.) 1998. *Young and Active? Young People and Health-enhancing Physical Activity – Evidence and Implications.* London: Health Education Authority.

25 Food Standards Agency. 2000. *Publication of National Diet and Nutrition Survey of Young People Aged 4-18. Press release, Thursday 1st June 2000. 2000/0013.* London: Food Standards Agency.

26 Department of Health. 2000. *The NHS Plan. A Plan for Investment. A Plan for Reform.* London: The Stationery Office.

27 HM Treasury. 2002. *Opportunities and Security for All: Investing in an Enterprising, Fairer Britain.* London: The Stationery Office.

28 Department of Health. 2000. *The NHS Plan. A Plan for Investment. A Plan for Reform.* London: The Stationery Office. Paragraph 13.7.

29 Lobstein T, Longfield J. 1999. *Improving Diet and Health through European Union Food Policies.* London: Health Education Authority.

30 Lang T. Food and nutrition. In: Weil O, McKee M, Brodin M, Oberle D. 1999. *Priorities for Public Health Action in the European Union.* Brussels: European Commission.

31 Commission of the European Communities. 2000. *White Paper on Food Safety, Com/99/719.* Brussels: Commission of the European Communities.

32 Société Française de Santé Publique. 2000. *Health and Human Nutrition: Elements for European Action. Collection Santé et Société No 10.* Vandoeuvre-les-Nancy: Société Française de Santé Publique.

33 World Health Organization Regional Office for Europe. 2000. *The Impact of Food and Nutrition on Human Health. The Case for a Food and Nutrition Policy and Action Plan for the European Region of WHO 2000-2005.* Copenhagen: World Health Organization.

Chapter 8

The determinants of young people's participation in physical activity, and investigation of tracking of physical activity from youth to adulthood

Nick Cavill

Cavill Associates

Professor Stuart Biddle

School of Sport and Exercise Sciences, Loughborough University

This chapter:

- reviews the evidence on the factors which can be classed as determinants of young people's participation in physical activity, or which correlate with physical activity participation
- reviews the evidence on the extent to which participation in physical activity among young people is likely to carry through into adulthood, and
- aims to provide a basis for policy guidance that will help to increase young people's participation in physical activity, and positively influence the likelihood of future adult participation in physical activity.

Key themes

- A number of factors have been shown to be related to levels of physical activity among children and adolescents.
- Non-modifiable factors (such as gender) give indications for the targeting of physical activity interventions, and indicate in particular the importance of targeting girls and adolescents.
- Modifiable factors which have been shown to be consistently related to physical activity participation should be emphasised and developed within policies and programmes. These include psychological, behavioural, social and environmental factors.
- Evidence for the 'tracking' of physical activity from childhood to adolescence and adulthood is not strong.
- Studies show that the nature of early life experiences in physical activity has a slightly stronger effect as a precursor of adult physical activity, but still this effect appears small, and may be the result of other factors.
- Research into tracking must account for the quality of childhood experiences in physical activity as well as the changes in activity levels during childhood, adolescence and adulthood.

Introduction

There is now strong evidence to support the relationship between physical activity and many aspects of adult health. Physical activity reduces morbidity and mortality from many of the leading causes of ill health, including coronary heart disease, as well as having positive effects on aspects of health such as body fat and weight control, depression and anxiety.[1]

The data on direct health benefits for young people are, however, not so conclusive. This is partly due to methodological problems, but is primarily because the main morbidities which affect adults, and which are caused at least in part by a sedentary lifestyle, have not had long enough to develop.[2] The main exception to this is childhood obesity, which can be considered a health problem in its own right, and which has increased in recent years.[3] It has been suggested that this, together with likely improvements in young people's psychological health, are sufficient reasons alone to justify efforts to assist all young people in developing regular physical activity habits.[4]

It is clear from national surveys that many young people are not meeting current recommended levels of physical activity. The most recent consensus conference on this issue[4] proposed two main recommendations, based on existing evidence and expert opinion:

- All young people should participate in physical activity of at least moderate intensity for one hour per day.

- Young people who currently do little physical activity should increase their level to at least half an hour of moderate intensity activity per day, as practising minimal physical activity is still beneficial, and highly preferable to practising little or none.

The National Diet and Nutrition Survey[5] showed that 39% of young males and 58% of young females did not achieve the recommendation for an hour a day of at least moderate intensity physical activity. The proportions achieving this level declined sharply with age. Other sources indicate that in the last five years or so, physical activity has begun to reduce in many aspects of a young person's life: at school,[6,7] on the way to school,[8] and as organised sport.[9]

This chapter reviews the evidence on the determinants of young people's participation in physical activity, and whether participation is likely to carry through into adulthood. The overall aim of the chapter is to provide a basis for policy guidance that will help to increase young people's participation in physical activity, and positively influence the likelihood of future adult participation in physical activity.

Methods of review

There have been a number of reviews on both the determinants of physical activity among children[10-16] and the 'tracking' of physical activity from youth into adulthood.[17] Most of the conclusions of this chapter are based on these reviews. In addition, searches were carried out using Medline and via manual searches of known papers and their references. Search terms included: 'reviews', 'physical activity', 'young people', 'children', 'determinants', and 'tracking'.

Correlates of physical activity in young people

A number of papers have reviewed the determinants or correlates of physical activity among children.[10-16] The term 'correlates' is generally preferred, because 'determinants' implies that causality can be inferred,[16] whereas most studies report only observed associations between factors. Reviews have ranged in the methodologies used, but have in the main tended to rely on narrative evaluations of the literature, and some have restricted the age of the participants studied or the range of variables included. The exceptions are the studies by Taylor, Baranowski and Sallis[13] and Sallis et al,[16] which were systematic in nature. The latter of these two papers[16] was a landmark study in this field because: it reviewed all published studies of correlates of young people's participation in physical activity; it included the entire range of potential correlates; it studied young people aged 3-18 years; it used a semi-quantitative methodology; and it analysed both younger children (3-12 years) and adolescents (13-18 years). As this study brings the entire field up to date, it will be used as the basis for this section of the chapter.

The literature on correlates is drawn largely from the US (three-quarters of papers), and covers both boys and girls. There is some research on racial or ethnic differences in determinants, but this is among the US populations so caution needs to be applied when considering implications for the UK context.[18]

A number of factors have been studied which have the potential to be related to physical activity levels in young people.[16] These include demographic and biological variables (such as age and sex), psychological variables (such as intention to be active), behavioural variables (such as diet), social variables (such as parental physical activity), and environmental variables (such as time spent outdoors). We have adopted these categories and drawn on the evidence provided by Sallis et al.[16] Additional comment will be provided to allow application to the UK context where appropriate. One note of caution is that Sallis et al considered a variable to be associated with physical activity if such a link was statistically significant. This could include small effect sizes for large samples and exclude moderate or large effects for small samples. Also it should be noted that Sallis et al included any variable that had been the subject of at least three studies, and reported a *consistent association* where the majority of studies supported the expected association. Therefore in some cases conclusions are drawn based on only two positive studies. Where fewer than half of the studies reported a consistent association, the variable is reported as *inconsistently related*. Where factors were studied but no association was found with physical activity levels, the factor is reported as *not related*.

Demographic and biological correlates

Table 1 ***Demographic and biological factors related to physical activity participation***

Factors consistently associated with physical activity among children
- **Gender.** Boys were more active than girls. (25/31 studies)
- **Parental weight.** Overweight parents tend to have more active children. (3/5 studies).

Factors consistently associated with physical activity for adolescents
- **Gender.** Boys were more active than girls. (27/28 studies)
- **Age.** (Negative correlation.) Older adolescents were less likely to be active. (19/27 studies)
- **Ethnicity.** White adolescents were more active than those from minority ethnic communities. (10/14 studies)

Source: See reference 16.

One of the strongest findings is that boys are more active than girls. This relationship begins at a young age, continues throughout adolescence, and is observed in many cross-sectional studies and longitudinal studies.[5, 9, 19] Age is consistently related to physical activity among adolescents only, supporting observations from cross-sectional studies that young children are habitually active, but that participation tends to decrease around adolescence.[5] Body weight and adiposity were frequently studied but were not found to be consistently related to physical activity. The finding that overweight adults tend to have more active children was surprising, but was supported by the majority of 3 out of 5 studies.

Inconsistent findings

Body weight and adiposity were frequently studied but there were inconsistent findings of associations with physical activity for both children and adolescents. Studies looking into age as a correlate within the 3-12 year age range also showed inconsistent findings.

Not related

Socioeconomic status was not related to physical activity for either children or adolescents.

Psychological correlates

Table 2 ***Psychological factors related to physical activity participation***

Factors consistently associated with physical activity among children

- Perceived barriers to physical activity. (Negative correlation.) Those who perceived more barriers to physical activity were less likely to be active. (3/3 studies)
- Intention to be physically active (3/5 studies)
- Preference for physical activity (3/5 studies)

Factors consistently associated with physical activity among adolescents

- Achievement orientation (5/6 studies)
- Perceived competence (2/3 studies)
- Intention to be physically active (6/8 studies)
- Depression (Inverse association.) Those with higher levels of depression were less likely to be active. (3/4 studies)

Source: See reference 16.

Perceived barriers to physical activity was the most consistently associated variable for children, but there were inconsistent findings among studies of adolescents. Intention to be physically active was seen as important for both age groups. Perhaps most surprising in this review was that self-efficacy (belief in one's ability to be able to do something) was found to be inconsistently related to physical activity, and self-esteem was found to have no relationship. The latter finding may be due to inappropriate measurement or lack of assessment of domains of self-esteem most likely to be associated with physical activity.

Inconsistent findings

Self-efficacy, perceived competence, and attitudes to physical activity were often studied but any associations with physical activity for children were inconsistent across studies. Attitudes to physical activity, barriers, self-efficacy, body image, attitudes, knowledge and enjoyment of physical activity were often studied but had inconsistent associations with physical activity for adolescents.

Not related

Body image, self-esteem, perceived benefits, attitudes to sweating, and after-school activity were often studied but had no association with physical activity for children. 'Talking loudly', external locus of control, self-esteem, self-motivation, enjoyment of exercise, and perceived stress were often studied but had no association with physical activity among adolescents.

Behavioural correlates

Table 3 ***Behavioural factors related to physical activity participation***

Factors consistently associated with physical activity among children
• Healthy diet (3/3 studies)
• Previous physical activity (5/6 studies)
Factors consistently associated with physical activity among adolescents
• Sensation seeking (3/3 studies)
• Previous physical activity (11/12 studies)
• Participation in community sports (7/7 studies)
• Sedentary behaviour after school and at weekends. (Inverse association with physical activity.) (3/3 studies)

Source: See reference 16.

Among the behavioural variables, healthy diet was found to be related to physical activity in children, but not in adolescents. Interestingly, previous physical activity was a frequent correlate for both age groups, implying that there is evidence for a 'tracking' effect throughout childhood. This is considered in more detail later. Sensation seeking and participation in community sports were also correlated with physical activity for adolescents, suggesting an effect for involvement based on perceived competence.

It is often assumed that large amounts of time spent in sedentary behaviour would be negatively correlated with overall physical activity but this is not supported by the majority of studies. This implies that young people may be able to spend a great deal of time being sedentary but may still be able to take part in adequate levels of physical activity. The exception is sedentary behaviour specifically after school and at weekends, which was found to be negatively associated with physical activity in the majority of studies of adolescents.

Inconsistent findings

Time spent in sedentary pursuits was the most frequently studied behaviour but studies did not consistently report an association with physical activity among children. Cigarette smoking was studied among adolescents but findings were inconsistent.

Not related

Alcohol use, healthy diet, and time spent in sedentary activity were found to be unrelated to physical activity in adolescents. Smoking, alcohol use and calorie intake were unrelated to children's physical activity.

Social correlates

Table 4 ***Social factors related to physical activity participation***

Factors consistently associated with physical activity among children
• None
Factors consistently associated with physical activity among adolescents
• Parental support (2/3 studies) • Direct parental help (3/4 studies) • Support from 'significant others' (4/4 studies) • Sibling physical activity (4/4 studies)

Source: See reference 16.

It is often assumed that parents have a large degree of influence on children's physical activity levels, but this was not found to be the case. Only 38% of the 29 studies that had investigated parents' physical activity found it to be correlated with children's physical activity. There were no variables with consistent associations for children. Among adolescents, however, concepts including support and help were important. Such findings need to be seen alongside environmental and socioeconomic constraints, such as parents driving children to school because of concern for their safety or unfavourable environmental conditions.

Inconsistent findings
Parental physical activity was the most frequently studied behaviour but studies did not find a consistent association between parental physical activity and physical activity in children. This was also found with parental participation in children's physical activity.

Perceived support from peers, subjective norms/social influence, and perceived attitudes of significant others were inconsistently related to physical activity in adolescents.

Not related
Parental physical activity, peer modelling and teacher or coach modelling showed no association with physical activity in adolescents.

Environmental correlates

Table 5 ***Environmental factors related to physical activity participation***

Factors consistently associated with physical activity among children
• Access to facilities and programmes (3/3 studies)
• Time spent outdoors (3/3 studies)
Factors consistently associated with physical activity among adolescents
• Opportunities to exercise (2/3 studies)

Source: See reference 16.

Access to facilities and programmes, and time spent outdoors, were found to be important for children's physical activity, and overall opportunities to exercise were found to be important for adolescents, supporting the need for environmental interventions.[20]

Inconsistent findings

Season and rural/urban location were found to be inconsistently related to children's physical activity.

Not related

Neighbourhood safety and parents providing transport to physical activity opportunities were unrelated to children's physical activity level. The influence of the sports media, and having equipment available were not related to adolescent physical activity, although there are relatively few studies in this area.

Conclusions on correlates for physical activity

A number of factors have been shown to be related to levels of physical activity among children and adolescents. The non-modifiable variables (such as gender and age) give indications for the targeting of physical activity interventions, and indicate in particular the importance of targeting girls and adolescents. Factors which have been shown to be consistently related to physical activity participation should be emphasised and developed within policies and programmes. These include psychological, behavioural, social and environmental factors. A number of implications for public policy are given at the end of this chapter.

One point of interest arising from this review is whether we should be promoting physically active behaviour, or a decrease in sedentary behaviour. Although many people assume that there is a strong relationship between time spent in sedentary pursuits (notably TV watching and playing computer games) and overall physical activity level,[21] this is generally not supported in the literature. This may be due to methodological problems, but is more likely to be due to the fact that it is quite possible for young people to achieve recommended levels of physical activity while still spending a large amount of the day inactive in front of a screen.[14] Whether this implies that targeting a reduction in sedentary behaviour may be more effective than promoting active behaviour remains unclear. Indeed, sedentary behaviour may be associated with increasing levels of obesity, making this an important area for future research. In addition, there is some evidence that sedentary behaviour may track better than physical activity, particularly for boys.[22]

Tracking of physical activity from youth to adulthood

Common sense suggests that you are more likely to be an active adult if you were active in childhood or adolescence. The well-cited US Surgeon General's Report[1] states that childhood and adolescence are 'pivotal times' for adults as well as youth. The report subscribes to the view that maintaining physical activity habits in youth helps prevent sedentary behaviour in adults. Similarly, the British Heart Foundation[21] says that "physically active children are more likely to be active adults". The National Heart Forum[23] has published quantified estimates of the strength of the tracking effect, reporting the claim that "active children are 10 times more likely than inactive children to be active adults".

Although this assumption is reasonable, evidence to substantiate it is mixed. Many factors in the transition to adult life are likely to affect the levels and patterns of physical activity and changes in the adult life cycle itself will affect the extent to which adults are active. Indeed, some have claimed that our understanding of the stability of physical activity during childhood, and from childhood into adulthood, is poor,[24] while others propose that the most important research priority in the area of youth physical activity is to "study the effects of childhood physical activity and its determinants as predictors of adult physical activity".[12] It is perhaps even worth asking why we should expect physical activity to track through such an unstable period as adolescence when physical activity is found to be a most unstable behaviour even among adults.

Conclusions from reviews of physical activity tracking

Powell and Dysinger[25] reviewed six studies that investigated the link between childhood participation in organised sport and physical education and adult physical activity. The most convincing support came from the Harvard Alumni Study. However, this involved predicting adult activity levels from sports participation at college age, a time when activity levels are likely to be more stable. In short, this was not a test of tracking from youth to adulthood but of tracking during adulthood. Powell and Dysinger identified several methodological weaknesses prevalent in the studies they reviewed, and hence they concluded that no firm data were available to support the view that childhood activity leads to a more active adulthood.

The most comprehensive review on physical activity tracking was conducted by Malina.[17] He concluded that the magnitude of tracking during adolescence and into adulthood is "low to moderate". In other words, there is not a strong likelihood that active young people will become active adults. Riddoch,[2] drawing on similar studies to Malina, arrived at the same conclusion and highlighted that the correlations for tracking are particularly weak when self-report measures are used. For example, Telama, Yang et al,[26] reporting data from the Cardiovascular Risk in Young Finns longitudinal study, showed correlations between measures of physical activity for 9, 12 and 15 year olds to be between 0.18 and 0.31 for 9-year follow-up, and 0.01 to 0.27 for 12-year follow-up. Stability was higher for 18 year olds after 9 years (0.41-0.47), but again very low after 12 years (0.21-0.26). From this study the greatest stability appears to be among those who took part in more intense sports club training. Telama, Leskinen et al[27] report three-year follow-up correlations as high as 0.78 for 18 year old boys, falling to 0.27 for 18 year old girls at six-year follow-up.

One of the few studies using more 'objective' measures of activity in tracking was reported by Pate, Baranowski et al.[28] Using heart rate measures, they reported correlations that were quite high (r = 0.57-0.66). However, this study investigated 3-4 year olds over a three-year period. This is a time when relatively little change in environmental, social and psychological factors is expected. Stability of behaviour, therefore, is likely.

Since Riddoch's review,[2] Pate, Trost et al[29] have reported tracking data for rural, predominantly African-American 10 year olds over three years using self-report measures. Stability was low-to-moderate for: vigorous physical activity (r = 0.36); moderate-to-vigorous physical activity (0.24); estimated after-school energy expenditure (0.41); and TV watching (0.41). This again raises the important issue of whether inactivity tracks better than activity. Twisk[30] suggests that the data are mixed on the tracking of sedentary behaviour and Malina[17] says that inactivity has not been studied often enough. This area requires further study.

Other markers of tracking

The conclusions so far have been drawn mainly from longitudinal studies that have calculated correlation coefficients across time. These have shown that tracking is generally low. Other studies have either addressed the issue of tracking without longitudinal data or have, within a longitudinal design, assessed likely determinants of the stability of physical activity participation.

Evidence from the Allied Dunbar National Fitness Survey (ADNFS) in England[31] provides some support, at least indirectly, for an association between early participation in physical activity and a greater likelihood of involvement later in life. Through interview, participants in the survey were asked to recall the moderate-to-vigorous physical activity they took part in at 16, 24 and 34 years of age. It was concluded that current participation in physical activity in later adult years was strongly associated with participation at an earlier age. For example, 25% of those stating that they were very active between the ages of 14 and 19 years were active currently, whereas only 2% of those who were currently active were inactive in the past during those teenage years. This was the basis for the claim made by the National Heart Forum that "active children are 10 times more likely than inactive children to be active adults".[23] In addition, about 30% of the adults in the survey remained in the same activity category across the three time periods studied. However, given that the earliest age of recall was 16 years, stability would be expected to be higher than, say, from early adolescence. The reliability of people's assessment of activity levels carried out some 10-20 years previously must also cast doubt on the validity of this study's conclusions on tracking.

Longitudinal data from Sweden support the view that activity in childhood is a predictor of activity in adulthood given the right circumstances. Engstrom[32] followed 2,000 Swedish youths from 15 to 30 years of age. The study allows for a wider consideration of tracking because potentially important determinants of the stability of activity were assessed. However, the liberal definition of 'activity' as weekly involvement in activity of the intensity of jogging was used and this weakens the study. To test for tracking effects from childhood to adulthood, Engstrom used three conditions as indicators of early (aged 15 years) activity involvement: at least four hours per week of sports or physical activities at age 15 years; being a member of a sports club at 15 years of age; and having a high grade in physical education in school year 8. An index of 'psychological readiness' at the age of 30 was calculated and results showed a clear relationship between the number of conditions fulfilled for activity involvement at 15 years of age and high psychological readiness at age 30. For example, for women fulfilling all three criteria at 15 years, 52% had a high psychological readiness at 30 years, whereas for those not fulfilling any of the criteria, only 17% had high readiness.

These data are supported by a relationship between psychological readiness at age 30 years and actual involvement in physical activity for both men and women. Engstrom[32] also analysed environmental circumstances and involvement in physical activity. Again, there was a clear relationship between the number of environmental conditions fulfilled at the age of 30 years, and current involvement in physical activity. For example for men who lacked environmental support, only 16% were currently active, whereas for men with a supportive environment, 80% were active. This begs the question whether it is the environmental support or the psychological readiness that predicts activity since both correlated highly with physical activity. Engstrom found that those with a positive environment, but low readiness, were more active than those with high readiness but a negative environment, suggesting a more dominant role for environmental circumstances.

Engstrom provides an interesting perspective on the issue of physical activity tracking, supporting the view that "early experience with physical activity during childhood and adolescence ... is of importance for the practice of keep-fit activities in adulthood". The important point to stress here is that the nature of the physical activity experience has been assessed, rather than physical activity *per se*, and it is the quality of experience that predicts future involvement. However, the criterion measure of activity was weak.

Similar to Engstrom, but using a retrospective design, Taylor et al attempted to identify different predictors of adult men's physical activity from measures recalled from childhood and adolescence.[33] Correlations between recalled childhood experiences in physical activity (e.g. enjoyment of activity, or being encouraged to exercise) and current weekly energy expenditure in exercise were all very low (range -0.20 to 0.17). When controlling for current fitness and sum of skinfolds, adult energy expenditure in exercise was predicted negatively by the frequency of being forced to exercise in the pre-teen years. This supports Engstrom's findings that if tracking does exist it is likely to be due to the quality of physical activity experiences in youth rather than involvement *per se*.

Finally, where evidence for tracking has been presented, it is slightly stronger for sports activities, again suggesting that it is important to look at the nature of the activity. Evidence from the Amsterdam Longitudinal Growth and Health Study shows that while organised sport activities contribute only small amounts to total weekly activity above an intensity of 4 METs (1 MET = 1 'metabolic equivalent', equal to the energy expenditure of sitting quietly), they contributed relatively more from the early 20s as other activities are dropped.[19] Early physical development usually offers an advantage in children's sports and such early success may be predictive of later involvement. For example, Taylor et al[33] found a small trend for teacher ratings of sport ability to be associated with adult activity involvement. Similarly, Telama et al[34] found that the best predictors of adult activity nine years after initial assessment in childhood were school grade for physical education and participation in organised sport.

Confounding factors

The discussion so far has suggested that the quality of physical activity experiences might be more important than involvement itself. This leads one into the study of socialisation experiences, which space does not permit here. One issue requiring a mention, however, is that tracking of activity from childhood into adulthood is confounded by changes that might occur *in* childhood and *in* adulthood. For example, Caspersen et al[35] show that for American adolescents, the greatest increase in physical inactivity and the greatest decline in regular vigorous activity is between 15 and 18 years for both boys and girls. For regular 'sustained light-to-moderate' activity, the greatest decline for girls is between 12 and 15 years but for boys it is between 15 and 18 years. Moreover, Mihalik et al[36] have shown that different activities 'expand' and 'contract' at different stages of the adult lifespan. These findings make it highly unlikely that activity at two life stages will be strongly associated.

Conclusions on tracking

Evidence from reviews and primary studies can be summarised as follows.

- Studies testing the statistical relationship between physical activity in adulthood and activity in childhood or adolescence show a low-to-moderate level of association, meaning that it is not highly probable that active children will become active adolescents or active adults.

- Studies show slightly stronger effects for the nature of early life experiences in physical activity as precursors of adult physical activity, but still these effects appear small.

- The small effects identified may be real or the result of other factors. For example, it is quite possible that a third variable – such as motor competence or early maturation – is the key influence, with children experiencing early success less likely to quit later on.

- Research into tracking must account for the *quality* of childhood experiences in physical activity as well as the changes in activity *levels* during childhood, adolescence and adulthood.

Policy implications

There are a number of implications for public policy that arise from an exploration of these correlates for physical activity, and the literature on tracking. These can best be seen in terms of the following principles that might be used in planning young people's physical activity programmes.

Target girls

Most studies show that girls are less active than boys. Girls need to be offered activities that are appropriate for their age, and that enable participation both in and beyond school.

Prioritise interventions aimed at older adolescents

Physical activity declines from the age of around 12 years in most studies. If activities can be designed and delivered in a way that they appeal to adolescents, it may increase the likelihood that activity is continued into adulthood. Youth clubs and community activities may offer the greatest potential for this age group.

Promote different types of activity for different age groups

Older children are more likely to want physical activity that develops factors like achievement, competence and sensation seeking – implying the need for more competitive sports and activities. Younger children are more likely to play spontaneously so they need space and opportunities to do so.

Make the environment safe, so that children can be outdoors whenever possible

Time spent outdoors is a strong correlate of physical activity for young children. Parks, open spaces, playgrounds and school playing fields need to be made more available and their use should be promoted. Parents should be encouraged to let children outdoors as much as possible as this increases the likelihood of them being physically active.

Enhance the provision of community sports and physical activity programmes and facilities

Studies show that if programmes and facilities are provided, physical activity participation will rise. Activities such as after-school clubs, sports clubs, and facilities for informal recreation (such as playgrounds, skate parks or basketball hoops) will be used if they respond to young people's needs.

Prioritise after-school and weekend activity, especially for older adolescents

These are key times for young people to be physically inactive, and allow for innovative interventions beyond the PE curriculum. The journey home from school is important here as it offers good opportunities to promote walking or cycling.

Encourage family activity

Parental support and direct help (though not parental activity level), and sibling activity are related to physical activity levels of young people. So, while parents should be physically active for their own health, they should not expect their children to follow their own example without direct help, such as encouragement to join a club, or practical help such as transportation.

Research priorities

This review has shown that there are a number of priorities for future research, including both investigations of the factors shown to be inconsistently related to physical activity levels, and further studies investigating the issue of tracking.

The key research priorities are:

- Longitudinal studies investigating the tracking of physical activity from childhood to adulthood.
- The long-term effect of programmes designed explicitly around the factors known to correlate with physical activity levels.
- Correlational studies of the factors found to provide inconsistent associations, especially psychological factors such as self-efficacy, knowledge and attitudes, and also parental physical activity.
- The role of sedentary behaviour: is it more effective to encourage physical activity or to discourage sedentary behaviour?
- Investigations into a number of broader social and environmental factors that are increasingly seen to be influencing young people's participation in physical activity.
- Data from minority ethnic populations.

Conclusions

In this review we have presented the evidence of the determinants or correlates of young people's physical activity participation, and have demonstrated that current evidence shows that physical activity does not track well from childhood or youth into adulthood. This latter finding may seem to question the commonly held view that physical activity interventions should be designed to 'catch 'em young'. It could be argued that if physical activity does not have a strong impact on young people's current health, and if we are unlikely to be successful in influencing future adult participation in physical activity, then maybe we should turn our attention away from young people as a priority target group.

This, however, ignores the evidence regarding the possible influence of the quality and nature of the childhood physical activity experience, which supports efforts to design interventions which aim to *maximise the possibility, however small*, that physical activity in youth may be continued into adulthood. In addition, there are a number of other compelling reasons to promote quality physical activity among young people, including its influence on psychological well-being, childhood obesity, and social development.

We have also presented a number of principles for promoting physical activity among young people that are based on the best available evidence of the factors that correlate with young people's current participation. Following these principles would be likely to improve current participation, but further research is needed to see whether following these principles could help to maximise the likelihood of active young people growing into active adults.

References

1 US Department of Health and Human Services. 1996. *Physical Activity and Health: A Report of the Surgeon General*. Atlanta, GA: Centers for Disease Control and Prevention.

2 Riddoch C. Relationships between physical activity and physical health in young people. In: Biddle S, Sallis J, Cavill N (eds.) 1998. *Young and Active? Young People and Health-enhancing Physical Activity: Evidence and Implications*. London: Health Education Authority: 17-48.

3 Chinn S, Rona RJ. 2001. Prevalence and trends in overweight and obesity in three cross sectional studies of British children, 1974-94. *British Medical Journal*; 322: 24-26.

4 Cavill N, Biddle S, Sallis JF. 2001. Health-enhancing physical activity for young people: Statement of the United Kingdom Expert Consensus Conference. *Pediatric Exercise Science*; 13: 12-25.

5 Gregory J, Lowe S, Bates CJ, Prentice A, Jackson LV, Smithers G, Wenlock R, Farron M. 2000. *National Diet and Nutrition Survey. Young People Aged 4 to 18 Years. Volume 1: Report of the Diet and Nutrition Survey*. London: The Stationery Office.

6 Physical Education Association of Great Britain and Northern Ireland. 1993. Report of the 4th meeting in Helsinki, 18-20 June 1993. *British Journal of Physical Education*; 24; 3: 26-27.

7 UNESCO. UNESCO survey of physical education in schools. Paper presented at a conference at the European College of Sport Science, Jyvaskyla, Finland, 2000.

8 Department of the Environment, Transport and the Regions. 1999. *Transport Statistics Bulletin: National Travel Survey 1996-98*. London: HMSO.

9 Sport England. 2000. *Young People and Sport in England 1999*. London: Sport England.

10 De Bourdeauhuij I. Behavioural factors associated with physical activity in young people. In: Biddle S, Sallis J, Cavill N (eds.) 1998. *Young and Active? Young People and Health-enhancing Physical Activity: Evidence and Implications*. London: Health Education Authority: 98-118.

11 Sallis JF. Determinants of physical activity behavior in children. In: Pate RR, Hohn RC (eds.) 1994. *Health and Fitness through Physical Education*. Champaign, IL: Human Kinetics: 31-43.

12 Sallis JF, Simons-Morton BG, Stone EJ, Corbin CB, Epstein LH, Faucette N et al. 1992. Determinants of physical activity and interventions in youth. *Medicine and Science in Sports and Exercise*; 24; 6 (suppl): S248-S257.

13 Taylor WC, Baranowski T, Sallis JF. Family determinants of childhood physical activity: A social cognitive model. In: Dishman RK (ed.) 1994. *Advances in Exercise Adherence*. Champaign, IL: Human Kinetics: 319-42.

14 Taylor WC, Sallis JF. Determinants of physical activity in children. In: Simopoulos AP, Pavlou KN (eds.) 1997. *Nutrition and Fitness: Metabolic and Behavioral Aspects in Health and Disease. World Review of Nutrition and Diet, 82*. Basel: Karger: 159-67.

15 Wold B, Hendry L. Social and environmental factors associated with physical activity in young people. In: Biddle S, Sallis J, Cavill N (eds.) 1998. *Young and Active? Young People and Health-enhancing Physical Activity: Evidence and Implications*. London: Health Education Authority: 119-32.

16 Sallis JF, Prochaska JJ, Taylor WC. 2000. A review of correlates of physical activity of children and adolescents. *Medicine and Science in Sports and Exercise*; 32: 963-75.

17 Malina RM. 1996. Tracking of physical activity and physical fitness across the lifespan. *Research Quarterly for Exercise and Sport*; 67; 3 (suppl): S48-S57.

18 Sallis JF, Patterson TL, Buono MJ, Atkins CJ, Nader PR. 1988. Aggregation of physical activity habits in Mexican-American and Anglo families. *Journal of Behavioral Medicine*; 11: 31-41.

19 Van Mechelen W, Twisk JWR, Post GB, Snel J, Kemper HCG. 2000. Physical activity of young people: The Amsterdam Longitudinal Growth and Health Study. *Medicine and Science in Sports and Exercise*; 32: 1610-16.

20 Owen N, Leslie E, Salmon J, Fotheringham MJ. 2000. Environmental determinants of physical activity and sedentary behavior. *Exercise and Sport Sciences Reviews*; 28: 153-58.

21 British Heart Foundation. 2000. *Couch Kids – The Growing Epidemic: Looking at Physical Activity in Children in the UK*. London: British Heart Foundation.

22 Janz KF, Dawson JD, Mahoney LT. 2000. Tracking physical fitness and physical activity from childhood to adolescence: The Muscatine study. *Medicine and Science in Sports and Exercise*; 32: 1250-57.

23 National Heart Forum. 1999. *Looking to the Future: Making Coronary Heart Disease an Epidemic of the Past*. London: The Stationery Office.

24 Baranowski T, Bouchard C, Bar-Or O, Bricker T, Heath G, Kimm SYS et al. 1992. Assessment, prevalence, and cardiovascular benefits of physical activity and fitness in youth. *Medicine and Science in Sports and Exercise*; 24; 6 (suppl): S237-S247.

25 Powell KE, Dsyinger W. 1987. Childhood participation in organized school sports and physical education as precursors of adult physical activity. *American Journal of Preventive Medicine*; 3 (5): 276-81.

26 Telama R, Yang X, Laasko L, Viikari J. 1997. Physical activity in childhood and adolescence as predictor of physical activity in young adulthood. *American Journal of Preventive Medicine*; 13: 317-23.

27 Telama R, Leskinen E, Yang X. 1996. Stability of habitual physical activity and sport participation: A longitudinal tracking study. *Scandinavian Journal of Medicine and Science in Sports*; 6: 371-78.

28 Pate RR, Baranowski T, Dowda M, Trost SG. 1996. Tracking of physical activity in young children. *Medicine and Science in Sports and Exercise*; 28: 92-96.

29 Pate RR, Trost SG, Dowda M, Ott AE, Ward DS, Saunders R et al. 1999. Tracking of physical activity, physical inactivity, and health-related physical fitness in rural youth. *Pediatric Exercise Science*; 11: 364-76.

30 Twisk JWR. 2001. Physical activity guidelines for children and adolescents: A critical review. *Sports Medicine*; 31: 617-27.

31 Sports Council and Health Education Authority. 1992. *Allied Dunbar National Fitness Survey: Main Findings*. London: Health Education Authority and Sports Council.

32 Engstrom L-M. Exercise adherence in sport for all from youth to adulthood. In: Oja P, Telama R (eds.) 1991. *Sport for All*. Amsterdam: Elsevier: 473-83.

33 Taylor WC, Blair SN, Cummings SS, Wun CC, Malina RM. 1999. Childhood and adolescent physical activity patterns and adult physical activity. *Medicine and Science in Sports and Exercise*; 31: 118-23.

34 Telama R, Laasko L, Yang X. 1994. Physical activity and participation in sports of young people in Finland. *Scandinavian Journal of Medicine and Science in Sports*; 4: 65-74.

35 Caspersen CJ, Pereira MA, Curran KM. 2000. Changes in physical activity patterns in the United States, by sex and cross-sectional age. *Medicine and Science in Sports and Exercise*; 32: 1601-09.

36 Mihalik B, O'Leary J, McGuire F, Dottavio F. 1989. Sports involvement across the life span: Expansion and contraction of sports activities. *Research Quarterly for Sport and Exercise*; 60: 396-98.

Chapter 9

The relationship between physical activity during childhood and adolescence and coronary heart disease risk factors in young adulthood

Dr Melvyn Hillsdon

Health Promotion Research Unit, London School of Hygiene and Tropical Medicine

Charlie Foster

British Heart Foundation Health Promotion Research Group, University of Oxford

This chapter:

- describes patterns of physical activity across the lifespan
- assesses the effect of childhood and adolescent physical activity on cardiovascular disease risk factors in young adults
- considers the implications for coronary heart disease prevention strategies, and
- considers the public health implications of intervention options.

Key themes

- The relationship between physical activity in childhood and adolescence and selected coronary heart disease risk factors in young adults is not strong.
- Physically active children and adolescents have lower body fat and higher fitness levels in early adulthood compared with less active children and adolescents.
- There is an urgent need for more studies investigating the long-term relationship between childhood physical activity and adult risk factors for coronary heart disease.
- Interventions that promote increased levels of physical activity in children need to be combined with other strategies to prevent the age-related decline in physical activity.
- To maximise the public health benefits of physical activity, a sustained multi-sector effort is required across the lifespan.

Introduction

A meta-analysis of studies of physical activity in the aetiology of coronary heart disease concluded that the relative risk of developing coronary heart disease (CHD) in the least compared with the most active was 1.9,[1] similar to that of smoking and hypertension. It has been estimated that if half of those adults who do occasional moderate intensity physical activity (e.g. brisk walking) increased it to at least five days a week, there would be a 7% reduction in CHD deaths.[2] The government recommends 30 minutes of moderate intensity physical activity on at least five days a week, or three periods per week of vigorous intensity physical activity of 20 minutes each.[3] In 1998 it was estimated that 61% of men and 76% of women in England were not active at these levels.[4] The former Health Education Authority recommended that "all young people (aged 5-18 years) should participate in physical activity of at least moderate intensity for one hour per day."[5] In 1997 the proportion of children aged 5-15 years participating in one hour or more of physical activity on at least five days of the week was 56% of males and 35% of females.[6]

It is argued that the prevention of coronary artery disease should start early in life[7] and that participation in physical activity at a young age is an important determinant of adult physical activity habits. This systematic review examines whether physically active children and adolescents have an improved CHD risk profile in young adulthood.

Methods

Computerised searches were carried out using Medline, Embase, Sport and SCISearch from 1966 to October 1999. Key words for searching included 'children', 'adolescence', 'young adults', 'adults', 'cohort study', 'longitudinal studies', 'cardiovascular disease', 'coronary heart disease', 'risk factors', 'exercise', 'exertion', 'fitness', 'physical activity', 'alcohol', 'blood pressure', 'body composition', 'diet', 'lifestyle', 'lipoproteins', 'nutrition' and 'smoking'. The search was limited to English language journals. Additional searches were carried out using the references from existing reviews[8-12] and the papers identified during our own scan of the literature. All identified studies were read by the two authors independently. The criteria for inclusion of studies in the review were:

- a prospective observational study
- subjects with a mean age at baseline of less than 16 years
- subjects with a mean age at follow-up of 16 years or over
- a measure of physical activity behaviour made at baseline
- at least one established risk factor for CHD was an outcome measure
- the relationship between baseline physical activity and CHD risk factor status at follow-up was reported
- a follow-up period of three years or more.

When there was more than one paper from the same study, all papers reporting different outcomes or a different approach to analysis were included. If the same data were reported for more than one follow-up period, the longest follow-up period was used.

The findings were summarised narratively.

Results

Over 1,300 abstracts were examined for possible inclusion and, from these, 49 papers were examined in detail. Eight papers were found to meet the inclusion criteria, and these came from two observational studies – the Amsterdam Growth and Health

Study (AGHS) and the Cardiovascular Risk in Young Finns Study (Young Finns study).[13-20] (See Table 1.) Other longitudinal studies: did not have a mean age of less than 16 years at baseline;[21] did not have a follow-up measure after the age of 16 years;[22-24] did not measure CHD risk factors in adulthood;[25] or did not report the relationship between physical activity at baseline and CHD risk factors in adulthood.[26] These papers were not included in the review.

Table 1 ***Young Finns study and Amsterdam Growth and Health Study***

Study	Population	Years of follow-up	Definition of physical activity	Method of physical activity assessment	Follow-up periods	CHD risk factors measured
Young Finns study[13,19]	961 male and female adolescents, aged 12-18 years at entry	6	Physical activity index based on the product of frequency, duration and intensity of physical activity	Questionnaire assessing leisure-time physical activity in previous month	Baseline, 3 and 6 years	Serum insulin and glucose, lipoproteins, smoking, skinfolds, BMI
Amsterdam Growth and Health Study[14-18]	181 males and females, aged 13 years at entry	15	METs per week	Structured interview measuring total time spent on physical activities including school and leisure time in the previous three months	Annually during the first 4 years, and then at 8 and 15 years	Lipoproteins, blood pressure, skinfolds, waist to hip ratio, VO_2max, smoking, BMI

Physical fitness

Physical fitness was assessed in the AGHS by a treadmill test until exhaustion and expressed as $V0_2max$ measured in millilitres of oxygen per kilogram bodyweight. Subjects were classified as at high or low risk of being unfit if their summary measure of physical activity was above or below the median score at baseline. Participants who were physically active and/or who became physically active were at a lower risk of being unfit compared to low activity participants (odds ratio = 0.67, 95% CI 0.53 to 0.83, p=0.01).[16]

Body composition

The relationships between physical activity and measures of body composition have been evaluated in both studies. In the Young Finns study, there was no significant difference in BMI between participants who were classified as 'active' at all three measurement intervals and those classified as sedentary.[13] Similarly, the AGHS found no significant relationship between the long-term variation in daily physical activity and BMI.[17] However, daily physical activity was positively associated with lean body mass (ß=0.04; 95% CI 0.02 to 0.06; p<0.01) in the AGHS.[17] This suggests that BMI is not a good indicator of body fatness in adolescence.

In the Young Finns study the subscapular skinfold site was measured, which indicates body fat of the trunk. Constantly active young men had lower subscapular skinfold values than constantly sedentary men (9.9 ± 4.4 vs. 12.1± 5.3; p=0.012). Similar observations were found for young women (10.5 ± 2.9 vs. 14.2 ± 5.6; p=0.005).[13]

In the AGHS the sum of four skinfold (SSF) measures was used. Long-term variance in daily physical activity was inversely related to the long-term variance of SSF (ß= -0.06; 95% CI -0.09 to -0.03; p<0.01) with no differences between men and women.[17] Univariate analysis showed that daily physical activity during adolescence only (13-16 years of age) was not associated with the adult sum of SSF. However, daily physical activity during adolescence and young adulthood (13-21 years of age) was inversely related to adult SSF for men and women (ß= -013; p=0.05) and the relationship was even stronger when exposure was measured over the entire period (ß= -019; p=0.01).[16] In multivariate analysis daily physical activity during adolescence and young adulthood remained inversely related to SSF after adjusting for other biological and lifestyle variables (ß= -013; p<0.01) as did the relationship between long-term exposure to daily physical activity and SSF (ß= -0.20; p<0.01).[16]

After a correction for neuromotor fitness, the long-term variance in daily physical activity remained a significant independent predictor of SSF (ß= -0.05; p=0.01).[20] Also, participants who were active and/or became more active during the study period were less likely to have high SSF (equivalent to 20% or more body fat for males, and 30% or more for females) in adulthood (OR 0.81; 95% CI 0.69 to 0.96; p=0.01).[15]

Waist and hip circumferences were assessed only in the AGHS and only measured at the last data collection point (mean age 27 years). Multivariate analysis of the relationship between mean values of behavioural variables during the study period and the waist circumference at age 27 showed no significant relationship between daily physical activity and waist circumference for men or women.[18] However, in women but not men, daily physical activity was positively related to the waist to hip ratio (WHR) for all three time periods. For adolescence, adolescence and young adulthood and the entire longitudinal period, the standardised regression coefficients for women were 0.51, 0.34 and 0.26 respectively.[16] They were all significant at the 1%

level. The authors suggested that this surprise observation was explained by physically inactive women accumulating more fat in the hip/thigh region.

The lack of a relationship between physical activity and BMI shows the limitations of BMI as a measure of body fatness in adolescents. Muscular males and females with relatively low body fat will produce high BMI values without correspondingly high SSF.

Lipoproteins

In the Young Finns study,[13] lipoprotein levels at the six-year follow-up were compared between young adults who were 'active' (approximately 2 hours or more per week of intense [10 METs] physical activity) and those who were 'sedentary' (i.e. approximately 1 hour or less of light aerobic activity per week) at all three data collection points.

Active women had lower serum triglyceride values than sedentary women (0.80 ± 0.25 vs. 0.97 ± 0.37, p=0.005) but there were no significant differences in total cholesterol (TC), high density lipoprotein cholesterol (HDL), low density lipoprotein cholesterol (LDL) or the HDL:TC ratio. In young men, concentrations of triglycerides were lower in the physically active compared to the sedentary (0.92 ± 0.37 vs. 1.05 ± 0.36, p=0.040). In addition, the physically active had higher HDL:TC ratios than sedentary men (0.30 ± 0.07 vs. 0.26 ± 0.06, p=0.033). There were no significant differences in other lipoprotein measures.

No statistically significant relationships between physical activity change and six-year change in lipoproteins were found for men or women.

In the AGHS, generalised regression equations were used to assess the relationship between the long-term variation in TC, HDL and the TC:HDL ratio and the long-term variation in daily physical activity.[14] Covariates included gender, biological age, body fatness, lean body mass, cardiopulmonary fitness, diet, smoking and alcohol consumption. Daily physical activity was a positive independent predictor of HDL (ß = 0.05; 95% CI 0.00 to 0.10; p=0.04), but not of TC or of the TC:HDL ratio.

In a second analysis, the relationship between physical activity and non-fasting lipoprotein levels over three different time periods was examined.[16] An average value of daily physical activity was calculated from baseline (mean age 13 years) to age 16, 21 and 29 years. Univariate analyses revealed no statistically significant relationships between daily physical activity and TC, HDL or the TC:HDL ratio for any of the three time periods. In multivariate analyses, which included the covariates used in the analysis at aged 16, a non-significant inverse relationship was observed between daily physical activity and the TC:HDL ratio (ß = -0.09; p=0.18 and ß = -0.10; p=0.12) for the periods up to age 21 and 29 years. The positive relationship between daily physical activity and HDL observed in the first analysis was not repeated in the second. This may be because in the second analysis daily physical activity was averaged for each of the time periods whereas in the first one it was not.

When 'neuromotor fitness' (muscle strength, flexibility, speed of movement and coordination) was added to the statistical model,[20] after correcting for the sum of skinfolds, daily physical activity was significantly related to HDL (ß=0.06; p=0.02). High skinfold measures were an important confounder in the relationship between the three measures of fitness and physical activity. No significant relationships were observed between long-term variation in daily physical activity and long-term variation in total cholesterol or the TC:HDL ratio.

In a further analysis, participants were divided into groups based on measures of CHD risk factors at each time point, and odds ratios were calculated of the risk of a high TC:HDL ratio (4.0 between 13 and 16 years of age; 5.5 at 21 and 27 years of age) and a low HDL value (1.1mmol/l or below between ages 13 and 16 years; 0.9mmol/l or below at 21 and 27 years of age) related to daily physical activity. After correcting for lifestyle and biological parameters, there was no significant relationship between daily physical activity and an unhealthy lipoprotein profile.[15]

In summary, there is some evidence that remaining active from adolescence through to young adulthood is associated with lower triglyceride levels compared with those who remain sedentary. Daily physical activity may be positively associated with HDL levels but the data are inconsistent. Only one of the studies showed a relationship between physical activity and the TC:HDL ratio and this was limited to men.[13] Neither of the studies showed any relationship between physical activity and TC.

Serum insulin

In the Young Finns study, constantly active men had lower serum insulin levels than constantly sedentary men (8.07± 4.40 vs. 9.24 ± 2.73; p=0.03). In multiple regression analysis six-year change in physical activity was a significant, independent predictor of change in serum insulin levels, even after adjustment for triglyceride levels (ß= -0.00076; $p<0.05$).[13]

Smoking

In the Young Finns study, self-reported smoking habits were determined at baseline and at six years. Those who smoked "once a day or more often" were considered as smokers. A higher proportion of continuously sedentary girls took up smoking than continuously active girls (25.9% vs. 4.6%, p=0.053) and a higher proportion of sedentary young women were smokers at six-year follow-up than active young women (45.5% vs. 8.7%, p=0.002). No active young boys took up smoking compared to 33% of sedentary young boys (p=0.001). Approximately five times more sedentary than active young men were smokers at follow-up (46.9% vs. 9.3%, p=0.0001).[13]

Blood pressure

In the AGHS, blood pressure was measured twice on the left arm with a sphygmomanometer, and the lowest value recorded. No significant relationship was found between daily physical activity and either systolic blood pressure or diastolic blood pressure in any of three periods of exposure.[16]

The longitudinal relationship between daily physical activity, cardiopulmonary fitness and neuromotor fitness was examined. No significant relationship was found between systolic blood pressure or diastolic blood pressure and physical activity in univariate or multivariate analysis.[20]

Clustering of risk factors

Cardiovascular disease risk factors have been shown to cluster in children and adolescents.[22] In the Young Finns study those in upper tertiles for total serum cholesterol, high density lipoprotein and diastolic blood pressure were defined as having a high risk cluster. Moving out of the high risk cluster between baseline and the six-year follow-up was associated with an increase in physical activity.[19] In the AGHS, daily physical activity was strongly inversely associated with the clustering of the TC:HDL ratio, mean arterial blood pressure, the sum of four skinfolds and $V0_2max$.[12]

Discussion

Most studies of physical activity and CHD risk factors in children have been cross-sectional and produced equivocal results.[9] In this chapter we have examined the evidence of a relationship between physical activity during childhood and adolescence and the presence of CHD risk factors in young adulthood. A major limitation of the review is that only two studies fulfilled our inclusion criteria. However, both studies were of high quality, were prospective and mainly used all measures from each interval in the analysis. The longitudinal design can also be a disadvantage, as the costs involved and the commitment required from participants can lead to relatively small sample sizes.

Physical activity was consistently inversely associated with body fat, while a positive association was found with cardiorespiratory fitness. Physical activity was also inversely related to serum triglycerides in both sexes, and insulin levels in males. The relationship between adolescent physical activity and other lipoprotein measures in adults was equivocal. (See Table 2.)

Central adiposity, measured using the waist to hip ratio, was weakly positively related to physical activity in women. This unexpected relationship may be explained by the higher distribution of body fat in the hip and thigh region in sedentary young females compared to more active ones.

Table 2 ***Summary of the relationship between physical activity during childhood and adolescence and cardiovascular disease risk factors during young adulthood***

Risk factor	Boys	Girls
Lipoproteins		
Total cholesterol	⇔	⇔
Triglycerides	⇩	⇩
HDL	⇔ ⇧	⇔ ⇧
LDL	⇔	⇔
TC:HDL ratio	⇔ ⇩	⇔
Body composition		
Body mass index	⇔	⇔
Sum of skinfolds	⇩ ⇩	⇩ ⇩
Serum insulin	⇩	⇔
Smoking	⇩ ⇩ ⇩	⇩ ⇩ ⇩
Blood pressure	⇔	⇔
Physical fitness	⇧ ⇧	⇧ ⇧

⇧ indicates that physical activity during childhood and adolescence is associated with a higher value in young adulthood.
⇩ indicates that physical activity during childhood and adolescence is associated with a lower value in young adulthood.
⇔ indicates that physical activity during childhood and adolescence is not associated with this risk factor in young adulthood.

⇧ or ⇩ = small effect
⇧ ⇧ or ⇩ ⇩ = medium effect
⇧ ⇧ ⇧ or ⇩ ⇩ ⇩ = large effect

Source: See references 13-20.

Neither study showed a relationship between physical activity and BMI, although the AGHS showed a positive relationship between daily physical activity and lean body mass. BMI is more a measure of overweight than adiposity and can be high due to either a high lean body mass or high body fat. The increased lean body mass associated with higher levels of physical activity reported in the AGHS suggests that BMI may be a poor measure of body fat in children. Measurement of waist and skinfolds may be the best indicators of adiposity in childhood and adolescence.

The significantly lower serum insulin levels observed in males who remained active for the duration of the Young Finns study warrants further investigation. An important finding in the Young Finns study was that active males and females smoke less and are less likely to take up smoking. This relationship may not be causal but may reflect differences in the children who opt to participate in physical activity.

However, encouraging physical activity during the early school years may reduce the likelihood that children become regular smokers.

The weak relationships between physical activity in young people and individual CHD risk factors in young adulthood may have been influenced by the method of assessing physical activity. Self-report recall measures of physical activity are prone to measurement error, especially in children and adolescents. Also, both studies had relatively low numbers for the multiple comparisons being made, which reduces the power of the study to detect relationships.

Both studies found that physical activity was inversely related to a high-risk cluster of CHD risk factors and concluded that physical activity should be the focus of CHD prevention strategies.

In both studies, activity declined with age from early teens to the late 20s[27, 28] with a greater decline in adolescence rather than adulthood. Males are more active than females during adolescence but show a greater rate of decline thereafter. In England, 62% of 12 year old boys are active at recommended levels, dropping to 48% at age 15 years, while the figures for girls are 26% dropping to 18%.[6] The AGHS study found that vigorous activity, and in particular non-organised sport, accounted for most of the decline in activity, whereas moderate intensity physical activity increased from the age of 13 years to 27 years.[28]

Lifetime decline in physical activity is of particular concern as the cardioprotective effect of activity is only associated with current physical activity.[29] A prospective study of British civil servants showed no relationship between past playing of 'vigorous' sports and coronary events in men.[30] In the Harvard Alumni Study, students who participated in sport at college but quit as adults had similar risks for CHD as those who never exercised. Also, alumni who became active in later life showed a reduced risk similar to that of those who had remained active.[31] Active children and adolescents who cease to be active on leaving full-time education therefore achieve no reduction in risk of future CHD. Interventions are required across the lifespan, not just during school years. The determinants of physical activity include intrapersonal, interpersonal and environmental factors.[32] Therefore, attempts at changing population levels of physical activity will need to be multi-factorial requiring cross-government department co-operation if effective action is to be achieved.

Conclusion

A physically active lifestyle during childhood and adolescence is associated with lower body fat and increased fitness in young adulthood. There is some evidence that active boys and girls are less likely to become regular smokers.

The promotion of physical activity during childhood and adolescence may be an essential part of CHD prevention, but will only be worthwhile if other strategies are able to tackle the age-related decline in physical activity.

The results of this review should be treated with caution, as the evidence on which they are based is limited. Larger scale studies are urgently required to examine further the relationship between physical activity during childhood and adolescence, and cardiovascular risk profiles in adults.

References

1 Berlin JA, Colditz GA. 1990. A meta-analysis of physical activity in the prevention of coronary heart disease. *American Journal of Epidemiology*; 132: 639-46.

2 Physical Activity Task Force. 1995. *More People, More Active, More Often*. London: Department of Health.

3 Department of Health. 1996. *Strategy Statement on Physical Activity*. London: Department of Health.

4 Department of Health. 2000. *Health Survey for England 1998*. London: The Stationery Office.

5 Biddle S, Sallis J, Cavill N (eds.) 1998. *Young and Active? Young People and Health-enhancing Physical Activity – Evidence and Implications*. London: Health Education Authority.

6 Department of Health. 1999. *Health Survey for England 1997*. London: The Stationery Office.

7 Van Horn L, Greenland P. 1997. Prevention of coronary artery disease is a pediatric problem. *Journal of the American Medical Association*; 21: 1779-80.

8 Caspersen CJ, Nixon PA, Durant RH. 1998. Physical activity epidemiology applied to children and adolescents. *Exercise and Sports Science Reviews*; 26: 341-403.

9 Sallis JF. 1993. Epidemiology of physical activity and fitness in children and adolescents. *Critical Reviews in Food Science and Nutrition*; 33: 403-08.

10 Malina RM. 1996. Tracking of physical activity and physical fitness across the lifespan. *Research Quarterly for Exercise and Sport*; 67; 3 (suppl): 48-57.

11 Riddoch C. Relationship between physical activity and physical health in young people. In: Biddle S, Sallis J, Cavill N (eds.) 1998. *Young and Active? Young People and Health-enhancing Physical Activity – Evidence and Implications*. London: Health Education Authority.

12 Twisk JW. Physical activity, physical fitness and cardiovascular health. In: Armstrong N, van Mechelen W. 2000. *Paediatric Exercise Science and Medicine*. Oxford: Oxford University Press: 253-63.

13 Raitakari OT, Porkka KV, Taimela S et al. 1994. Effects of persistent physical activity and inactivity on coronary risk factors in children and young adults. The Cardiovascular Risk in Young Finns study. *American Journal of Epidemiology*; 140: 195-205.

14 Twisk JW, Kemper, HC, Mellenbergh GJ et al. 1996. Relation between the longitudinal development of lipoprotein levels and lifestyle parameters during adolescence and young adulthood. *Annals of Epidemiology*; 6: 246-56.

15 Twisk JW, Kemper, HC, van Mechelen W et al. 1997. Which lifestyle parameters discriminate high- from low-risk participants for coronary heart disease risk factors? Longitudinal analysis covering adolescence and young adulthood. *Journal of Cardiovascular Risk*; 4: 393-400.

16 Twisk JW, van Mechelen W, Kemper HC et al. 1997. The relation between 'long-term exposure' to lifestyle during youth and young adulthood and risk factors for cardiovascular disease at adult age. *Journal of Adolescent Health*; 20: 309-19.

17 Twisk JW, Kemper HC, van Mechelen W et al. 1998. Body fatness: longitudinal relationship of body mass index and the sum of skinfolds with other risk factors for coronary heart disease. *International Journal of Obesity*; 22: 915-22.

18 Van Lenthe FJ, van Mechelen W, Kemper HC, Post GB. 1998. Behavioral variables and development of a central pattern of body fat from adolescence into adulthood in normal-weight whites: The Amsterdam Growth and Health Study. *American Journal of Clinical Nutrition*; 67: 846-52.

19 Raitakari OT, Porkka KVK, Rasanen L, Ronnenaa T. 1994. Clustering and six year cluster tracking of serum cholesterol, HDL-cholesterol and diastolic blood pressure in children and young adults. The Cardiovascular Risk in Young Finns Study. *Journal of Clinical Epidemiology*; 47: 1085-93.

20 Twisk JW, Kemper, HC, van Mechelen W. 2000. Tracking of activity and fitness and the relationship with cardiovascular disease risk factors. *Medicine and Science in Sports and Exercise;* 32: 1455-61.

21 Andersen LB. 1996. Tracking of risk factors for coronary heart disease from adolescence to young adulthood with special emphasis on physical activity and fitness. *Danish Medical Bulletin;* 43: 407-18.

22 Boreham C, Twisk J, van Mechelen W, Savage M, Starin J, Cran G. 1999. Relationships between the development of biological risk factors for coronary heart disease and lifestyle parameters during adolescence: The Northern Ireland Young Hearts Project. *Public Health;* 113: 7-12.

23 Myers L, Strikmiller PK, Webber LS, Berenson GS. 1996. Physical and sedentary activity in school children grades 5-8: the Bogalusa Heart Study. *Medicine and Science in Sports and Exercise;* 28: 852-59.

24 Janz KF, Dawson JD, Mahoney LT. 2000. Tracking physical fitness and physical activity from childhood to adolescence: the Muscatine study. *Medicine and Science in Sports and Exercise;* 32: 1250-57.

25 Dennison BA, Straus JH, Mellits ED, Charney E. 1988. Childhood physical fitness tests: predictor of adult physical activity levels? *Pediatrics;* 82: 324-30.

26 Beunen G, Ostyn M, Simons J, Renson R, Claessens AL, Vanden Eynde B et al. 1997. Development and tracking in fitness components: Leuven longitudinal study on lifestyle, fitness and health. *International Journal of Sports Medicine;* 18; suppl 3: S171-78.

27 Telama R, Yang X. 2000. Decline of physical activity from youth to young adulthood. *Medicine and Science in Sports and Exercise;* 32: 1617-22.

28 Van Mechelen W, Twisk JW, Post GB, Snel J, Kemper HCG. 2000. Physical activity of young people: The Amsterdam Longitudinal Growth and Health Study. *Medicine and Science in Sports and Exercise;* 32: 1610-16.

29 Sherman SE, D'Agostino RB, Silbershatz H, Kannel WB. 1999. Comparison of past versus recent physical activity in the prevention of premature death and coronary artery disease. *American Heart Journal*; 138: 900-07.

30 Morris JN, Clayton DG, Everitt MG, Semmence AM, Burgess EH. 1990. Exercise in leisure time: coronary attack and death rate. *British Heart Journal;* 63: 325-34.

31 Paffenbarger RS, Hyde RT, Wing AL, Steinmetz CH. 1984. A natural history of athleticism and cardiovascular health. *Journal of the American Medical Association*; 252: 491-95.

32 Sallis JF, Bauman A, Pratt M. 1998. Environmental and policy interventions to promote physical activity. *American Journal of Preventive Medicine;* 15: 379-97.

Chapter 10

Policy implications for reducing smoking in young people

Dr Ann McNeill

Honorary Senior Lecturer in Psychology, St George's Hospital Medical School, London University, and independent consultant in public health

Professor Anne Charlton

Emeritus Professor of Cancer Health Education, The University of Manchester

This chapter:

- examines the extent to which we should focus on reducing young people's smoking rather than concentrating on reducing adult smoking prevalence
- discusses the role of the tobacco industry in young people's smoking and what must be done to curb its influence
- considers other factors that predict young people's smoking, and
- reviews some of the interventions which have so far been implemented to counter these influences.

Key themes

- Young people's smoking is strongly related to that of adults, so reducing adult smoking prevalence may be the best way to influence youth. However, delaying the onset of smoking in children may reduce the likelihood of becoming addicted, of smoking heavily later in life, and of future substance use disorders. Early understanding of the health risks of smoking might increase the inclination of smokers to stop and help to protect them against the ploys of the tobacco industry. It also reduces the risks of the immediate and future health problems which become established in young smokers. Addiction can quickly develop in young smokers.

- In spite of its claims not to want children to smoke, the tobacco industry relies on recruiting young smokers, and internal documents of the tobacco industry confirm this. Young people are susceptible to cigarette advertising and to a wide range of promotions, including sports, concerts, free gifts, films and attractive cigarette packaging.

- Availability of cigarettes to young people, price, and sociodemographic, personal and behavioural factors can also play a part in a young person's decision to smoke or not to smoke.

- School-based interventions have generally proved ineffective in reducing smoking prevalence among young people. Most promising at present appear to be community-based programmes involving adults and youth. A global approach is needed to tackle young people's smoking as part of well resourced, comprehensive campaigns aimed principally at reducing adult smoking.

Introduction

Reducing smoking among young people continues, for some, to be the holy grail of tobacco control. Over 80% of those who ever smoke daily start before the age of 18[1,2] so if young people could be dissuaded from taking up smoking, then the problem would be largely solved. Traditionally therefore, governments focused on preventing smoking uptake as the key to reducing the smoking epidemic. However, success was hard to come by.

Thankfully, in recent years, the failure of such a single-minded approach has been recognised and governments around the world are beginning to implement multi-faceted strategies in which preventing uptake is only one prong. As a result, there are now some successes in reducing young people's smoking, for example in California[3] where there have been well resourced, comprehensive campaigns.

The smoking prevention literature is extensive and ever-increasing and there have been many excellent and comprehensive reviews of it.[1, 2, 4-11] This chapter is therefore an update of this literature base, emphasising the implications of recent findings and identifying the remaining gaps in our knowledge, rather than a comprehensive review.

The chapter begins by examining a current hot topic – to what extent we should focus on reducing young people's smoking rather than concentrating on reducing adult smoking. It then looks at the role of the tobacco industry in young people's smoking and what must be done to curb its influence. Next it examines other factors that predict young people's smoking and the interventions that have so far been implemented to counter them, making recommendations about the way forward in each section.

Youth smoking in England

Regular surveys of smoking prevalence among 11-15 year old secondary school pupils began in 1982.[12] Since then, overall prevalence has fluctuated around the 10% line. Early surveys found similar prevalence of regular smoking (at least one cigarette per week) among boys and girls, namely 11% in 1982 and 13% in 1984, but since then, girls' smoking prevalence has always been the higher.[13] In the 1988 survey, regular smoking in this age group appeared to be at an all-time low, but it rose over the next few years to reach 13% again in 1996. Since then it has decreased again. The 1998, 1999, 2000 and 2001 surveys found that 9%, 8%, 9% and 8% of boys, and 12%, 10%, 12% and 11% of girls smoked regularly. Among 15 year olds, prevalence of regular smoking was 28% in boys and 33% in girls in 1996, giving an overall prevalence of 30%. By 2001, smoking prevalence among 15 year olds had decreased to 22%.[13] It is important to view these recent decreases with caution. Similar falls have happened before, in the late 1980s and early 1990s and were followed by a sharp rise. Short-term fashion changes, sampling or simply the statistical variations which might be expected in a series of cross-sectional surveys, might underlie the fluctuations. It is, however, tempting to hope that smoking is falling out of favour with young people and it is hoped that future surveys will show a continued downward trend.

Charlton and Bates hypothesised that the decrease in smoking prevalence among youth might be due to the rise in mobile phone use.[14] They postulated that the link could be due to money being spent on mobile phones that would otherwise have been spent on cigarettes, or that the phones satisfied similar needs to smoking. However, this was based on correlational evidence only and the phenomena could be unrelated or explained by another factor linking them both. A similar relationship has not been observed elsewhere.[15]

The recent decrease might also be due to changes in smoking policy, or more effective education, or to the diffusion of innovations process postulated by Rogers and Shoemaker.[16] It would make sense to see smoking as an innovation which was taken up by men, then boys, women and girls. Equally it would make sense to see non-smoking as an innovation taken up in the same pattern. Certainly the decrease among adult males has been the most dramatic, namely from 51% in 1974 to 28% in 1998,[17] followed by the decrease among boys from 34% in year 10 (14-15 year olds) in 1966 [18] to 17% in 1998.[19] Women's smoking prevalence has fallen less steeply, from 41% in 1974 to 26% in 1998. There is no corresponding baseline for girls but, from the evidence available, it appears that girls' smoking prevalence might now be at the very beginning of its decline. The WHO Global Youth Tobacco Surveys indicate that the processes in the developing world are similar but at a much earlier stage; there, the innovation is smoking, rather than non-smoking.[20]

Until very recently teenage smoking levels were relatively high compared with other European countries. In 1997/98 England joined the Health Behaviour of Schoolchildren Study (HBSC) for the first time. The HBSC had been regularly measuring smoking prevalence among schoolchildren in a number of countries. In 1997/98, England had the seventh highest prevalence of daily smoking among school children out of 28 European countries.[21]

How much emphasis should be put on preventing young people from starting to smoke?

The debate still rages as to whether young people should remain the 'prime' target or whether focusing on adults would have a greater impact.[22, 23] If the diffusion of non-smoking hypothesis is correct, moving on the adult quitting process would pave the way for young people doing the same. Peto and Doll and others have emphasised the importance of cessation in acquiring short-term impacts on public health given that reducing smoking uptake in teenagers would not have a public health impact for more than 50 years (for example[24]). They argue that what is important is that young people who smoke stop in early middle age before much of the harm is done. This makes good common sense; experimentation with cigarettes will be hard to eliminate as adolescence is a period in which young people learn about their world by, inter alia, trying things. As will be seen later in this chapter, very few interventions focusing solely on teenagers have been effective.

Further support for this approach comes from the influence that adult smoking role models have on young people's smoking.[1] In addition, a Californian study[25] has recently demonstrated that parental smoking cessation discourages adolescent smoking. Adolescents whose parents had quit smoking were less likely to be ever-smokers than those with a parent who still smoked. Also, adolescent ever-smokers whose parents quit smoking were more likely to have quit than those who had a parent who still smoked. Parental quitting was most effective in reducing initiation if it occurred before the child reached nine years of age.

Many studies over the past few decades have shown that young people whose parents smoke are at increased risk of taking up smoking themselves and that parents' disapproval reduces that risk.[26]

Other adults' smoking is also being seriously considered in relation to young people. For example, a study of exposure of children and childminders to smoke is proposed, to advise the government by December 2003 as to whether or not current guidelines should be amended.[27]

Doll and Peto's approach makes good common sense. Reducing adult smoking will have a more immediate health impact than reducing teenage smoking would, and it would also mean a reduction in adult smoking role models that might impact on teenage smoking patterns. The main difficulty with this adult-focused approach is the difficulty of encouraging and supporting smokers to stop smoking in middle age. Even with the advent of proven behavioural and pharmacological treatments, stopping smoking is still very difficult and the majority fail.

However, there are still obvious benefits to be reaped from maintaining efforts to stop young people from starting.

First, if it were possible to delay the age of onset of smoking, this would be likely to have a positive public health impact as earlier onset is related to heavier smoking, a lower likelihood of stopping and more smoking-related diseases.[2] Recently, Everett and colleagues in the US found that delaying the onset of smoking may affect the likelihood of becoming addicted to nicotine and smoking heavily.[28] There is also some evidence of a relationship between earlier age of smoking onset and future substance use disorders.[29] DuRant and colleagues[30] in a US study found that even after allowing for sociodemographic factors, earlier age of onset of cigarette use was the strongest correlate of the number of health risk behaviours in which the young adolescents had engaged.

Secondly, unless a good understanding of the risks of smoking is reinforced over the years, some smokers might feel less inclined to stop later on.

Third, without primary prevention efforts, the adolescent will be left entirely at the beck and call of the tobacco industry. This might mean a rise in young people's smoking rates.

Finally there is evidence of a variety of health effects resulting from smoking (other than addiction) even at this young age.[1, 31-33] Although many of the serious health risks of smoking do not manifest themselves until later in life, teenage smokers are already damaging their health, by initiating changes which lay the foundations for these later diseases or by causing immediate health effects.[1] In the first of these categories come heart and circulatory diseases, cancers, emphysema and other respiratory problems. Recently, Wiencke and colleagues' research[34] suggested that smoking during adolescence may produce physiological changes that lead to increased DNA adduct persistence. As DNA adducts may be involved in carcinogenesis, their presence may indicate a high risk of lung cancer. Similarly, Rowland and Harding[35] found a higher frequency of sister chromatid exchange in young women smokers which they postulated may be indicative of initial damage to the DNA already having occurred, thus causing an increased risk of developing cancer later in life.

Children with low blood pressure and slow pulse rate were found in one study to be at increased risk of becoming smokers, perhaps because smoking raises their blood pressure sharply, giving them the boost they feel they need.[36] This hypothesis might also be supported by the finding that young people with depressive symptoms were at increased risk of smoking.[37] However, these rapid and strong increases in blood pressure every time a cigarette is smoked place a strain on the heart, causing serious health risks both immediately and in the future.

Regarding immediate effects, young smokers have, among many other health problems, more respiratory diseases, increased blood coagulability, reduced fitness, increased risk of subarachnoid haemorrhage, reduced immunity and more menstrual problems.[38] These and other health problems cause increased risk of absence from school,[39] which in turn can lead to lack of progress and becoming less 'engaged' with education. Young smokers are also at increased risk of truancy which might, in part, be related to this feeling of isolation from learning, under-achievement and consequent rejection of school values.

In conclusion, therefore, there are considerable risks of smoking in adolescence and so it is still ethically important to continue work in this area. However, adolescence should never be the main focus of tobacco control campaigns as this would only emphasise the definition of tobacco as adult and may enhance its appeal to young people.[40] The emphasis and resources should therefore remain largely on adults with comprehensive strategies. This approach has been emphasised in the Health Development Agency's guidance on the National Service Framework for coronary heart disease.[41]

Recommendation

Teenage smoking should be tackled as part of a comprehensive strategy aimed principally at adults but including all target groups. The emphasis within the strategy should be on reducing adult smoking. Reducing teenage smoking should be a secondary objective.

The role of the tobacco industry in young people's smoking

Any discussion of young people's smoking must examine the role of the tobacco industry. New smokers are the tobacco industry's lifeblood, as without recruiting new smokers, the tobacco business would fail. The industry's awareness of this is revealed in the thousands of private industry documents made available through the discovery process resulting from litigation trials in the US.[42] There is evidence that the tobacco industry has been monitoring young people and their smoking for years and quotations from these industry documents refer to youth as a source of sales which is fundamental to the industry's survival.[43, 44]

Tobacco industry marketing

There is convincing evidence that tobacco advertising influences young people's smoking. Although the tobacco industry outwardly claims that they do not want young people to smoke and that their advertising is aimed at adult smokers to encourage brand-switching, there is constant evidence that their advertising and promotion appeal to youth. Research has shown that children can see tobacco advertising as generic i.e. that it advertises smoking rather than a brand of cigarettes.[45] Thus they are encouraged to smoke and at first take any available brand. When regular smoking is established, adolescents smoke the most heavily advertised brands and brand loyalty is established early in a smoker's career. Children report that their brand choice is influenced by advertising, promotion, package design and labelling.[46] The introduction of tobacco advertisements that appealed to young people in the US has been demonstrated to be associated with increases in young people's smoking uptake and use of the advertised brands.[47, 48] Advertising also influences susceptibility to tobacco use.[49, 50] Pollay and colleagues in the US have estimated that teenagers are three times more sensitive to advertising than adults.[51]

Promotion of sports (such as motor racing, snooker and rugby), concerts, and photography are all used by tobacco companies as a means of advertising. Some of these activities, especially Formula 1 motor racing, appeal strongly to young people. One study showed that young teenage boys who named motor racing as one of their favourite television sports were twice as likely as those who did not, to become regular smokers during the next year.[52]

Several studies have now shown the association between awareness of and involvement with tobacco promotions and being susceptible to tobacco use or using tobacco products[53-55] including one study which was carried out in the North East of England.[55] Current voluntary agreements to protect young people from smoking are not working. Statutory regulations are needed.

Packaging of cigarettes is also a form of advertising and young people are very aware of cigarette packs. For example, they prefer to carry the most advertised and expensive brand packs, even going to the extent of filling these with cheap cigarettes.[56] Recent research in Australia, where tobacco advertising is banned in all the media and, in most states, at point of sale, has found that cigarette manufacturers are modifying their logos on cigarette packets to make them more appealing and interesting.[57]

Another example of the pervasiveness of the tobacco industry is candy cigarettes.[58] Many of these have brand names, logos and packaging that resemble real cigarettes and there is evidence from internal industry documents "that tobacco companies cooperated with manufacturers of candy cigarettes in designing candy products that would effectively promote smoking to children" and "unfavourable research sponsored by the US candy cigarette industry was suppressed".[58]

Pierce and colleagues analysed the proportion of new experimenters who had started because of cigarette advertising and promotional activities. For example, they estimated that between 1988 and 1998 there would have been 7.9 million new experimenters in the US because of tobacco advertising and promotional activities.[59]

The UK Tobacco Advertising and Promotion Bill was published in 2000 by the government after the annulment of the EU Directive. It aimed to ban all advertising and promotion of tobacco, including sponsorship, and to place restrictions on display. In 2001, the Bill fell out due to lack of time before the election and did not feature in the Queen's Speech after the election. It was reintroduced as a Private Member's Bill in the House of Lords in November 2001. After successful passage through the House of Lords, the government announced in March 2002 that it would formally support the Bill, which should have become law by mid-2002, but might be delayed due to EC notification requirements.[60]

In February 2002, the *Warsaw Declaration for a Tobacco-free Europe* was produced at a WHO Ministerial Conference.[61] It commits all ministers and representatives of the European states to developing and adopting the Fourth Action Plan for a Tobacco-free Europe, which includes a focus on young people and other especially vulnerable groups.

Recommendation

Support should be given for speedy and comprehensive implementation of the ban on advertising and promotion of tobacco including all aspects of marketing and promotions currently going through the UK Parliament. Although enforcement aspects have recently been strengthened, vigilance will still be needed in enforcing this.

Tobacco industry youth prevention programmes

The major multi-national tobacco companies adopt an anti-youth smoking posture and are implementing youth prevention programmes in many countries around the world. The insidiousness and disingenuity of this was recently comprehensively reviewed by ASH and the Cancer Research Campaign.[40] This report found that:

- The internal industry documents indicate that tobacco industry youth prevention programmes have been developed "to forestall serious regulation and garner better PR, rather than to reduce sales or the number of potential customers".

- The industry's positioning of tobacco as adult enhances the images of the cigarette as forbidden fruit, and smoking as rebellious.

- The types of youth prevention strategies favoured by the tobacco companies – age restrictions, ID cards, age-related warnings and retailer schemes – are generally ineffective (see page 223) especially because the industry never advocates embedding them in comprehensive strategies involving measures such as taxation or advertising bans, which are known to be effective.

- Tobacco companies involve figures of authority such as parents or teachers in their programmes, but use "heroic aspirational role models such as racing drivers, actors and rock stars in promoting tobacco".

- Focus group work with adolescents indicated that measures favoured by the tobacco industry could enhance the appeal of tobacco to them.

Some tobacco companies have introduced their own education programmes for young people. Their main approaches are school-based lessons and media advertising with plain messages such as "Think. Don't smoke", which is used by Philip Morris. A study was carried out to find out what young people thought of the Philip Morris message and of the Massachusetts anti-smoking advertisements for youth.[62] The outcome was that the young people did not see the "Think. Don't smoke" message as effective in preventing them from smoking because it did not discuss illness. Messages and approaches used by the tobacco industry are unlikely to be effective. Health educators could learn from this.

Recommendation

The tobacco industry should not be allowed to be involved in any anti-smoking programmes anywhere in the world.

Other environmental factors influencing smoking in youth

Portrayal of smoking in the media

Several studies have demonstrated the portrayal of smoking in Hollywood films.[63, 64] One recent content analysis indicated that smoking was highly prevalent in Hollywood films featuring popular actresses and could influence youngsters to smoke.[65] Another analysis of a 10-year sample of contemporary films found that tobacco-brand appearances were common in films and were becoming increasingly endorsed by actors.[66] The findings of a comprehensive study in the US suggested that the portrayal of smoking in films particularly by stars who were admired by adolescents, contributed to adolescent smoking.[67]

A campaign involving print advertisements was launched by Stan Glantz in the US in March 2002 to influence the amount of smoking in Hollywood films.[68]

Recommendation

Advocate further to encourage film-makers to reduce tobacco use in films. The US campaign could be broadened, and supported in the UK.

Price of cigarettes

Although the evidence on price and young people's smoking has been somewhat mixed, most believe that teenagers are at least as sensitive to price as adults, and possibly more so. Most young smokers who try smoking at first get their cigarettes from friends and relatives, so onset is unlikely to be affected much by price increases. However, once smoking is established, many adolescents buy their cigarettes from shops and are then sensitive to cigarette prices.[69] Indeed, a recent review concluded that "substantial sustained cigarette tax increases are potentially the most effective means of achieving long-run reductions in smoking in all segments of the population".[70]

The government recently reneged on its 1997 announcement to increase tobacco duties on average by at least 5% in real terms a year. In the March 2001 budget, the Chancellor announced a 6p increase in a packet of 20 cigarettes, a decrease in real terms after adjusting for inflation. Again in the March 2002 budget, the increase was just 6p per packet of 20. Tobacco control groups greeted this with disappointment and every effort must be made to influence higher price rises in the future. Health organisations lobbied the Chancellor to link tobacco pricing to the National Health Service, specifically for 2p in the pound to be channelled back to help smokers quit. This would provide £152 million from the £7.6 billion currently raised in tobacco duties.[71, 72]

Recommendation

It is crucially important to advocate for price rises over and above inflation each year.

Availability of cigarettes and retailer programmes

The general availability of cigarettes and offers from siblings and parents have been found to predict tobacco onset.[73]

There has been much attention focused on restrictions on tobacco sales as a means of cutting off the supply of cigarettes to young people and hence reducing their smoking, although lessons from the illegal drugs field would suggest that this will not be easy. Although it is illegal to sell cigarettes to under 16 year olds, many children who smoke regularly still say they buy their cigarettes from shops, demonstrating that the law is not strictly enforced. Research in Atlanta, in the US, has highlighted the importance of young smokers getting someone else to buy cigarettes for them and 'borrowing' cigarettes from friends. Only 23.5% of the regular smokers under the age of 18 years in this Atlanta study usually purchased their cigarettes from shops.[74]

Enforcing the law will require considerable time and resources. How much attention and focus should be given to reducing illegal sales has therefore been another hotly debated topic in the smoking field over the years. Although intensive efforts combining both educational campaigns and law enforcement have been demonstrated to reduce illegal sales and in some cases reduced smoking prevalence,[75] there is no consistent evidence of a substantial effect on tobacco consumption or prevalence among children.[76]

Rigotti and colleagues' recent study[77] showed that although enforcement of illegal sales laws improved compliance by shopkeepers and reduced illegal sales to minors, it did not affect adolescents' perceptions of their access to tobacco or their smoking. However, a computer simulation model, *Simsmoke*, suggests that a well-enforced policy has the potential to reduce youth smoking prevalence. (Levy et al[78] developed *Simsmoke,* which they describe as: "a model of youth access policies based on empirical research and a theory of perceived risk. The model incorporates substitution into other sources as retail sales are restricted, and is used to project the number of smokers and smoking-related deaths". The study evaluated various policies to limit youth access to cigarettes.) The Cochrane Review shows that interventions with retailers can lead to substantial decreases in the number of outlets selling tobacco to adolescents.[79, 80] Giving retailers information was less effective in reducing illegal sales than active enforcement and/or multi-component education strategies. However, few of the communities studied in the review achieved sustained levels of high compliance, which probably explained why there was limited evidence for this intervention affecting youth's perception of their ease of access to tobacco or their smoking behaviour. The idea of ID cards is proving very popular at present in many regions but evaluations of their effectiveness have not yet been completed.

Reducing under-age access to cigarettes is one of the main prongs of the tobacco industry's approach to reducing teenage smoking.[40] They advocate minimum age laws, youth access programmes, ID cards, retailer schemes and warnings on packs. The motivation for the industry's focus lies in shifting "the responsibility to others – retailers and kids themselves – and a distraction from the companies' own role in building the demand".[40] The tobacco industry documents support this – they show that the industry had a strategy to undermine law enforcement efforts, including encouraging legislation to undermine successful prosecutions and outlawing the use of compliance tests.[81]

Recommendation

Restricting youth access may only be important because of the message it sends out to young people about the dangers of tobacco. Reducing youth access in reality, as opposed to during research studies, is too expensive and difficult in practice, and is likely to have only a minimal effect.

Sociodemographic, personal and behavioural factors

A number of sociodemographic, personal and behavioural factors[9] influence uptake – for example genetic factors, age, gender, sibling smoking, lack of parental support during adolescence and peer influence.[82, 83]

The genetics of smoking is being increasingly investigated. Swan[84] in a recent review concluded that genetic factors play an important role in the initiation and maintenance of tobacco use, but it remains unknown which psychoneurogenetic elements are affected and which gene-environment interactions influence regular smoking uptake. Koopmans and colleagues' recent study indicated that genetic factors play a role in both initiation and the quantity of cigarettes smoked.[85]

Unfortunately some publications about genes which predispose to early onset of smoking and increased risk of lung cancer in later life, have been used by the tobacco industry to create a controversy about the health effects of smoking. A recent review has set out to clarify the facts.[86] Their conclusion is that twin, adoption and other studies suggest that all stages of tobacco use and dependence are partially under genetic control, but that genetic research does not support the hypothesis that there is a common genetic cause for smoking and lung cancer.

Low academic achievement, rebelliousness, alienation from school, the perception that tobacco use is the norm, and the belief that smoking confers future advantages in social life also predict onset. Smoking may also be used by teenage girls as self-medication for depression and anxiety[87] although two recent studies have given conflicting results as to whether mental health problems predict smoking in young people.[88, 89] Finally, a lack of skills to resist offers, and low self-esteem were found to be important.

Protective factors have also been shown to be important. Such factors (illustrating the concept of resilience) include autonomy, self-regulation, problem-solving, family characteristics and community characteristics and the availability of opportunities at major life transition points.[90]

An association between active participation in sport and non-smoking status in young people has long been taken for granted. A recent study of 16,262 school students has confirmed this association.[91] When all other factors were controlled for, those who were highly involved in sport were least likely and those not involved at all were most likely to smoke cigarettes. However, the athletes were most likely to have used smokeless tobacco and cigar smoking was unrelated to sports participation.

Peers are important in a young person's decision to smoke or not to smoke, but the association is not as clear-cut as it was once thought to be. Peer pressure is probably a misnomer. Peer bonding might be a more appropriate term. School students can take up smoking because they belong to a group which smokes or because they want to join a particular group.[92] A recent study found that in schools where prevalence of current smoking was highest among popular students, prevalence was also high in the school as a whole.[93]

A recent study suggested that smoking is a communicable disease as it found that the risk of incident smoking in schoolchildren was independently increased by exposure to other ever-smokers in school tutor groups. They suggested that it could be partly prevented by policies that reduce exposure to smoking at school.[94]

A number of types of intervention have been developed to influence young people not to smoke and a summary of these follows.

Education programmes

Although initially school smoking education programmes focused on the health hazards of smoking, these did not affect smoking behaviour, and were followed in the 1980s by school smoking programmes based on social learning theory which focused on the development of personal and social skills to resist social pressures to smoke. Some of these programmes delayed the onset of smoking for 4-10 years. However, they were implemented under experimental conditions and when implemented under real life conditions using ordinary classroom teachers they were shown to be relatively ineffective.[4, 95]

These disappointing findings were supported very recently in a publication from the most rigorous randomised trial that could be implemented in this field: the Hutchinson Smoking Prevention Project (HSPP) which was conducted in the US from 1984 to 1999. The intervention was a theory-based, social-influences intervention on smoking beginning in grade 3 and sustained throughout the period of smoking acquisition, up to grade 12. The study involved 40 geographically and demographically diverse school districts in Washington and over 8,000 children randomised by school district. Ninety four per cent of the students were followed up and the programme was implemented comprehensively. No significant difference in prevalence of daily smoking or other smoking outcomes was observed between control and experimental districts. The authors concluded that there was no evidence that a school-based social-influences approach was effective in the long-term deterrence of smoking among youth.[96] They suggested that more theoretical and empirical research was needed to understand smoking initiation and intervention strategies.

An associated editorial suggested that the social cognitive learning approach "may be virtually useless in explaining what causes some people to smoke."[97] They also thought that there might be other important factors that were not currently being measured such as early experiences with tobacco and the emergence of symptoms of dependence (see page 231). They felt that a transdisciplinary perspective was needed in the future.

Negative results were also found in a recent Canadian study that involved a 'Healthy Hearts' Programme in Montreal[98] aimed at preparing children to acquire healthier eating habits, engage in sport, and avoid smoking. After five years, the programme was apparently successful in the first two goals but not the third, with boys and girls in the experimental programmes being more likely to use tobacco than the controls. The tobacco phase has since ended and a meeting is scheduled to discuss the 'unexpected paradox'. Similarly negative results have recently been found in a school-based computerised prevention programme implemented in the UK.[99]

There has been much discussion about the utility of school-based educational approaches to smoking prevention over the years. Some believe that individual components of the social influences programme might still be effective. Others believe that starting school programmes even earlier might be more appropriate[9] (although there is little evidence for this and younger children anyway tend to have very strong anti-smoking opinions). Another key problem with school-based interventions is that they do not reach high-risk youth. Young people who smoke are often away from school and therefore miss school-based smoking interventions. They are also more likely to reject school-based information.[100] Health education is not seen as important by many young people, as is evidenced by the high failure rate in examinations.[101] Also, teachers might not be trained in the methods needed for affective topics such as tobacco control.

A recent review in the US investigated the approaches and extent of school-based smoking control education in schools: short-term health consequences, normative education ('most people in my age group are non-smokers'), reasons why young people smoke and refusal skills training.[102] They found lower prevalence of current smoking among those who had received a multi-strategy programme (8.4%) compared with those whose programme was not multi-strategy (12.5%).

The five-year EC-funded multi-strategy European Smoking-prevention Framework Approach (ESFA) programme evaluation ended in 2002 and analysis of the outcomes is in preparation. The intervention, which was carried out in seven European centres, including the North West and Midlands of England, had four main components: individual school-based education; school policy; parental; and community/out of school.[103]

Many experts believe, however, that it was wrong to expect tobacco education programmes in isolation of other factors to work in the long term. Most experts believe that few single approaches would work, but that comprehensive approaches were needed, including price increases.[104]

It remains possible that educational approaches might have more impact in developing countries that are at an early stage in tobacco control activities, where there is very little information other than that provided by ubiquitous tobacco industry promotion.

Comprehensive school programmes dealing with a range of substance use or health effects may have greater efficacy.[4] Similarly whole school approaches including smoking policies (see page 229) should be supported, such as the UK government's National Healthy School Standard and the European Network of Health Promoting Schools.

Recommendation

School tobacco prevention programmes should continue but only be invested in within the broader context of other tobacco control activities. School tobacco prevention programmes should be embedded within comprehensive school programmes which include school smoking policies.

Media interventions

The Cochrane Centre review in this area examined 63 studies of which only six met their criteria for inclusion. Of the two of these that reported significant effects of the media influencing smoking behaviour of young people, both had a solid theoretical basis, used formative research in designing the campaign messages, and messages were broadcast at a reasonable intensity over extensive periods of time.[105] The reviewers concluded that there was some evidence that the mass media could be effective in preventing smoking uptake, but overall the evidence was not strong.

Increasing the duration and frequency of the advertisements will be costly but an analysis of one of the successful campaigns carried out at the University of Vermont indicated that it was still cost-effective and compared favourably with other preventive and therapeutic strategies.[106]

Another recent review of mass media interventions to prevent smoking also concluded that only a few studies had been conducted in this area and there was a need for more adequately resourced multi-disciplinary approaches to using the mass media to prevent smoking.[107]

Siegel and Biener[108] more recently examined the impact of an anti-smoking media campaign on progression to established smoking in a four-year longitudinal survey of around 600 adolescents in Massachusetts who were aged 12-15 years at the outset in 1993. Those 12-13 year olds (but not 14-15 year olds) who were exposed to television anti-smoking advertisements at baseline were significantly less likely to progress to established smoking. They concluded that the television component of the Massachusetts anti-smoking media campaign may have reduced the rate of progression to established smoking among the young adolescents. This comprehensive anti-smoking campaign – the Massachusetts Tobacco Control Programme – is one of the oldest and best funded.[109] It has three elements with regard to youth: community activities supporting the passage and enforcement of legislation on youth access to tobacco; school-based programmes; and media strategies. Prevalence surveys showed significant decreases in all types of smoking between 1996 and 1999, including a drop in current cigarette use from 30.7% to 23.7% in grades 7 to 12, reversing the earlier increase seen in the first half of the 1990s.

Similarly encouraging results on the initiation of smoking have also been demonstrated in a short-term analysis of television advertisements from the Florida 'Truth' campaign,[110, 111] a campaign which included an aggressive stance against the tobacco industry. The 200 million dollar programme, funded from Florida's settlement with the tobacco companies, involved young people in developing counter-advertising to cigarettes. Between 1998 and 2001, the period of the campaign, the percentage of youth having used tobacco during the previous 30 days fell from 18.5% to 11.1% in middle school, and from 27.4% to 22.6% in high school.[112] Analyses in the US[113] have indicated that tobacco industry manipulation and second-hand smoke are the most effective strategies for advertising campaigns, but it is not known whether UK audiences would react in a similar way.

One of the most promising programmes at present is the Australian National Tobacco Campaign.[114] Aimed not at youth, but at 18-40 year old smokers, which includes the younger parental generation, and with a focus on cessation, the campaign used three advertising messages: artery, showing fatty deposits being squeezed out of a human aorta; lung, showing emphysema damage; and tumour, showing how the p53 tumour suppressor gene works. The effects were dramatic. Smoking prevalence in the age group fell from 23.5% to 22.1% by the end of the campaign, namely 190,000 fewer smokers.[115] Although other factors could be operating, it is a remarkable decrease.

A difficulty with community-wide campaigns is how they can best be evaluated. A report of a meeting held at the Johns Hopkins Bloomberg School of Public Health recommended both quantitative and qualitative methods. Their report provides valuable guidelines for anyone planning community-based interventions.[116]

The use of unpaid publicity and media advocacy has been shown to be a cost-effective way of increasing adult cessation and of influencing public opinion and that of decision-makers. It may well also influence teenage smoking although this has not been studied in controlled trials.

Recommendation

The use of mass media could be effective but it cannot yet be recommended as not enough is known about what elements would contribute to effectiveness. It would be useful to carry out research into the use of unpaid publicity and media advocacy.

Primary care interventions

A recent general practice intervention in the UK (following an exploratory trial carried out in Australia[117]) sought to maintain non-smoking status in young people by the local GP sending out information about smoking, certificates and posters to 10-15 year old non-smokers. This intervention significantly reduced smoking uptake among young people, particularly boys, one year after the initial contact.[118]

Recommendation

Primary care professionals should reinforce anti-smoking messages with young people, although further research is needed in this area.

Smoking policies

There is evidence of a relationship between smoking policies in schools and young people's smoking but this has not always been consistent and the policies are often poorly enforced.[4] A review of policy implications was recently published by the Control of Adolescent Smoking (CAS) Project, based on a study in eight European regions.[119] Based on the findings of their study, the authors present a useful set of recommendations for establishing and monitoring smoke-free school policies. Research in Gran Canaria found compliance, or otherwise, with anti-smoking rules to be the main factor in predicting smoking.[120] A study in Wales found that policy strength and enforcement were associated with pupils' smoking prevalence after controlling for other factors. Smoking prevalence was 9.5% in schools with a written smoke-free policy, and 30.1% in schools which did not have one.[121] Workplace and public place restrictions have been shown to be associated with reductions in young people's smoking,[122] but again not all analyses have demonstrated this.[75] Another recent study suggested that restrictions on smoking at home, more extensive bans on smoking in public places, and enforced bans on smoking at school may reduce teenage smoking.[123]

The National Healthy School Standard was introduced in 1999. Smoking control policies in schools are included in its remit.[124]

Recommendation

Smoking policies reinforce smoking as socially unacceptable and have been demonstrated to be effective in reducing adult smoking. Smoking policies are desirable and should be actively encouraged.

Comprehensive community-wide interventions

Community-wide interventions aim to change tobacco use in populations, not at the individual level. By implementing a range of strategies (including the interventions listed above) they aim to change the social norms surrounding tobacco use.

Early community-wide interventions were implemented in Minnesota (the Minnesota Heart Health Program Class of 1989 Study), the North Karelia programme in Finland and the Stanford five-city programme. The findings of these regarding teenage smoking were mixed.[7]

In a recent review of community-wide interventions in tobacco control (not those aimed specifically at young people), Cummings[125] indicated that there was evidence of effectiveness in the US. Sharper declines in tobacco consumption have been observed in those US states that have invested in comprehensive tobacco control campaigns. However, he also commented that the reports from randomised controlled trials (RCTs) have been disappointing in that they have not demonstrated large changes in tobacco use. He suggested that, given that community-wide interventions encompass entire populations and change over time, the gold standard RCT model might not be appropriate.

The Cochrane review of community interventions[126] which examined the evidence for community campaigns influencing teenage smoking also found the evidence mixed. Thirteen studies were included in their review. They concluded by finding some limited support for the effectiveness of community interventions in helping prevent the uptake of smoking in young people.

As indicated above, however, the evidence from those US states that have implemented comprehensive community-wide interventions is quite compelling.[8] A consistent effect on teenage smoking is observed. For example, the first programme initiated was in California. Current smoking rates in California for grades 6-8 are now the lowest in the US at 6.7%.[3] Between 1995 and 1999 the prevalence of cigarette use among youth dropped by 43% in California. Similarly, drops in youth smoking have recently been observed in Massachusetts (the second state-wide programme to be implemented, beginning in 1993). There was a 70% reduction in current smoking among 6th graders between 1996 and 1999.[3]

Wakefield and Chaloupka[8] identified level of funding as one of the critical factors in programme success, "and the degree to which this is undermined by the tobacco industry and other competitors for funding". Tobacco price increases were also important factors predicting success. Reductions in adult smoking prevalence were also observed in three of the five states that had, at the time of the review, implemented comprehensive tobacco control programmes.

In 1997, Florida began implementing a comprehensive tobacco control programme which was particularly aimed at reducing tobacco use among youth. A major part of the programme was the 'Truth' campaign – a media campaign aimed at teenagers (see page 228). Changes in cigarette use and intentions were observed two years after implementation[127] but longer term follow-up has yet to be carried out.

Recommendation

Comprehensive community-wide campaigns show promise but the results are not always consistent. Young people's views on the appropriateness of intervention messages aimed at them within these comprehensive campaigns should be canvassed. Given that comprehensive community-wide campaigns impact also on adult smoking, their implementation should be actively supported. Adequate resourcing will be critical for their success.

The development of dependence on smoking

One study among a sample of a low-income birth cohort in the US has demonstrated that prenatal tobacco exposure might have a significant role in the early initiation to tobacco among exposed offspring.[128] The authors suggested that this might be due to the damaging effects of tobacco exposure on the brain of the developing foetus, which may then create a vulnerability in the child's personality that might contribute to poorer adolescent adjustment and hence a greater likelihood of smoking uptake at an early age. Alternatively the prenatal nicotine exposure caused increases in nicotine receptors in the developing foetus that might increase susceptibility to tobacco use later on. The authors speculated that these findings might help in targeting adolescent prevention programmes at those most at risk.

The development of dependence on smoking has been extensively reviewed in a series of articles in a special supplement of the journal *Drug and Alcohol Dependence*.[129] This supplement contained reviews on measuring nicotine dependence among youth,[130] initial tobacco use episodes in young people,[131] and whether adolescent smokers were dependent on nicotine.[132]

The review of initial tobacco experiences[131] illustrated that very little is known about these and concluded that there was some evidence that people who become regular smokers may be less sensitive to nicotine's dysphoric effects than those who remain non-smokers. This could either reflect a difference in physiological response to nicotine and/or a more rapid development of tolerance to the dysphoric effects.[133]

Experiments with adolescent rats injected regularly with nicotine are beginning to examine the impact of nicotine on their development. They found that the number of receptors dedicated to nicotine increased to twice as much as in the adults.[134] (Nicotine attaches to proteins called nicotine receptors which are found on the surface of nerve cells. This causes the transmission of a chemical message which triggers a variety of different actions depending on the type of receptor involved.) A follow-up study showed that adolescent nicotine exposure also caused permanent behavioural problems, especially in females.[135]

Adolescents who experiment with smoking are highly likely to become regular smokers.[136] Inhalation is quickly established and young smokers inhale substantive doses of nicotine.[137] Nicotine can therefore play an active role in reinforcing smoking very early in the smoker's career and many adolescent smokers show symptoms of nicotine dependence early in their smoking careers.[138] The majority of young smokers perceive themselves to be dependent on their cigarettes, want and have tried to give up, and experience difficulties when they try.[7] A study in Canada found nicotine dependence to be a function of current frequency of cigarette use in adolescents, and even non-daily smokers had subjective behavioural consequences of abstinence.[139] A recent longitudinal study of a cohort of young smokers aged 12-13 years found symptoms of tobacco dependence developing rapidly after the onset of intermittent smoking and there did not appear to be a minimum nicotine dose or duration of use as a pre-requisite for symptoms to appear.[140] As a result of a new conceptualisation of nicotine dependence, the Autonomy Theory has been proposed.[141] Research in New York found that adolescents who smoked had higher levels of perceived stress and less use of cognitive coping methods than non-smokers had.[142] They recommended that interventions for inner city adolescents should target these particular young people.

The terms 'mild' and 'light' cigarettes are misleading.[143] One recent review makes the point that 'virtuous' brand names, high tech imagery, ineffective filters and menthol have all been used by the tobacco industry to present low tar machine yield brands of cigarette to make them appear safer.[144]

In May 2001 the EU Tobacco Product Directive became law. It determined, among other things, maximum tar yield, disclosure by the tobacco industry of ingredients and additives, and removal of the terms 'mild' and 'light'. It was planned that some of its provisions would come into force in September 2002 but others would not apply until 2007.[145]

Cessation programmes aimed at adolescent smokers

Given the inherent difficulties in preventing young people from experimenting with cigarettes, it has been suggested that more attention should be given to encouraging teenage smokers to quit.[146]

There have not been many studies examining predictors of smoking cessation in young people. One small-scale study in the Netherlands[147] looked at longitudinal predictors of young people's cessation. They found that motivation to quit was affected by smoking-related cognitions and habitual factors. Further analyses indicated that difference in attitudes and self-efficacy predicted whether subjects had no motivation to quit or had actually quit over a three-year follow-up period.

A Norwegian study looked at adolescent occasional smokers and found differences between these and daily smokers (for example, occasional smokers were more engaged in organised activities and sports) and suggested that these differences could be used for targeted smoking cessation programmes.[148]

Studies to date have shown that smoking cessation programmes aimed at young people have had low success rates because of low recruitment and retention, and low quit rates.[4, 149, 150] For example, a recent study examining a computerised expert system based on the transtheoretical model found no evidence that it was effective either in smoking prevention or cessation for young people.[99]

Smoking cessation in young people was the subject of an international expert seminar hosted by the Health Development Agency.[151] This reviewed the evidence that suggested that there was considerable demand for smoking cessation support from young people. For example, data on the number of calls to Scottish Smokeline, a free telephone helpline for adults, suggested that a substantial minority of young Scottish smokers were calling the Smokeline for help.

There is currently a debate among experts around giving nicotine replacement therapies (NRT) to young smokers. A UK seminar concluded that young people should be encouraged to try to stop smoking without NRT in the first instance, but that NRT would be less harmful than cigarettes and should not be discouraged as a replacement for them. Little research has so far been carried out on young people and

NRT use.[152, 153] A trial of NRT use in children is currently on-going in the Nottingham area.[154]

Some smoking cessation campaigns for young people are already being implemented in the UK and elsewhere – for example, Quit's 'Break Free' campaign. Health professionals may also have a role to play.[155] Research is on-going in this area in the UK.

Recommendation

There is a demand from adolescent smokers for cessation support that is currently not being met. Further research is needed in this area, and this should include canvassing adolescents' views. In the meantime, the NHS could offer support to smokers based on what is known to work with adults. However, it would not be wise currently to allocate too many resources to teenage cessation at the expense of implementing known effective interventions. The emerging evidence on the effects of prenatal exposure to tobacco shows the need for a strong focus on reducing smoking in pregnancy.

Conclusions

The aetiology of smoking uptake is a very complex area. A review by Flay and colleagues[156] described this well when it indicated that:

"…sociocultural, social/interpersonal and intrapersonal factors act through mediated chains of ultimate, distal and proximal influences. Some influences moderate the effect of others. Once tobacco is used, feedback mechanisms modify prior causes that in turn alter subsequent tobacco use behaviour."

It seems not surprising therefore that longitudinal studies do not explain much of the variance in smoking uptake. Engels and colleagues[157] found that although cross-sectional analyses showed strong associations between the predictors and smoking behaviour, only 8% of the variance (from non-smoking to regular smoking) was explained in a longitudinal study over a period of five years. They suggested that factors may change quickly in ways that make them of little predictive value. Brynin's study of a panel survey of 11-15 year olds supports this.[158] He found that although some young people could be seen to be predisposed to smoke, in terms of their family background "some of the key explanatory factors in smoking initiation were seen to be temporary, psychological states", confirming "that adolescent smoking is in large measure an adaptive response to immediate concerns and feelings".

This probably also explains the difficulty of designing programmes to prevent people from starting to smoke and indeed cessation programmes.

However, the picture is not so gloomy and the research database is rapidly growing. Sophisticated research methodologies are being used, particularly in the US, to focus on these issues and sub-groups of adolescent smokers are being examined. For example, Chassin and colleagues found that psychosocial characteristics significantly distinguished between early stable smokers, late stable smokers, experimenters and quitters.[159] Lewinsohn and colleagues also looked at predictors in different groups.[160]

But, more importantly, we know a lot about what does work. A recent report of the US Surgeon General[2] commented that "although our knowledge about tobacco control remains imperfect, we know more than enough to act now" and "our lack of greater progress in tobacco control is more the result of our failure to implement proven strategies than it is the lack of knowledge about what to do."

The evidence points to tackling young people's smoking as part of well resourced, comprehensive campaigns aimed principally at reducing adult smoking. This fits well with what is known about the epidemiology of diseases.[161] Knowledge and interventions are needed on all of the following:

- the agent (i.e. tobacco products)
- the host (i.e. users and potential users of tobacco products)
- the incidental host (i.e. involuntary smokers)
- the vector (i.e. tobacco product manufacturers)
- the environment (e.g. historical, economic, cultural and political influences).[162]

This will require a global effort, and support should therefore be given to the World Health Organization's developing Framework Convention on Tobacco Control which will provide a framework internationally for tobacco control interventions aimed at all relevant factors, to be implemented in countries around the world.

References

1 Royal College of Physicians of London. 1992. *Smoking and the Young. A Report of a Working Party of the Royal College of Physicians*. London: Royal College of Physicians.

2 Department of Health and Human Services. 1994. *Preventing Tobacco Use Among Young People: A Report of the Surgeon General*. Atlanta: US Department of Health and Human Services, Public Health Service, Centers for Disease Control and Prevention, National Center for Chronic Disease Prevention and Health Promotion, Office on Smoking and Health.

3 US Centers for Disease Control. *Investment in Tobacco Control – State Highlights 2001*. Available at: http://www.cdc.gov/tobacco/statehi/statehi 2001.htm

4 Reid DJ, McNeill AD, Glynn TJ. 1995. Reducing the prevalence of smoking in youth in Western countries: an international review. *Tobacco Control*; 4: 266-77.

5 Lynch BS, Bonnie RJ. 1994. *Growing Up Tobacco Free. Preventing Nicotine Addiction in Children and Youths*. Washington: National Academy Press.

6 Stead M, Hastings G, Tudor-Smith C. 1996. Preventing adolescent smoking: A review of options. *Health Education Journal*; 55: 31-53.

7 McNeill A. Preventing the onset of tobacco use. In: Bolliger CT, Fagerstrom KO (eds.) 1997. *The Tobacco Epidemic. Progress in Respiratory Research*. Vol 28. Basel: S Karger AG: pp 213-29.

8 Wakefield M, Chaloupka F. 2000. Effectiveness of comprehensive tobacco control programmes in reducing teenage smoking in the USA. *Tobacco Control*; 200; 9: 177-86.

9 NHS Centre for Reviews and Dissemination. 1999. Preventing the uptake of smoking in young people. *Effective Health Care Bulletin*; 5 (5). Available at: http://www.york.ac.uk/inst/crd/ehc55.pdf

10 Nicotine and Tobacco Research. 1999. *Proceedings from 'New Partnerships and Paradigms for Tobacco Prevention Research', Sundance, Utah, 6-9 May 1997*. Middleton, WI: Society for the Research on Nicotine and Tobacco; 1; Suppl 1: S1-S136.

11 Jacobson PD, Lantz PM, Warner KE, Wasserman J, Pollock HA, Ahlstrom AK. 2001. *Combating Teen Smoking: Research and Policy Strategies*. Ann Arbor: The University of Michigan Press.

12 Dobbs J, Marsh A. 1983. *Smoking among Secondary School Children*. London: Her Majesty's Stationery Office.

13 Department of Health. 2002. Drug use, smoking and drinking among young people in England in 2001. Available at: http://www.doh.gov.uk/public/press15march02.htm

14 Charlton A, Bates C. 2000. Decline in teenage smoking with rise in mobile phone ownership: hypothesis. *British Medical Journal*; 321: 1155.

15 Jones T, Invernizzi G, Lee C-Y et al. 2001. Smoking and use of mobile phones. *British Medical Journal*; 322: 616-17.

16 Rogers EM, Shoemaker FF. 1971. *Communication of Innovations*. New York: Free Press.

17 Office for National Statistics. 2000. *Living in Britain: Results from the 1998 General Household Survey: An Inter-departmental Survey Carried Out by the Office for National Statistics between April 1998 and March 1999*. London: The Stationery Office.

18 Bynner J. 1969. *The Young Smoker*. London: Her Majesty's Stationery Office.

19 Office for National Statistics. 1999. *Smoking, Drinking and Drug Use among Young Teenagers in 1998. Volume 1: England*. London: The Stationery Office.

20 Warren CW, Riley L, Asma S, Erikson MP, Green L, Blanton C, Loo C, Batchelor S, Yach D. 2000. Tobacco use by youth: a surveillance report from the Global Youth Tobacco Survey project. *Bulletin of the World Health Organization*; 78: 868-76.

21 Available at http://www.ruhbc.ed.ac.uk/hbsc/downlad/hbsc.pdf

22 Hill D. 1999. Why we should target adult smoking first. *Tobacco Control*; 8: 333-35.

23 Myers ML. 1999. Adults versus teenagers: a false dilemma and a dangerous choice. *Tobacco Control*; 8: 336-38.

24 Peto R, Darby S, Deo H, Silcocks P, Whitley E, Doll R. 2000. Smoking, smoking cessation, and lung cancer in the UK since 1950: combination of national statistics with two case-control studies. *British Medical Journal*; 321: 323-29.

25 Farkas AJ, Distefan JM, Choi WS, Gilpin EA, Pierce JP. 1999. Does parental smoking cessation discourage adolescent smoking? *Preventive Medicine*; 28: 213-18.

26 Withers NJ, Low JL, Holgate ST, Clough JB. 2000. Smoking habits in a cohort of UK adolescents. *Respiratory Medicine*; 94: 391-96.

27 House of Commons Education and Skills Committee. 2002. *The Work of OFSTED: First Session Report 2001-2002*. London: House of Commons.

28 Everett SA, Warren CW, Sharp D, Kann L, Husten CG, Crossett L. 1999. Initiation of cigarette smoking and subsequent smoking behaviour among US high school students. *Preventive Medicine*; 29: 327-33.

29 Lewinsohn PM, Rohde P, Brown RA. 1999. Level of current and past adolescent cigarette smoking as predictors of future substance use disorders in young adulthood. *Addiction*; 94: 913-21.

30 DuRant RH, Smith JA, Kreiter SR, Krowchuk DP. 1999. The relationship between early age of onset of initial substance use and engaging in multiple health risk behaviors among young adolescents. *Archives of Pediatrics and Adolescent Medicine*; 153: 286-91.

31 Machuca G, Rosales I, Lacalle JR, Machuca C, Bullon P. 2000. Effect of cigarette smoking on periodontal status of healthy young adults. *Journal of Periodontology*; 71: 73-78.

32 Lubinski W, Targowski T, Frank-Piskorska A. 2000. [Evaluation of the influence of tobacco smoking on pulmonary function in young men]. *Pneumonologia i Alergologia Polska*; 68: 226-31.

33 Altarac M, Gardner JW, Rose M, Popovich RM, Potter R, Knapik JJ, Jones BH. 2000. Cigarette smoking and exercise-related injuries among young men and women. *American Journal of Preventive Medicine;* 18 (3 Suppl): 96-102.

34 Wiencke JK, Thurston SW, Kelsey KT, Varkonyi A, Wain JC, Mark EJ, Christiani DC. 1999. Early age at smoking initiation and tobacco carcinogen DNA damage in the lung. *Journal of the National Cancer Institute*; 91: 614-19.

35 Rowland RE, Harding KM. 1999. Increased sister chromatid exchange in the peripheral blood lymphocytes of young women who smoke cigarettes. *Hereditas*; 131: 143-46.

36 Charlton A, While D. 1995. Blood pressure and smoking: observations on a national cohort. *Archives of Disease in Childhood*; 73: 90-107.

37 Simantov E, Schoen C, Klein JD. 2000. Health compromising behaviours: why do adolescents smoke and drink? *Archives of Pediatrics and Adolescent Medicine*; 154: 1025-33.

38 Charlton A, While D. 1996. Smoking and menstrual problems. *Journal of the Royal Society of Medicine*; 89: 193-95.

39 While D, Kelly S, Huang W, Charlton A. 1997. Causes of absence from school related to children's and their parents' smoking. *Tobacco Control*; 6: 150-51.

40 ASH/Cancer Research Campaign. 2000. *PR in the playground. Tobacco industry initiatives on youth smoking*. Available at: www.ash.org.uk

41 Health Development Agency. 2000. *Coronary Heart Disease. Guidance for Implementing the Preventive Aspects of the National Service Framework*. London: Health Development Agency.

42 Perry CL. 1999. The tobacco industry and underage youth smoking: tobacco industry documents from the Minnesota litigation. *Archives of Pediatrics and Adolescent Medicine*; 153: 935-41.

43 Cummings KM, Morley CP, Horan JK, Steger C, Leavell NR. 2002. Marketing to America's youth: evidence from corporate documents. *Tobacco Control*; 11; Suppl 1: 118-31.

44 Lovell G. 2002. *You are the Target. Big Tobacco: Lies, Scams – Now the Truth.* Vancouver: Chryan Publications.

45 While D, Kelly S, Huang W, Charlton A. 1996. Cigarette advertising and the onset of smoking in children: a questionnaire survey. *British Medical Journal*; 313: 398-99.

46 DiFranza JR, Eddy JJ, Brown LF, Ryan JL, Bogojavlensky A. 1994. Tobacco acquisition and cigarette brand selection among youth. *Tobacco Control*; 3: 334-38.

47 Pierce JP, Gilpin EA. 1995. A historical analysis of tobacco marketing and the uptake of smoking by youth in the United States: 1890-1977. *Health Psychology*; 14: 500-08.

48 Pierce JP, Lee L, Gilpin EA. 1994. Smoking initiation by adolescent girls, 1944 through 1988: an association with targeted advertising. *Journal of the American Medical Association*; 217: 608-11.

49 Pierce JP, Choi WS, Gilpin EA, Farkas AJ, Merritt KK. 1996. Validation of susceptibility as a predictor of which adolescents take up smoking in the US. *Health Psychology*; 15: 355-61.

50 Evans N, Farkas A, Gilpin E, Berry C, Pierce JP. 1995. Influence of tobacco marketing and exposure to smokers on adolescent susceptibility to smoking. *Journal of the National Cancer Institute*; 87: 1538-45.

51 Pollay R, Siddarth S, Siegel M, Haddix A, Merritt RK, Giovino GA, Eriksen MP. 1996. The last straw? Cigarette advertising and realized market shares among youths and adults, 1979-1993. *Journal of Marketing*; 60: 1-16.

52 Charlton A, While D, Kelly S. 1997. Boys' smoking and cigarette-brand-sponsored motor racing. *The Lancet*; 350: 1474.

53 Altman DG, Levine EW, Coeytaux R, Slade J, Jaffe R. 1996. Tobacco promotion and susceptibility to tobacco use among adolescents aged 12 through 17 years in a nationally representative sample. *American Journal of Public Health*; 86: 1590-93.

54 Feighery E, Borzekowski DL, Schooler C, Flora J. 1998. Seeing, wanting, owning: the relationship between receptivity to tobacco marketing and smoking susceptibility in young people. *Tobacco Control*; 7: 122-28.

55 MacFadyen L, Hastings G, MacKintosh AM. 2001. Cross sectional study of young people's awareness of an involvement with tobacco marketing. *British Medical Journal*; 322: 513-17.

56 Deppe B. 1996. *An exploration of the social image of smoking held by adolescent girls.* MSc Thesis, Department of Public Health and Health Promotion, School of Epidemiology and Health Sciences, The University of Manchester.

57 Wakefield M, Letcher T. 2002. My pack is cuter than your pack. *Tobacco Control*; 11: 154-56.

58 Klein JD, St Clair S. 2000. Do candy cigarettes encourage young people to smoke? *British Medical Journal*; 321: 362-65.

59 Pierce JP, Gilpin EA, Choi WS. 1999. Sharing the blame: smoking experimentation and future smoking-attributable mortality due to Joe Camel and Marlboro advertising and promotions. *Tobacco Control*; 8: 37-44.

60 Action on Smoking and Health (ASH). 2002. *Factsheet No.19: Tobacco Advertising and Promotion. April 2002.* London: ASH.

61 WHO European Ministerial Conference for a Tobacco-free Europe, Warsaw, 18-19 February 2002. *Warsaw Declaration for a Tobacco-free Europe*. Copenhagen: World Health Organization.

62 Biener L. 2002. Anti-tobacco advertisements by Massachusetts and Philip Morris: what teenagers think. *Tobacco Control*: 11; suppl 11: ii43-ii46.

63 Teti TS, Glantz SA. 1998. Smoking in movies remained high in 1997. *Tobacco Control*; 7: 441.

64 Shields DLL, Carol J, Balbach ED, McGee S. 1999. Hollywood on tobacco: how the entertainment industry understands tobacco portrayal. *Tobacco Control*; 8: 378-86.

65 Escamilla G, Cradock AL, Kawachi I. 2000. Women and smoking in Hollywood movies: a content analysis. *American Journal of Public Health*; 90: 412-14.

66 Sargent JD, Tickle JJ, Beach ML, Dalton MA, Ahrens MB, Heatherton TF. 2001. Brand appearances in contemporary cinema films and contribution to global marketing of cigarettes. *The Lancet*; 357: 29-32.

67 Tickle JJ, Sargent JD, Dalton MA, Beach ML, Heatherton TF. 2001. Favourite movie stars, their tobacco use in contemporary movies, and its association with adolescent smoking. *Tobacco Control*; 10: 16-22.

68 Available at: http://smokefreemovies.ucsf.edu

69 Emery S, Gilpin EA, White MM, Pierce JP. 1999. How adolescents get their cigarettes: implications for policies on access and price. *Journal of the National Cancer Institute*; 91: 184-86.

70 Chaloupka FJ. 1999. Macro-social influences: the effects of prices and tobacco-control policies on the demand for tobacco products. *Nicotine and Tobacco Research*; 1; Suppl 1: S105-09.

71 Action on Smoking and Health (ASH). 2002. Budget: Tobacco tax frozen in real terms. *Burning Issues*; April 2002.

72 Wanless D. 2002. *Securing Our Future Health: Taking a Long-term View.* London: The Treasury.

73 Conrad KM, Flay BR, Hill D. 1992. Why children start smoking cigarettes: Predictors of onset. *British Journal of Addiction*; 87: 1711-24.

74 Everett Jones S, Sharp DJ, Husten CG, Crossett LS. 2002. Cigarette aquisition and proof of age among US high school students who smoke. *Tobacco Control*; 11: 20-25.

75 Lewit EM, Hyland A, Kerrebrock N, Cummings KM. 1997. Price, public policy, and smoking in young people. *Tobacco Control*; 6; Suppl 2: S17-S24.

76 Glantz SA. 1996. Editorial: Preventing tobacco use – the youth access trap. *Tobacco Control*; 86: 156-58.

77 Rigotti NA, DiFranza JR, Chang Y, Tisdale T, Kemp B, Singer DE. 1997. The effect of enforcing tobacco-sales laws on adolescents' access to tobacco and smoking behaviour. *New England Journal of Medicine*; 337: 1044-51.

78 Levy DT, Friend K, Holder H, Carmona M. 2002. Effect of policies directed at youth access to smoking: results from the *Simsmoke* computer simulation model. *Tobacco Control*; 10: 108-16.

79 Stead LF, Lancaster T. 2000. Interventions for preventing tobacco sales to minors. *Cochrane Database Systematic Review*; (2): CD001497.

80 Stead LF, Lancaster T. 2000. A systematic review of interventions for preventing tobacco sales to minors. *Tobacco Control*; 9: 169-76.

81 DiFranza JR, Godshall W. 1996. Tobacco industry efforts hindering enforcement of the ban on tobacco sales to minors: Actions speak louder than words. *Tobacco Control*; 86: 156-58.

82 West P, Sweeting H, Ecob R. 1999. Family and friends' influences on the uptake of regular smoking from mid-adolescence to early adulthood. *Addiction*; 94: 1397-411.

83 Derzon JH, Lipsey MW. 1999. Predicting tobacco use to age 18: a synthesis of longitudinal research. *Addiction*; 94: 995-1006.

84 Swan GE. 1999. Implications of genetic epidemiology for the prevention of tobacco use. *Nicotine and Tobacco Research*; 1; Suppl 1: S49-56.

85 Koopmans JR, Slutske WS, Heath AC, Neale MC, Boomsma DI. 1999. The genetics of smoking initiation and quantity smoked in Dutch adolescent and young adult twins. *Behavior Genetics*; 29: 383-93.

86 Hall W, Madden P, Lynskey M. 2002. The genetics of tobacco use: methods, findings and policy implications. *Tobacco Control*; 11: 119-24.

87 Patton GC, Hibbert M, Rosier MJ, Carlin JB, Caust J, Bowes G. 1996. Is smoking associated with depression and anxiety in teenagers? *American Journal of Public Health*; 86: 225-30.

88 Sonntag H, Wittchen HU, Hofler M, Kessler RC, Stein MB. 2000. Are social fears and DSM-IV social anxiety disorder associated with smoking and nicotine dependence in adolescents and young adults? *European Psychiatry*; 15: 67-74.

89 McGee R, Williams S, Stanton W. 1998. Is mental health in childhood a major predictor of smoking in adolescence? *Addiction*; 93: 1869-74.

90 Braverman MT. 1999. Research on resilience and its implications for tobacco prevention. *Nicotine and Tobacco Research*; 1; Suppl 1: S67-72.

91 Melnick MJ, Miller KE, Sabo DF, Farrell MP, Barnes GM. 2001. Tobacco use among high school athletes and nonathletes: results of the 1997 Youth Risk Behaviour Survey. *Adolescence*; 36: 727-47.

92 Michell L. 1997. Loud, sad or bad: young people's perceptions of peer groups and smoking. *Health Education Research*; 12: 1-14.

93 Alexander CA, Piazza M, Mekos D, Valente T. 2002. Peers, schools and adolescent cigarette smoking. *Journal of Adolescent Health*; 29: 22-30.

94 Molyneux A, Lewis S, Antoniak M, Hubbard R, McNeill A, Godfrey C, Madeley R, Britton J. 2002. Is smoking a communicable disease? Effect of exposure to ever smokers in school tutor groups on the risk of incident smoking in the first year of secondary school. *Tobacco Control*; 11: 241-45.

95 Nutbeam D, Macaskill P, Smith C, Catford J. 1993. Evaluation of two school smoking prevention programmes under normal classroom conditions. *British Medical Journal*; 306: 102-07.

96 Peterson AV, Kealey KA, Mann SL, Marek PM, Sarason IG. 2000. Hutchinson Smoking Prevention Project: Long-term randomised trial in school-based tobacco use prevention. Results on smoking. *Journal of the National Cancer Institute*; 92: 1979-91.

97 Clayton RR, Scutchfield FD, Wyatt SW. 2000. Hutchinson Smoking Prevention Project: a new gold standard in prevention science requires new transdisciplinary thinking. *Journal of the National Cancer Institute*; 92:1964-65.

98 Available at: http://www.ledevior.com/san//2000a/taba220400.html

99 Aveyard P, Cheng KK, Almond J, Sherratt E, Lancashire R, Lawrence T, Griffin C, Evans O. 1999. Cluster randomised controlled trial of expert system based on the transtheoretical ('stages of change') model for smoking prevention and cessation in schools. *British Medical Journal*; 319: 948-53.

100 Charlton A. 2000. Why are school-based, youth-centred smoking interventions not as effective as we hoped? Some ideas for research. *International Journal of Health Promotion and Education*; 38: 124-28.

101 Northern Examinations and Assessments Board. 1999. *Annual Report 1998.* Manchester: Northern Examinations and Assessments Board.

102 American Legacy Foundation. 2002. *Legacy First Look Report No. 8: Using Multiple Strategies in Tobacco Use Prevention Education.* Washington: American Legacy Foundation.

103 Kremers SPJ, Mudde AN, De Vries H. 2000. Measuring the effectiveness of ESFA: towards best practices in smoking prevention research. In: Norheim L, Waller M (eds.) *Best Practices: A Selection of Papers on Quality and Effectiveness in Health Promotion.* Helsinki: Finnish Centre for Health Promotion.

104 Reid D. 1996. Tobacco control: overview. *British Medical Bulletin*; 52: 108-20.

105 Sowden AJ, Arblaster L. 2000. Mass media interventions for preventing smoking in young people. *Cochrane Database Systematic Review*; (2): CD001006.

106 Secker-Walker RH, Worden JK, Holland RR, Flynn BS, Detsky A. 1997. A mass media programme to prevent smoking among adolescents: costs and cost effectiveness. *Tobacco Control*; 6: 207-12.

107 Worden JK. Research in using mass media to prevent smoking. 1999. *Nicotine and Tobacco Research*; 1; Suppl 1: S117-S121.

108 Siegel M, Biener L. 2000. The impact of an antismoking media campaign on progression to established smoking: results of a longitudinal youth study. *American Journal of Public Health*; 90: 380-86.

109 Soldz S, Clark TW, Stewart E, Celebucki C, Klein Walker D. 2002. Decreased youth tobacco use in Massachusetts 1996 to 1999: evidence of tobacco control effectiveness. *Tobacco Control*; 11; Suppl 11: ii14-ii19.

110 Sly DF, Hopkins RS, Trapido E, Ray S. 2001. Influence of a counteradvertising media campaign on initiation of smoking: the Florida 'Truth' campaign. *American Journal of Public Health*; 91: 233-38.

111 Hicks JJ. 2001. The strategy behind Florida's 'Truth' campaign. *Tobacco Control*; 10: 3-5.

112 Sly DF, Heald GR, Ray S. 2001. The Florida 'Truth' anti-tobacco media evaluation: design, first year results and implications for planning future state media evaluations. *Tobacco Control*; 10: 9-15.

113 Goldman L, Glantz S. 1998. Evaluation of antismoking advertising campaigns. *Journal of the American Medical Association*; 279: 772-77.

114 Research and Evaluation Committee of the National Expert Advisory Commission on Tobacco. 1999. *Australia's National Tobacco Campaign. Summary. Evaluation Report Volume 1. Every Cigarette is Doing You Damage.* Melbourne: Anti Cancer Council of Victoria.

115 Australian National Campaign Research and Evaluation Committee. 2000. *Australia's National Tobacco Campaign. Evaluation Report Volume 2.* Melbourne: Anti Cancer Council of Victoria.

116 Institute for Global Tobacco Control, Johns Hopkins Bloomberg School of Public Health. 2002. Conference Report: Evaluating comprehensive tobacco control interventions: challenges and recommendations for future action. *Tobacco Control*; 11: 140-45.

117 Jamrozik KD, Tait RJ. 1998. A new health education strategy to reduce smoking among young people. *Tobacco Control*; 8: 194.

118 Fidler W, Lambert TW. 2001. A prescription for health: a primary care based intervention to maintain the non-smoking status of young people. *Tobacco Control*; 10: 23-26.

119 Kannas L, Schmidt B. 2001. Policy implications and recommendations for a smoke-free school. *International Study Control of Adolescent Smoking. CAS Factsheet 3, June 2001.* University of Jyvaskyla, Finland.

120 Pinilla J, Gonzales B, Barber P, Santana Y. 2002. Smoking in young adolescents: an approach with multilevel discrete choice models. *Journal of Epidemiology and Community Health*; 56: 227-32.

121 Moore L, Roberts C, Tudor-Smith C. 2001. School smoking policies and smoking prevention among adolescents: multilevel analysis of cross-sectional data from Wales. *Tobacco Control*; 10: 117-23.

122 Wasserman J, Manning WG, Newhouse JP, Winkler JD. 1991. The effect of excise taxes and regulations on cigarette smoking. *Journal of Health Economics*; 10: 43-64.

123 Wakefield MA, Chaloupka FJ, Kaufman NJ, Orleans CT, Barker DC, Ruel ER. 2000. Effect of restrictions on smoking at home, at school, and in public places on teenage smoking: cross sectional study. *British Medical Journal*; 321: 333-37.

124 Wired for Health. *National Healthy School Standard*. Available at http://www.wiredforhealth.gov.uk/healthy/healsch.html

125 Cummings KM. 1999. Community-wide interventions for tobacco control. *Nicotine and Tobacco Research*; 1; Suppl 1: S113-116.

126 Sowden A, Arblaster L. 2000. Community interventions for preventing smoking in young people. *Cochrane Database Systematic Reviews*; (2): CD001291.

127 Bauer UE, Johnson TM, Hopkins RS, Brooks RG. 2000. Changes in youth cigarette use and intentions following implementation of a tobacco control program: findings from the Florida Youth Tobacco Survey, 1998-2000. *Journal of the American Medical Association*; 284: 723-28.

128 Cornelius MD, Leech SL, Goldschmidt L, Day NL. 2000. Prenatal tobacco exposure: is it a risk factor for early tobacco experimentation? *Nicotine and Tobacco Research*; 2: 45-52.

129 Clayton RR, Merikangas KR, Abrams DB (guest editors.) 2000. Tobacco, Nicotine and Youth (Supplement title). *Drug and Alcohol Dependence*; 59; Suppl 1.

130 Colby SM, Tiffany ST, Shiffman S, Niaura RS. 2000. Measuring nicotine dependence among youth: a review of available approaches and instruments. *Drug and Alcohol Dependence*; 59; Suppl 1: S23-S39.

131 Eissenberg T, Balster RL. 2000. Initial tobacco use episodes in children and adolescents: current knowledge, future directions. *Drug and Alcohol Dependence*; 59; Suppl 1: S41-S60.

132 Colby SM, Tiffany ST, Shiffman S, Niaura RS. 2000. Are adolescent smokers dependent on nicotine? A review of the evidence. *Drug and Alcohol Dependence*; 59; Suppl 1: S83-S95.

133 Perkins KA, Grobe JE, Fonte C, Goettler J, Caggiula AR, Reynolds WA, Stiller RI, Scierka A, Jacob RG. 1994. Chronic and acute tolerance to subjective, behavioural and cardiovascular effects of nicotine in humans. *Journal of Pharmacology and Experimental Therapeutics*; 270: 628-38.

134 Slotkin TA, Orband-Miller L, Queen KL. 1987. Development of [H3] nicotine binding sites in brain regions of rats exposed to nicotine prenatally via maternal injections or infusions. *Journal of Pharmacology and Experimental Therapeutics*; 242: 232-37.

135 Slotkin TA, Cho H, Whitmore WL. 1987. Effects of prenatal nicotine exposure on neuronal development. Selective actions on central and peripheral catecholaminergic pathways. *Brain Research Bulletin*; 18: 601-11.

136 Patton GC, Carlin JB, Coffey C, Wolfe R, Hibbert M, Bowes G. 1998. The course of early smoking: a population-based cohort study over three years. *Addiction*; 93: 1251-60.

137 McNeill AD, Jarvis MJ, Stapleton JA, West RJ, Bryant A. 1989. Nicotine intake in young smokers: longitudinal study of saliva cotinine concentrations. *American Journal of Public Health*; 79: 172-75.

138 DiFranza JR, Rigotti NA, McNeill AD, Ockene JK, Savageau JA, St Cyr D, Coleman M. 2000. Initial symptoms of nicotine dependence in adolescents. *Tobacco Control*; 9: 313-19.

139 Corrigall WA, Zack M, Eissenberg T, Belsito L, Scher R. 2001. Acute subjective and physiological responses to smoking in adolescents. *Addiction*; 96: 1409-17.

140 DiFranza JR, Savageau JA, Rigotti NA, Fletcher K, Ockene JK, McNeill AD, Coleman M, Wood C. 2002. Development of symptoms of tobacco dependence in youths: 30 month follow up data from the DANDY study. *Tobacco Control*; 11: 228-35.

141 DiFranza JR, Savageau JA, Fletcher K, Ockene JK, Rigotti NA, McNeill AD, Coleman M, Wood C. 2002. Measuring the loss of autonomy over nicotine use in adolescents: the DANDY Development and Assessment of Nicotine Dependence in Youths (DANDY) Study. *Archives of Pediatrics and Adolescent Medicine*; 156: 397-403.

142 Siqueira LM, Rolnitzky LM, Rickert VI. 2001. Smoking cessation in adolescents: the role of nicotine dependence, stress and coping methods. *Archives of Pediatrics and Adolescent Medicine*; 155: 489-95.

143 Leavell N-R. 1999. The low tar lie. *Tobacco Control*; 8: 433-39.

144 Pollay RW, Dewhirst T. 2002. The dark side of marketing seemingly 'Light' cigarettes: successful images and failed fact. *Tobacco Control*; 11; Suppl 1: 118-31.

145 European Union Tobacco Product Directive. *The Guardian*: 16th May 2001.

146 Lamkin L, David B, Kamen A. 1998. Rationale for tobacco cessation interventions for youth. *Preventive Medicine*; 27: A3-8.

147 Engels RC, Knibbe RA, de Vries H, Drop MJ. 1998. Antecedents of smoking cessation among adolescents: who is motivated to change? *Preventive Medicine*; 27: 348-57.

148 Holmen TL et al. 2000. Adolescent occasional smokers – a target group for smoking cessation? The Nord-Trondelag Health Study, Norway, 1995-1997. *Preventive Medicine*; 31: 682-90.

149 Moolchan ET, Ernst M, Henningfield JE. 2000. A review of tobacco smoking in adolescents: treatment implications. *Journal of the American Academy of Child and Adolescent Psychiatry*; 39: 682-93.

150 Sussman S, Lichtman KA, Ritt, A, Pallonen UE. 1999. Effects of 34 adolescent tobacco use cessation and prevention trials on regular users of tobacco products. *Substance Use and Misuse*; 34: 1469-503.

151 Foulds J. 2000. *Smoking Cessation in Young People. Should We Do More to Help Young Smokers to Quit?* London: Health Development Agency.

152 Smith TA, House RD, Croghan IT, Gauvin TR, Colligan RC, Offor KP, Gomez-Dahl LC, Hurt RD. 1996. Nicotine patch therapy in adolescent smokers. *Pediatrics*; 98: 659-67.

153 Hurt RD, Croghan GA, Beede SD, Wolter TD, Croghan IT, Patten CA. 2000. Nicotine patch therapy in 101 adolescent smokers: efficacy, withdrawal symptom relief, and carbon monoxide and plasma cotinine levels. *Archives of Pediatrics and Adolescent Medicine*; 154: 31-37.

154 Details from: http://science.cancerresearchuk.org/research/ (Search for researcher J Britton.)

155 Townsend J, Wilkes H, Haines A et al. 1991. Adolescent smokers seen in general practice: health, lifestyle, physical measurements, and response to antismoking advice. *British Medical Journal*; 303: 947-50.

156 Flay BR, Petraitis J, Hu FB. 1999. Psychosocial risk and protective factors for adolescent tobacco use. *Nicotine and Tobacco Research*; 1; Suppl 1: S59-65.

157 Engels RC, Knibbe RA, Drop MJ. 1999. Predictability of smoking in adolescence: between optimisim and pessimism. *Addiction*; 94: 115-24.

158 Brynin M. 1999. Smoking behaviour: predisposition or adaptation? *Journal of Adolescence*; 22: 635-46.

159 Chassin L, Presson CC, Pitts SC, Sherman SJ. 2000. The natural history of cigarette smoking from adolescence to adulthood in a Midwestern community sample: multiple trajectories and their psychosocial correlates. *Health Psychology*; 19: 223-31.

160 Lewinsohn PM, Brown RA, Seeley JR, Ramsey SE. 2000. Psychosocial correlates of cigarette smoking abstinence, experimentation, persistence and frequency during adolescence. *Nicotine and Tobacco Research*; 2: 121-31.

161 Giovino GA. 1999. Epidemiology of tobacco use among US adolescents. *Nicotine and Tobacco Research;* 1; Suppl 1: S31-40.

162 Orleans CT, Slade J. 1993. In: Orleans CT, Slade J (eds.) *Nicotine Addiction: Principles and Management.* New York: Oxford University Press: ix-xi.

Chapter 11

Health promotion for young people in primary care: what works, and what doesn't work

Dr Aidan Macfarlane

International independent consultant on the strategic planning of child and adolescent health services

This chapter:

- examines the links between foetal life, child and adolescent behaviours and adult heart disease
- considers whether health-related behaviours in adolescence form the basis for health-related behaviours in adults, and
- examines the factors that influence young people's health-related behaviours such as smoking, diet and physical activity, whether there is evidence that there are interventions that are effective in altering these behaviours, and whether these interventions should be used.

Key themes

- Health promotion for adolescents is based on the premise that certain adult health-related behaviours that affect adults' cardiac disease are laid down during adolescence.
- There are two ways to approach health promotion during adolescence:
  a) addressing issues which society generally should be responsible for so that adolescent health-related behaviours can be improved, and
  b) addressing issues that the individual adolescent could take responsibility for. The major emphasis should be on the former.
- Young people do not 'risk take'. They learn from experimenting with the huge menu that life experiences have to offer.
- Effective interventions into adolescent health-related behaviours have to match the complex mix of factors which influence young people's behaviours.
- To be effective, health promotion interventions for adolescents have to be carried out simultaneously at governmental, community, and more local levels.

Introduction

"What should I be doing about my health?" is not going to be the first thought passing through a teenager's mind when he or she wakes up each morning. It is more likely to be: "Headache. Drank too much last night. Did I use contraception? What homework have I got to have in today? Hell, it can't be that time already," etc.

Health promotion to this age group has two main emphases: that of society's responsibilities (for example the availability of cigarettes, their legality, their pricing and how they are advertised); and that of the individual young person's responsibility (for example for deciding whether to smoke or not) which assumes a concept of 'free will' and 'equity of choice' for the individual young person. It is the balance between these two that is important, with primary health care playing a role in both areas, although overall the emphasis should be on the role of society, allowing teenagers to get on with the more important things in their lives – such as their education, their relationships, and their creativity.

Both the 'society' approach and the 'individual' approach are traditionally used, but the question of emphasis remains of paramount importance. It is the suggestion here that, for young people, by far the stronger emphasis should be on society providing them with a safe environment within which to experiment and explore, without at the same time placing excessive medical pressures on their individual lives.

It seems unlikely that there will be total consensus among readers as to the exact definitions of any of the terms set out above, or about the reasons for interfering in young people's lives at all, or the methodologies involved. This will arise partly from the personal beliefs of the readers, partly from their political inclinations, partly from the cultural background from which they come, and partly from their professional perspectives.

The approach in this chapter will therefore be to take a broad look at what is known about 'effective health promotion to young people' in general terms, and then to concentrate on three specific areas of adolescent behaviours – smoking, diet and physical activity – and how they relate to heart disease in the adult and to prevention of the disease.

Adolescent/young person/teenager Young people from the beginning of their 10th year to the end of their 19th year.

Health The ability to resist the strains and stresses of a physical, mental and social nature, so that they do not lead to a reduction in lifespan, function or well-being.

Health promotion Any deliberate intervention aimed at increasing 'the ability to resist the strains and stresses of a physical, mental and social nature, so that they do not lead to a reduction in lifespan, function or well-being'.

'Effective' health promotion intervention Where there is some research evidence that such an intervention has a significant effect on health in the direction desired at some time during the entire lifespan of the recipient of such an intervention.

Links between foetal life, child and adolescent behaviours and adult heart disease

In relation to cardiovascular disease the main rationale of health promotion to young people is premised on the hypothesis that there are a number of health-related factors in early life which either directly or indirectly impinge upon the future cardiovascular health of the individual adult.

Although this chapter examines this hypothesis for the age group of young people from the beginning of their 10th year to the end of their 19th year there is, of course, evidence for associations from much earlier in life. (See Chapter 1.)

Direct evidence that factors during childhood and adolescence have an adverse effect on the cardiovascular system comes from the post mortem studies looking at the cardiovascular systems of young American soldiers killed in the Korean and Vietnam wars which seem to indicate that fatty deposition in the walls of the coronary arteries starts at an early age.[1, 2] Interestingly the amount of these fatty deposits showed a marked decrease across time between the two sets of post mortems, lending support to the idea that there were factors in growing Americans, early in their lives, which had changed so as to improve these cardiovascular post mortem outcomes between the 1940s and the 1950s/60s.

The evidence for various health-related behaviours in young people having a more indirect effect on adult cardiovascular outcomes is based around the theory that certain adult behaviours that have been found to be related to adult cardiovascular disease – such as smoking, diet and physical activity (see Chapters 10, 7 and 9) – are all behaviours which are established during adolescence or earlier in life and continue thereafter into adult life. The 'adolescent health promotion intervention' rationale is therefore based on the idea that we can, by early intervention into young people's lives, prevent or change aspects of their behaviours and that this will prevent such behaviours continuing into adult life, and therefore decrease the prevalence of these risk factors in adults overall.

Added to this is the health promotion specialist's more direct reasons for intervening in adolescent health-related behaviours which is that some immediate aspects of adolescent well-being will also be improved by such interventions. Drinking, smoking and physical inactivity are all associated with young people feeling less healthy than those who do not partake in these behaviours.[3, 4]

However, in the field of prevention of cardiovascular disease, there are a number of very real problems, for those involved in health promotion, in deciding whether they are justified in putting these concepts into practice. Throughout the rest of this chapter examples given will, in the main, be related to smoking, diet and physical activity as being the more obvious factors associated with adult cardiovascular disease, with particular emphasis on smoking as it is better researched than the other two factors.

What is the evidence that health-related behaviours in adolescence form the basis for health-related behaviour in adults?

Smoking

For smoking the evidence is fairly straightforward: over 80% of those young people who are regular smokers by the age of 20 began smoking before the age of 16.[5] This, coupled with the knowledge of just how addictive tobacco is, makes a clear case for trying to decrease the uptake of smoking in young people, by one means or another.

Diet, obesity and physical activity

For diet, obesity and physical activity the evidence is more complicated. We know that two out of three obese children will go on to become obese adults, but we also know that the majority of obese adults were not obese as children. Adult obesity is associated with a large number of adverse outcomes including so called metabolic or insulin resistance syndrome which is itself strongly associated with cardiovascular mortality (see Chapter 1). Furthermore, there is evidence that those obese adults who were obese as children are significantly more likely to suffer the *consequences* of obesity than those who were not obese as children.[6]

However, there is little evidence that the present increasing prevalence of obesity in children and young people is due to increased calorie intake, which leaves open the possibility (and probability) that it may be due to a decrease in physical activity. On average 15 year old girls take 2.4 hours of exercise per week, and boys take 3.6 hours. There is evidence that older girls are, over the years, becoming less fit and that by the age of 14-15 only 25% of girls see themselves as fit.[7]

Further evidence for the influence of diet in childhood and adolescence on adult cardiovascular disease is given by the American post mortem studies mentioned on page 248.

Other factors

Alcohol intake appears to be another possible area where young people's behaviour is sometimes linked with adult behaviour, and which may have a protective effect for cardiovascular disease. One might therefore propose an intervention where encouraging young people to drink wine would have a beneficial effect. However, there is at present no research evidence that young people who start by drinking wine as teenagers continue to drink wine as adults, although it would be reasonable to assume that the social drinking of wine within families in wine-drinking countries such as France may affect what type of alcohol is drunk as adults. This area of research could, in the long run, be fruitful, in that one might look at the long-term outcomes, in terms of cardiovascular disease, of trying to persuade beer-drinking adolescents to become wine-drinking adolescents. However it is doubtful, at the present stage of health promotion in the UK, that an intervention encouraging young people to drink wine, even at the expense of beer-drinking, would be either socially or politically acceptable.

There is no evidence at present that illegal drug-taking or sexual activity in adolescence is linked to adult cardiovascular disease.

Health promotion interventions related to the behaviours of young people

'Health' as defined in this chapter is a concept which will inevitably be deemed more important and of higher priority by those working in the field of 'health promotion' (because their livelihood depends on it), than to young people or the rest of the population. Adolescents, who may be inexperienced but are not illogical, may be perfectly able to grasp many of the concepts of what is good for their 'health' both in the short and long term. But the logic and priorities that young people use when they are dealing with health-related information may not be the same as that used by adults – whether these 'adults' be their parents or professionals with whom they come into contact.

To give an example of these alternative logics and priorities – take a 14 year old girl who has just spent her week's pocket money on the latest fashion in vest tops. She goes out to a party on a coldish night with a vest top, jeans, pants, socks and shoes but little else. She thinks "I look terrific. I want people to see that I look terrific. I want people to see my new top." Her parents think "She will catch cold. She is looking too sexually explicit. Some man will want to have sex with her." Both points of view are perfectly reasonable; they are just based on totally different sets of logic with different priorities. Apart from other considerations, this makes it dangerous to extrapolate from evidence that – because an intervention works with adults – it will also work with adolescents.

Nor, in the field of health promotion interventions, is it useful to conceive of young people's behaviours as 'risk-taking' – mainly because the young people themselves do not see their behaviours as 'risk-taking'. Yes, it is a fact that some of the behaviours that young people experiment with do carry increased health risks, but this experimentation and exploration is also part of the *normal learning process*, not only for young people, but for us all even as adults. This is true over a whole range of behaviours – the music people play, the clothes they wear, the sex they have, the alcohol they use, the drugs they choose to try, the food they eat, the tobacco they smoke, and the exercise they take.

Therefore if as adults, whether parents or professionals involved in health promotion, we undertake to interfere with these normal behaviours in some way, it is our responsibility to ensure that we are having a positive effect. It is not enough just to look at controlled trials and say that, by doing X in the way of an intervention, we can see that Y happens as an outcome. We have to ensure that the actual 'side effects' of the intervention, in terms of changing other behaviours, does not mean that overall the outcomes are worse. Take for example, the young girl and her vest top. If her parents say "We won't let you go out to this party if you are wearing that vest top" they may dis-empower their daughter, and lower her self-esteem and, if the threat is carried through, decrease her chances of normal successful social interaction. How should we weigh that against the risks the parents perceive in her behaviour?

Thus, as adults, we may know that the long-term effects of smoking are going to be bad for young people's health, that the kind of foods that they are eating are clogging up their arteries, that their lack of physical activity will lead to obesity, but do we know what priority this knowledge should have within a young person's own particular life at this particular time in terms of his or her social relationships, his or her economic circumstances, and his or her need to learn and to survive?

If young people *are* inexperienced but not illogical then perhaps the only two interventions that young people should be offered are:

1) knowledge about the short-term and long-term outcomes of certain behaviours, and

2) equality and ease of access to changing to alternative 'healthier' lifestyles.

If we (adults or society) are unable to provide these, should we be interfering at all?

Because of this, and other factors, and with the provisos given above, it is also true that trying to promote the health *of* young people is less confrontational than trying to promote health *to* young people. Trying to promote health *to* adolescents is fraught with paternalistic dilemmas; young people may perceive that such health promotion interventions are based on the concept that adults think that they are wiser and 'know what is better'. In contrast, trying to promote the health *of* adolescents, although based on the same premise, is more subversive and is less confrontational on an individual basis. Both methods do however carry the possibility that not only do the interventions fail but that they may actually be harmful.

Yet there is an obvious dilemma. For instance we do know (and so do by far the majority of young people) that in the long run smoking *is* harmful to health. We also know that after smoking a few cigarettes, and some would suggest as few as five or fewer, there is a very high chance of continuing to smoke cigarettes regularly thereafter because of their extremely addictive nature.

A further dilemma, in the wider perspective, and one that does not belong solely to health promotion to this age group but to health promotion to all age groups, is that of other vested interests – particularly that of political imperatives. Before looking at possible areas of intervention, we therefore need to understand both the complexity of factors influencing young people's behaviours and who the major stakeholders are in influencing the health of young people.

What influences young people's behaviours?

Part of the present singular lack of success in the field of trying to alter health-related behaviours in young people has been the naivety of the approaches and the lack of understanding as to what factors influence adolescent behaviours. The more research that is done in the field, the greater the complexity of the interactive factors which we need to include:

- genetic influences on both physique and behaviours
- the need for survival in a very rapidly changing society
- the socioeconomic environment in which the child or adolescent grows up
- cultural factors relating to the child's or adolescent's background and present environment
- physical and psychological changes relating to puberty
- the influences of the media and advertising
- parental influences
- influences relating to gender
- peer group influences.

Who are the major stakeholders in the behaviour of young people?

There are many stakeholders in the behaviour of young people, and their different influences vary in subtlety, as do the vested interests which are frequently at conflict with one another when it comes to promoting adolescent health. They include:

- young people themselves
- parents
- other members of society

- the government and a variety of government departments
- companies with direct financial interests in young people as a potential market, e.g. for cigarettes, clothes, toys, electronic games, foods, magazines, books
- television
- schools
- primary, secondary and tertiary health care providers, and
- those in any of these areas or other areas, whose livelihood depends on health promotion to or for young people.

What do we know about effective interventions?

None of the evidence available for effective interventions in the field of adolescent health is particularly strong. In fact, where there is evidence, in broad terms almost all discrete single-issue interventions in the field seem not to work. In the field of tobacco use and food intake by young people, what evidence there is would suggest that the most effective interventions are those which involve:

- pricing policies
- advertising policies
- simultaneous multi-dimensional inputs at a national, local and individual level.

Smoking and tobacco

Because of the huge financial interests involved, the extremely serious and deleterious long-term outcomes, and the highly addictive nature of tobacco, the amount of research undertaken in this area is much greater than in the areas of diet, obesity and exercise.

Facts that need to be taken into account in relation to the initiation and continuation of smoking by young people

Presently available facts indicate the following.

- The factors influencing the initiation of smoking in young people are extremely complex.

- There is a sharp rise in smoking in young people between the ages of 12 and 15 and, while many young people are firmly opposed to smoking up to this age span, there is a marked change of attitude thereafter.[7]

- By the age of 16, approximately one-third of young people in the UK will never have smoked, one-third will have tried smoking and stopped, and one-third will have started smoking and will be regular smokers.

- Different factors have different influences on initiation of smoking in the two sexes.

- Some of the factors include family influences – whether the parents smoke, and particularly the mother's attitude towards smoking.[8]

- There may be a genetic factor influencing addictive behaviour but this area is in need of further research.

- The peer groups with which the young person associates have an influence on initiation and continuation of smoking.[9]

- During adolescence there is a more variable smoking pattern of beginning and stopping smoking than is found in adults.

- It may take only five cigarettes or fewer to have a profoundly addictive effect on young people.

- Where or when cigarette advertising is directly or subtly aimed at promoting cigarettes to young people, this has an effect on cigarette smoking in young people.[10]

- As with adults, there is some evidence that pricing of cigarettes affects the continuation of smoking by young people.[11]

- Many young people, having started smoking, wish to give it up.[7,12]

What evidence is there that specific interventions concerning the initiation and maintenance of smoking during adolescence are effective?
(The first three points below were made in a review of the effectiveness of interventions to change health-related behaviours.[13])

1 *"The evidence, at the present time, that school-based programmes for the prevention of smoking uptake by young people are effective is limited. However, programmes which include re-enforcement of social norms and which also include curricular components relating to short-term health outcomes of smoking combined with programmes which give*

information on the social influences which lead to smoking seem more effective than the traditional 'knowledge based' programmes. These again need to be combined with training on how to resist pressures to smoke."

2 *"There is some limited support for the effectiveness of community interventions in helping prevent the uptake of smoking in young people."* [13]

3 *"There is little evidence that local ordinances alone reduce the prevalence of smoking in young people, who can easily obtain tobacco from other sources."* [13]

4 The effectiveness of pharmacological agents (including nicotine replacement therapy) for smoking cessation has been mainly researched in adults where it has been found to be moderately effective. It is possible that this form of intervention may help some young people to stop smoking. A randomised controlled trial under way in Nottingham and funded by Cancer Research UK, is looking at the effectiveness of nicotine replacement therapy in smoking cessation among 12-18 year olds. The results of this year-long trial are expected in 2003.

5 Among adults it appears that education campaigns (such as No Smoking Day) and continued advice and encouragement from health professionals have a small but significant (positive) effect on tobacco cessation. There is limited research into the effectiveness of such interventions in young people except in the case of No Smoking Day, which appears to appeal in particular to younger smokers (aged 16-34).[14]

6 *"Most programmes have targeted 11-17 year olds. However, attitudes towards smoking and experimentation with cigarettes may already be established by this time. Programme implementation before regular patterns of smoking behaviour are formed should be considered. This may involve targeting children as young as 4-8 years of age."* (From *Preventing the Uptake of Smoking in Young People.*[15])

Diet, exercise and obesity

Obesity in young people is the result of several factors – genetics, diet, and physical activity – which are themselves controlled by a number of other factors including availability of different foods, access to exercise facilities, advertising, parental attitudes, etc. Evidence for the effectiveness of specific interventions concerning diet in young people is limited, as pointed out by Jones et al:[16]

"Programmes that have been found to be effective in the USA are those aimed at reducing young people's consumption of saturated fat in snack foods. A variety of interventions are used together – including skills training, practice in menu planning and resisting peer pressure.[17] *Most UK school-based interventions have not yet been proven to have a positive effect. There is, as yet, no evidence of any effective primary care based interventions with young people in relation to diet."*

For physical activity their conclusions were much the same:

"In Australia a 'healthy heartbeat' school initiative produced significant gains in fitness in 11-12 year olds, despite the fact that the initiative did not produce any measurable effects on knowledge, attitudes or behaviours.[18] In adults, the evidence on interventions to increase physical activity suggests that personal instruction, continued support, and participation in an activity which does not necessitate attendance at a special fitness centre, are all important factors in the encouragement of continued participation.[19] There are no fully evaluated studies to suggest whether the same factors are pertinent to young people."

Conclusion

How best to promote the health of young people? It is better to promote health *for* them rather than *to* them, on a number of different levels from government downwards. Preaching does not work, and health professionals are at their most effective a) when we are advocates on behalf of the health of young people, and b) when we provide young people and their carers with the most relevant and up-to-date evidence-based information we can, using the appropriate methods or technologies to make this information available in the most accessible ways, for example through websites such as www.teenagehealthfreak.org or www.doctorann.org.

Recommended action

National government

- Continue to increase greatly the price of cigarettes.
- Ban all cigarette advertising.
- Make nicotine replacement therapy free for all adolescents, if the trial mentioned on page 255 proves it to be successful for smoking cessation in this age group.
- Subsidise the vegetables and fruits available for school meals.

Local government

- Encourage young people to walk or cycle to school by giving priority to pedestrians and cyclists over motor vehicle users.
- Ensure that all state schools have access to proper sports facilities.
- Ensure that all local communities have access to sports facilities.

Primary care

- Provide nicotine replacement therapy free to adolescents.

- Regularly discuss 'smoking' with young people when they attend for related health problems such as chest infections.

- Highlight the many benefits of regular physical activity for young people (for decreasing stress, increasing concentration, increasing the 'feel good' factor, etc), for example through posters in general practice.

- Act as advocates in local communities for access to appropriate sports facilities.

- Act as advocates in local communities for pedestrian and cycle paths to take precedence over motor vehicles.

Others involved in health promotion

- Examine very carefully what has and has not been shown to be useful health promotion to young people and undertake pilot studies before mainstreaming initiatives.

- Promote young people's access to health information that is appropriate to their needs – for example to websites such as www.teenagehealthfreak.org.

References

1 Enos WF, Holmes RH, Beyer J. 1953. Coronary disease among United States soldiers killed in action in Korea: preliminary report. *Journal of the American Medical Association*; 152: 1090-93.

2 McNamara JJ, Molot MA, Stremple JF, Cutting RT. 1971. Coronary artery disease in combat casualties in Vietnam. *Journal of the American Medical Association*; 216: 1185-87.

3 Currie C, Hurrelmann K, Settertobulte W, Smith R, Todd J (eds.) 2000. *Health and Health Behaviour among Young People. WHO Policy Series: Health Policy for Children and Adolescents. Issue 1.* Copenhagen: World Health Organization.

4 Haselden L, Angle H, Hickman M. 1999. *Young People and Health – Health Behaviour of School-aged Children. A Report of the 1997 Findings.* London: Health Education Authority.

5 Thomas M, Walker A, Wilmot A, Bennet N. 1998. *Living in Britain. Results from the 1996 General Household Survey.* London: The Stationery Office.

6 Vanhala M, Vanhala P, Kumpusalo E, Halonen P, Takala J. 1998. Relation between obesity from childhood to adulthood and the metabolic syndrome: population based study. *British Medical Journal*; 317: 319.

7 Balding J. 1999. *Young People in 1998.* Exeter: University of Exeter Schools Health Education Unit.

8 Tyas SI, Pederson IL. 1988. Psychosocial factors related to adolescent smoking: a critical review of the literature. *Tobacco Control*; 7: 409-20.

9 West P, Sweeting H, Ecob R. 1999. Family and friends' influences on the uptake of regular smoking from mid-adolescence to early adulthood. *Addiction*: 94 (9): 1397-1412.

10 Plence JP, Lee I, Gilpin FA. 1994. Smoking initiation by adolescent girls 1944 through 1988. An association with targeted advertising. *Journal of the American Medical Association*; 271: 608-11.

11 Chaloupka I-J, Wechsler H. 1997. Price, tobacco control policies and smoking among young adults. *Journal of Health Economics*; 16: 359-73.

12 Aggleton P. 1996. *Health Promotion to Young People.* London: Health Education Authority.

13 Jepson R. 2000. *The Effectiveness of Interventions to Change Health Related Behaviours: A Review of Reviews. MRC Social and Public Health Sciences Unit. Occasional Paper No 3, May 2000.* Glasgow: MRC Social and Public Health Sciences Unit.

14 McIntyre D. 2001. *No Smoking Day 2001: Awareness and Participation Results.* London: No Smoking Day.

15 NHS Centre for Reviews and Dissemination. 1999. *Preventing the Uptake of Smoking in Young People. Effective Health Care. Volume 5.* London: Royal Society of Medicine Press.

16 Jones R, Coleman J, Dennison C. 2000. *Community Health Provision for Young People: Indicators for Use in Evaluation. A Working Paper for the Trust for the Study of Adolescence.* Brighton: Trust for the Study of Adolescence.

17 King A. 1988. Promoting dietary change in adolescents: a school-based approach for modifying and maintaining healthful behaviour. *American Journal of Preventative Medicine*; 4: 68-74.

18 Plotnikoff R, Williams P, Fein A. 1999. Effects of a school capacity-building intervention on children's health: Evaluation of Coalfields Healthy Heartbeat school project in New South Wales, Australia. *Health Education Journal*; 58; 4: 389-400.

19 Almond L, McGeorge S, Healy C, Laventure B. 1997. *Young People and Physical Activity: A Literature Review.* London: Health Education Authority.

Chapter 12

Synopsis of government policies and initiatives

Louise Sarch

Dr Alison Giles

National Heart Forum

This chapter provides a summary of policies and initiatives, implemented under the UK government since 1997, which have a direct or indirect effect on the heart health of children and young people.

The purpose of this synopsis was to map recent policies and initiatives which influence children and young people's immediate and long-term heart health prospects. It was used as a working paper for the development of recommendations in the National Heart Forum's policy framework document *Towards a Generation Free from Coronary Heart Disease: Policy Action for Children's and Young People's Health and Well-being* to identify gaps, inconsistencies and overlaps in existing policy.

This synopsis is not exhaustive but charts the major policies and initiatives throughout the UK. Efforts have been made to make it reflect developments in Wales, Scotland, Northern Ireland and England but this was not always possible owing to the different policy setting agendas and time frames of the devolved administrations. Most initiatives listed apply to England, but note that each of the devolved administrations may have a similar initiative. For more information, refer to the relevant administration's website. (A list of these is provided on page 281.)

Work is currently under way to tailor the policy framework document *Towards a Generation Free from Coronary Heart Disease: Policy Action for Children's and Young People's Health and Well-being* more appropriately to the needs and developments in Northern Ireland, Scotland and Wales. This includes work on specific policy synopses for each of the devolved administrations.

The initiatives have been grouped in the following sections:

- For children of all ages
- For the under-5s and families
- For children and young people of school age
- For the community
- NHS policies
- Other initiatives

There is a complete index of the initiatives on page 282.

For children of all ages

Children's Commissioner

Northern Ireland – The Committee of the Centre endorsed the appointment of an independent Commissioner for Children in June 2001 and the Commissioner for Children Bill was introduced into the Assembly in June 2002. The Committee of the Centre has since heard oral evidence and will publish its report in due course.

Scotland – The Commissioner for Children and Young People (Scotland) Bill was introduced to the Scottish Parliament in December 2002. The Bill will create a new, unique post, providing a focused approach to the promotion of the rights of children and young people, able to influence decision-making at the highest level. It is expected that the Bill will go forward for Royal Assent in 2003.

Wales – A Commissioner was appointed in March 2001. The Commissioner's functions apply to all children, giving him the power to review proposed legislation and policy from the Welsh Assembly Government considering the potential effect that it might have on children, and to make representations to the Welsh Assembly Government about any matter that affects children.

England – A decision about whether to have a Children's Commissioner for England has not yet been made.

www.childpolicy.org.uk/features/index.cfm?ccs=1681&cs=1172

Children's Rights Director

Appointed by the National Care Standards Commission to safeguard vulnerable children living in children's homes, foster care, boarding schools and in residential family centres.

www.carestandards.org.uk

Children and Young People's Unit

Established in the Department for Education and Skills to support cross-government work on child poverty and youth disadvantage and to establish the principles for involving children in policy development, looking across the full 0-19 age range. Also responsible for implementing and managing the Children's Fund (see page 266). In 2001-02 the Unit consulted on a strategy for children and young people.

www.cypu.gov.uk/corporate/index.cfm

Children's Trusts

The Children at Risk Spending Review 2002 identified that there can be structural barriers to improving the coordination of services for children and young people. In

2003, the Department of Health and the Department for Education and Skills will pilot Children's Trusts, new models for the management of children's services. These Trusts will offer opportunities for local agencies, including education, health and social services, to come together on a voluntary basis in a new structure for joint planning, commissioning and delivery of services.

www.doh.gov.uk/childrenstrusts

Local Preventative Strategy

Chief Executives of all upper tier and unitary local authorities, on behalf of their councils which take the lead on delivering services to children and young people, are to agree a coordinated local preventative strategy by April 2003. The strategy will provide a new mechanism for agencies to work together to achieve better outcomes for children and young people at risk of social exclusion. Interim guidance was issued by the Children and Young People's Unit in December 2002.

www.cypu.gov.uk/corporate/services/preventive.cfm

Children at Risk green paper

In October 2002, preparation of a cross-departmental green paper on Children at Risk was announced by the Prime Minister. The green paper will look at improving services for children and young people at risk of social exclusion, and set out measures to reduce the levels of educational underachievement, offending, anti-social behaviour, teenage pregnancy and ill health. It will be overseen by a new Cabinet Sub-Committee and will have close links to the strategy for children and young people being developed by the Children and Young People's Unit.

www.number-10.gov.uk

For the under-5s and families

Children's Tax Credit/Child Tax Credit

The Children's Tax Credit was an income tax relief scheme to provide extra help for people who have a child or children aged under 16 living with them. It could reduce the amount of income tax paid by up to £529 a year or £10.17 a week in 2002-03. From April 2003, it was replaced by the Child Tax Credit, payable directly to the person mainly responsible for looking after the children, rather than through PAYE.

www.inlandrevenue.gov.uk/menus/credits.htm

Working Families' Tax Credit/Working Tax Credit

The Working Families' Tax Credit aimed to give working families with children a better deal by giving extra help to more families on low and middle incomes. In April 2003, it was replaced by the Working Tax Credit which includes a childcare tax credit element payable to households who are working and have to spend money on childcare.

www.inlandrevenue.gov.uk/menus/credits.htm

Welfare to Work strategy – New Deal

New Deal is individually-tailored practical help and support to improve job prospects among long-term unemployed people.

New Deal for Young People aims to improve job prospects for 18-24 year olds who have been unemployed for six months or more.

New Deal for Lone Parents is available to all lone parents who are not working or working less than 16 hours a week. The scheme provides help with training, looking for work, and finding childcare, including some financial assistance with transport costs and registered childcare while the person is in the scheme.

www.dwp.gov.uk/lifeevent/benefits/index.htm#n

National Family and Parenting Institute

Set up in 1999 under the government's Supporting Families programme to raise awareness of the importance of parenting and the family, particularly among low-income groups. It aims to encourage families to be able to seek help, and to promote a family-friendly society. The Institute runs a 24-hour helpline.

www.nfpi.org

Meeting the Childcare Challenge – a National Childcare Strategy
This provides the framework within which the government is developing good quality and affordable childcare across the country. The aim is to ensure a range of good quality, affordable childcare for children aged 0-14 in every neighbourhood. This includes formal childcare, such as playgroups, out-of-school clubs and childminders, and support for informal childcare, for example relatives or friends looking after children.

www.dfes.gov.uk/childcare

Early Years Development and Childcare Partnerships (EYDCPs)
Part of the National Childcare Strategy, EYDCPs have been set up by every local education authority to map out and develop plans for early education and childcare services for children aged 0-14 in their area. They are responsible for developing and coordinating an ongoing strategy and support structure for sustaining high quality local provision.

www.dfes.gov.uk/eydcp

Free nursery education
Free part-time early education places for all 3 year olds has been set as a 'long-term' target by the government. There are already places for all 4 year olds, and the government has promised that by 2004 there will be places for all 3 year olds. EYDCPs oversee the development of places.

www.surestart.gov.uk/newsShow.cfm?id=103

Neighbourhood Nurseries initiative
This initiative aims to reduce unemployment and child poverty in the most disadvantaged areas by offering childcare services that help parents return to work, and also aims to improve the life chances of children through offering quality childcare and early learning in good environments. Early Years Development and Childcare Partnerships are responsible for developing the neighbourhood nurseries.

www.surestart.gov.uk/infoDocs/neighbourhood_nurseries_guidance1.doc

Sure Start
A cross-government initiative which began as a strategy for children under 4 and their families in areas of disadvantage to promote the health and well-being of pre-school children by providing universal free early education, more and better childcare, increased support through the Working Families' Tax Credit, Children's Centres, and ongoing support for Sure Start local programmes. A Sure Start Unit was established in 2002 and the service was extended to provide support for families from pregnancy

until children are 14. Sure Start will cover a third of all children living in poverty by 2004.

www.surestart.gov.uk/home.cfm

Early Excellence Centre programme

Provides a one-stop shop, giving education and day care for young children up to 5, and services and opportunities for parents, carers, families and the wider community. The aim is to break down the barriers between health and education. In future, these will be linked up locally with Sure Start and Neighbourhood Nurseries to become the Children's Centres (see below).

www.earlyexcellence.org

Children's Centres

These will link up local Sure Start programmes, Neighbourhood Nurseries and Early Excellence Centres to provide a one-stop-shop for childcare, family support and health services, to benefit up to 650,000 children in disadvantaged areas by 2006. They form part of the £1.5 billion combined childcare, early years and Sure Start package outlined in the inter-departmental childcare review, *Delivering for children and families*, published in 2002.

www.strategy.gov.uk/2002/childcare/report/index.htm

Welfare Foods Scheme/Healthy Start

The Welfare Foods Scheme is the state provision of vitamin and milk tokens to families with young children who are living on a low income. In 2004 the Welfare Foods Scheme will be renamed Healthy Start and will be reformed so that resources are more effectively used to ensure that children in poverty have access to a healthy diet, including the provision of healthy weaning foods and increased support for breast feeding and parenting.

www.doh.gov.uk/healthystart/

Extension of the National Curriculum in England to include the foundation stage

The Education Act 2002 extended the National Curriculum for England to include the foundation stage. This means that, from the point at which a child receives government-funded early years education, on or after his or her third birthday, to the end of the school year in which the child is 5 years old, they will be formally taught in the areas of: personal, social and emotional development; communication, language and literacy; mathematical development; knowledge and understanding of the world; physical development; and creative development.

For children and young people of school age

Children's Fund

The Children's Fund of £450 million over 2001-04 is to help prevent vulnerable children and young people from falling into poverty and disadvantage. £380 million of the fund will go on prevention work with children. The fund works in partnership with local authorities and others, including the voluntary sector. Other funding will be available through the Children's Fund Local Networks. The fund will primarily target 5-13 year olds at risk of social exclusion. The Fund is overseen by the Children and Young People's Unit (see page 261).

www.cypu.gov.uk/corporate/childrensfund/index.cfm

Excellence in Cities

Tackles the particular problems facing children in cities. It aims to raise the aspirations and achievements of pupils and to tackle disaffection, social exclusion, truancy and ill-discipline and improve parents' confidence in cities.

www.standards.dfes.gov.uk/excellence

Quality Protects programme

Quality Protects is an initiative which aims to improve services for children in need, including those looked after by local authorities. Between 1999 and 2004, £885 million will be provided to enhance the effectiveness of services for children in need, and an additional £20m has been announced for children and young people's access to modern information technology.

www.doh.gov.uk/qualityprotects/

Beacon Schools scheme

The Beacon School scheme plays a key role in the government's drive to raise standards within education. Beacon Schools are specifically designed to help raise standards in schools through the sharing and spreading of good practice.

www.standards.dfes.gov.uk/beaconschools/

Infant class sizes

Part of the government's drive to raise standards in schools. From September 2001 the School Standards and Framework Act 1998 placed a duty upon local education authorities and governing bodies to limit the size of infant classes for 5, 6 and 7 year olds taught by a single qualified teacher to 30 and below.

www.dfes.gov.uk/governor/faqs.cfm?FCID=7

National Curriculum – Science

From Key Stage 1 through to Key Stage 4, pupils should be given opportunities to consider ways in which science is relevant to their personal health, for example starting with developing an understanding of the relationship between science and personal health, and leading to a more complex understanding of nutrition and the structure of the human digestive system.

www.nc.uk.net/home.html

National Curriculum – Personal, Social and Health Education

Personal, Social and Health Education is a non-statutory subject. It includes guidelines to help pupils live healthily and deal with the spiritual, moral, social and cultural issues they face. The aim is to develop pupils' well-being and self-esteem.

www.nc.uk.net/home.html

National Curriculum – Physical Education (PE)

The National Curriculum specifies general requirements that apply to teaching of all PE lessons across all key stages. Among these are the following requirements which promote physical activity for heart health: pupils should be taught to be physically active, to engage in activities that develop cardiovascular health, flexibility, muscular strength and endurance, and to warm up for and recover from exercise. The Prime Minister has made a commitment that all children will have an entitlement to two hours of high quality PE and school sport a week within and outside the curriculum.

www.nc.uk.net/home.html

Healthy Schools Programme

The Healthy Schools Programme is a joint venture between the Department of Health and Department for Education and Skills to improve standards of health and education and to tackle health inequalities. The aim of this programme is make everyone – young people, teachers, parents and communities – aware of the ways that schools can improve health.

www.wiredforhealth.gov.uk/healthy/healint.html

National Healthy School Standard (NHSS)

A joint initiative of the Department for Education and Skills and Department of Health to support the development of healthy schools in England through an accreditation process for local education and health partnerships. Part of the Healthy Schools Programme, the overall aim of this work is to help schools become healthier and address health inequalities.

www.hda-online.org.uk/html/improving/nhss.html

See also **School nurses** on page 278.

Nutritional standards for school lunches

The Education (Nutritional Standards for School Lunches) (England) Regulations stipulate the minimum provision of foods from the different food groups for lunches served in nurseries, primary and secondary schools maintained by local authorities.

www.dfes.gov.uk/schoollunches/default.shtml

School Meals (Scotland) Bill 2001

This Bill was defeated in Parliament in 2001, but stimulated the setting-up of an expert panel on school meals which spans the education, health and social justice departments. The panel will provide costed recommendations and a fully developed implementation strategy to establish nutritional standards for school meals, improve the take-up of school meals, and eliminate the stigma attached to taking free school meals.

www.scotland.gov.uk/education/schoolmeals/

National School Fruit Scheme

The NHS Plan proposed that every child in nursery and aged four to six in infant schools will be entitled to a free piece of fruit each school day, as part of a national campaign to improve the diet of children, subject to the success of current pilot programmes. The Scheme is being piloted for practicality before national roll-out in 2004.

www.doh.gov.uk/schoolfruitscheme/prevention.htm

Cooking for Kids programme

Cooking for Kids is a partnership between government, the Royal Society of Art's Focus on Food campaign, the Food Foundation and the National Association of Teachers of Home Economics. The programme, which is run in the school holidays, supports the teaching of basic cooking and food preparation skills, and provides facts about nutrition and food hygiene for children. No sustained funding is available.

www.doh.gov.uk/target33/targ33c.pdf

Safer Travel to School – school travel plans

The Department for Transport, the Department for Education and Skills and the Department of Health established the School Travel Advisory Group (STAG) in 1998 to spread best practice and identify practical ways of reducing car use while improving children's safety on the journey to school. A key recommendation was that schools should develop comprehensive travel plans in partnership with their local authority, the police and the health authority, putting forward a package of measures to improve safety and reduce car use. Bursaries and a programme of site-specific advice to help schools develop their travel plans are available.

www.local-transport.dft.gov.uk/schooltravel/index.htm

Active Schools programme

Launched as part of the Sport England lottery strategy, this comprises two national accreditation schemes – Activemark/Activemark Gold (for primary schools) and Sportsmark/Sportsmark Gold (for secondary schools). The awards are made in recognition of a school's commitment to providing a quality programme of physical education and school sport. The scheme is linked to the British Heart Foundation's *Active School* resource packs.

www.sportengland.org/active_schools/index.htm

Active Sports

Introduced to help address inequalities and the under-representation of young females, young people from minority ethnic groups and young people from disadvantaged areas in sport participation, through partnerships between local authorities, governing bodies of sport, and schools. Funding is provided by the Sport England Lottery Fund. Active Sports is the link between Sport England's Active Schools programme (see above) and the Active Communities programme (see page 274).

www.activesports.org/main.asp?page=0

Sale of school playing fields

Approval of the Secretary of State for Education is now needed for any state school to change the use of any field which has been used for school sports in the last five years.

www.dfes.gov.uk/pess

See also **Sale of public playing fields** on page 275.

Out of School Hours childcare

Funding from the New Opportunities Fund has been allocated to fund the provision of good quality, affordable and accessible out of school hours childcare in a range of settings which may involve the public, private and voluntary sectors. Some of this money is available for integrated childcare and learning schemes, which will link into both educational and childcare needs.

www.nof.org.uk/x_text_filter.cfm?loc=edu&inc=index

Out of School Hours learning
Funding from the New Opportunities Fund to enable at least half of all secondary schools, half of all special schools, and a quarter of all primary schools to offer regular out of school hours education activities.

www.nof.org.uk/x_text_filter.cfm?loc=edu&inc=index

School Sports Coordinator programme
A programme established in urban and rural areas of disadvantage. Coordinators work with the families of children attending primary, secondary and special schools to increase sports participation – particularly among girls, ethnic minorities, the disabled and low-income groups – and to improve standards of performance, motivation and achievement in all aspects of school life. The programme involves the Department for Education and Skills, the Department for Culture, Media and Sport, Sport England and the Youth Sport Trust. It is funded by the New Opportunities Fund.

www.dfes.gov.uk/pess

Space for Sports and Arts programme
A programme in primary schools in deprived areas, both urban and rural, to improve the quality of sport and arts provision for curricular and community use. The programme is a collaboration of the Department for Education and Skills, the Department for Culture, Media and Sport, Sport England, the New Opportunities Fund, and the Arts Council of England.

www.sportengland.org/about/reg_offices/briefings/Space_for_sport_arts.htm

Sure Start Plus
Aims to reduce the risk of long-term social exclusion and poverty from teenage pregnancy. The scheme's objectives are to improve the health of pregnant teenagers and teenage parents, to improve learning of teenage parents and their children, to strengthen families and communities, and to improve social and emotional well-being. The scheme has strong links with the Teenage Pregnancy strategy (see page 279), the Connexions service (see below), Health Action Zones (page 278) and Early Years Development and Childcare Partnerships (page 264).

www.surestart.gov.uk/infoDocs/SS__conference_handout.doc

Connexions service
Connexions is the government's new support service for all young people aged 13-19 in England. The service aims to provide integrated advice, guidance and access to personal development opportunities for this group and to help them make a smooth transition to adulthood and working life.

www.connexions.gov.uk/

Educational Maintenance Allowance

Financial assistance to encourage people from low-income households to remain in education after 16. The scheme will be national in 2004.

www.dfes.gov.uk/ema/what.shtml

For the community

Neighbourhood Renewal Strategy and Neighbourhood Renewal Fund
The aim of the strategy is to 'arrest' the decline of deprived neighbourhoods, to reverse it and to prevent it from recurring. It draws on the work of the 18 Policy Action Teams set up by the Social Exclusion Unit to help develop policies to address the needs of deprived neighbourhoods. The strategy focuses on four imperatives: reviving the local economy; reviving and empowering the community; improving key public services, particularly schools, health and the police; and leadership and joint working.

www.neighbourhood.gov.uk/publicationsdetail.asp?id=89

Neighbourhood Renewal Unit (NRU)
At national level, the Neighbourhood Renewal Strategy (see above) is implemented by the NRU which is part of the Office of the Deputy Prime Minister. The unit is responsible for driving progress across government.

www.neighbourhood.gov.uk

Financial services and local shops
Part of the Neighbourhood Renewal Strategy. A fund is available over three years to sustain and improve post offices and associated retail facilities in deprived urban areas (Commitment 15 of the strategy). Extra help is also available for rural post offices. Local strategic partnerships and neighbourhood management pathfinders (see *Neighbourhood management* below) are experimenting with the idea of local retail strategies (Commitment 16).

www.socialexclusionunit.gov.uk/publications/reports/html/action_plan/04.htm

Local Strategic Partnerships (LSPs)
To join up action locally, to bring together local authorities and other public services as well as residents' groups, local businesses and voluntary and community sector organisations. LSPs will identify which neighbourhoods should be prioritised, find the root cause of neighbourhood decline, develop ideas on how organisations and individuals can improve links, and implement agreed actions. Neighbourhood Renewal Fund money is being made available to help the 88 most deprived local authority areas.

www.neighbourhood.gov.uk/partnerships.asp

Neighbourhood management
The goals of neighbourhood management are to bridge the gap between the country's most deprived neighbourhoods and the average, and to improve outcomes in deprived neighbourhoods in terms of less long-term worklessness, less crime, better

health and better qualifications. Local communities will be able to identify local problems, decide what to do about them and ensure that this gets done. A neighbourhood manager will have overall responsibility at the neighbourhood level.

Neighbourhood management is being tested through 'pathfinders' rather than pilot schemes. Pathfinders afford a commitment from a wide variety of sources and a longer timeframe than pilot schemes. Sufficient pathfinders are being run to allow a number of different approaches to be tried, and to test the idea in a range of different areas and tenure mixes.

www.socialexclusionunit.gov.uk/publications/pat/pat4/01.htm

5 A DAY

Five local 5 A DAY pilot initiatives were set up to test the feasibility and practicalities of community approaches to improving access to and increasing consumption of fruit and vegetables. Since then, the New Opportunities Fund has given £10 million to support the establishment of other local 5 A DAY initiatives across the country. Lessons learnt from the first five pilots are set out in two Department of Health publications, which offer practical advice on the planning, setting up and running of an effective local 5 A DAY initiative.

www.doh.gov.uk/fiveaday/

Positive Futures

A joint partnership between Sport England, the Youth Justice Board and the UK Anti-Drugs Coordination Unit. The aim is to use sport to reduce anti-social behaviour, crime and drug use among 10-16 year olds within local neighbourhoods.

www.sportengland.org/active_communities/programmes/positive_futures.htm

Home Zones

At present there is no specific legislation supporting Home Zones in the UK. However, central government has given its support to nine pilot Home Zone schemes across England and Wales and the Scottish Parliament will be initiating three pilots in Scotland. The aim is to improve quality of life in residential streets by making them places for people, and not just traffic. Home Zones are designed to meet the needs of the local community and can provide areas for children to play and encourage environmental improvements.

www.homezonenews.org.uk

Business Impact Task Force

The Business Impact Task Force was established in 1998. Its objective was to establish a framework for businesses to measure and report their impact on society. Members of the Task Force include senior people from industry, government, the voluntary sector and others. The Task Force published its report, *Winning with Integrity*, in 1999.

www.corporate-impact.org/about.asp

Community Empowerment Fund

The Community Empowerment Fund provides funding to set up community networks in the 88 Neighbourhood Renewal Fund districts. It is administered by local community/voluntary sector 'lead organisations'. The networks will bring together the whole range of local organisations in the area, especially those representing the most deprived neighbourhoods and most marginalised groups (e.g. black and minority ethnic groups, and youth). They will bring together the community and voluntary sector, and ensure that they are properly represented on the Local Strategic Partnership.

www.neighbourhood.gov.uk/cef.asp

Education Action Zones (EAZs)

Education Action Zones have been established in areas (urban and rural) where there is a mixture of social deprivation and under-performing schools. The aim is to support schools by bringing them together with local businesses, local councils and others in an action forum. Each EAZ has between 15-25 schools and has a life span of three to five years. At the end of their statutory terms, the EAZs will be brought together with the Excellence in Cities schemes (see page 266).

www.standards.dfes.gov.uk/eaz/

Active Communities

Active Communities is a 'framework' comprising services, products and sources of funding provided by Sport England, often in partnership with other organisations and agencies, to help individuals and organisations to create their own active communities. Positive Futures (see page 273) and Sport Action Zones (page 275) fall under its umbrella.

www.sportengland.org/active_communities/default.htm

Playing Fields and Community Green Spaces

A scheme which aims to enable communities to have access to playing fields, green spaces, and community play areas. The scheme, which is overseen by Sport England, is part of the New Opportunities Fund Green Spaces and Sustainable Communities programme.

www.nof.org.uk/index.cfm?loc=env&inc=gssc

Urban parks and green spaces

Published in 2002, the report *Living Places – Cleaner, Safer, Greener* set out the government's vision for public space, outlining progress to date and signalling their future plans. It proposed the establishment of an inter-departmental ministerial team to improve coordination of policies and programmes across government, and the setting up of a new unit for urban spaces, attached to the Commission for Architecture and the Built Environment, to deliver a comprehensive programme of work for improving urban parks and green spaces.

www.urban.odpm.gov.uk/greenspace/living/pdf/lp_doc.pdf

Planning guidance PPG17 – Open space, sport and recreation

Provides guidance on a new and more effective planning framework for providing, protecting and enhancing open spaces.

www.planning.odpm.gov.uk/ppg/ppg17/index.htm

Sale of public playing fields

The Office of the Deputy Prime Minister now has the power to call for a ministerial decision in planning changes to public playing fields where it would result in a shortage of playing fields for the wider community and where Sport England have objected to the applications.

www.planning.odpm.gov.uk

See also **Sale of school playing fields** on page 269.

Sport Action Zones

The Sport Action Zone (SAZ) programme was launched in January 2000 to address sports deprivation in 12 of the most socially and economically deprived areas in England. Sport England is providing lottery funding of £70,000 a year over a five-year period to provide a manager in each zone whose role is to work with numerous partners to create effective sporting infrastructures and to contribute towards local economic regeneration by adopting more community-driven sporting initiatives. A further 18 SAZs were announced in 2002.

www.sportengland.org

Sport Direct

A telephone and internet advice service proposed in *Sporting Future for All: The Government's Plan for Sport*, published by the Department for Culture, Media and Sport. The service would operate in a similar way to NHS Direct, providing advice on sports and recreation facilities based on a recent nationwide audit.

www.culture.gov.uk/sport

Access to Open Land – Countryside and Rights of Way Act 2000
Introduced to give people better access to open land such as mountains and moorlands, thus offering the opportunity for physical activity. Introduced in November 2000 by the Department for Environment, Food and Rural Affairs.

www.defra.gov.uk/wildlife-countryside/cl/index.htm

NHS policies

The NHS Plan

The *NHS Plan*, published in 2000, set out the government's plan for reforms of and investment in, the health service over the following 10 years. The *NHS Plan* covers both health services and community health aspects. A core principle of the plan is to ensure a healthy population and to work to reduce health inequalities.

www.doh.gov.uk/nhsplan/

Shifting the Balance of Power

Department of Health documents outlining proposed structural changes to the NHS. Recommends that each strategic health authority, primary care group and primary care trust should have a senior member of staff responsible for planning and commissioning local children's healthcare services and that each NHS Trust that provides services for children should have a designated Executive Director with responsibility for protecting children's interests.

www.doh.gov.uk/shiftingthebalance/index.htm

Children's Taskforce

The Children's Taskforce was created in November 2000 to take forward the *NHS Plan* and coordinate health and social care provision for children. The mission of the Taskforce is to improve the lives and health of children through the delivery of needs-led, integrated, effective, and evidence-based services. To deliver this, their work is divided into a number of key projects, one of the most important being the remit to produce the National Service Framework for Children (see below).

www.doh.gov.uk/childrenstaskforce/

National Service Framework for Children

The National Service Framework for Children, due to be published at the end of 2004, will develop new national standards for services for children across both the NHS and social services. The new standards will help to ensure better access and smoother progression in the provision of services for children, from initial contact with the NHS, via a GP surgery or NHS hospital, through to social services support. Children will have access to modern health and social care services which are designed to meet their needs and which involve them and their carers in choices about their care. The framework also covers maternity services.

www.doh.gov.uk/nsf/children.htm

Health Action Zones

Partnerships between the NHS, local authorities, community groups and the voluntary and business sectors. Established in areas of deprivation and poor health to tackle health inequalities and modernise services through local innovation. They aim to develop and implement a health strategy that reduces inequalities, and delivers within their areas measurable improvements in public health and health outcomes, and in quality of treatment and care.

www.haznet.org.uk/

Health Improvement and Modernisation Plans (HIMPs)

The HIMP is the main focus for partnership working between the NHS, local agencies and communities. Led by primary care trusts, they set out a three-year strategic framework for improving health, reducing inequalities and delivering NHS modernisation. They focus on the main healthcare requirements of local people, and how local services should be developed to meet these.

www.doh.gov.uk/pricare/pdfs/nsf_partnershipworking.pdf

Health Visitors, Nurses and Midwives strategy

A strategy developed for nurses, midwives and health visitors to help strengthen the public health aspects of their roles and tackle health inequalities. The strategy will lead to more nurse-led primary care services and give midwives wider responsibility for women's health.

www.doh.gov.uk/pub/docs/doh/nurstrat.pdf

Health Visitor and School Nurse Development programme

A three-year programme to develop family-centred public health roles for health visitors and child-centred public health roles for school nurses. The programme aims to explore and support new innovative programmes of work. Toolkits for school nurses and health visitors have been developed giving examples of best and innovative practice in the public health role to help tackle health inequalities.

www.innovate.hda-online.org.uk

School nurses

The Department of Health document *Making a Difference* set out a child-centred public health role for school nurses, working with individual children, young people and families, schools and communities. The National Healthy School Standard (see page 267) provides a framework for strengthening and delivering the public health role of school nurses within schools.

www.wiredforhealth.gov.uk/new/school_nursing.pdf

NHS Direct
NHS Direct is a confidential telephone advice line staffed by nurses, open 24 hours a day, 365 days of the year. The aim of NHS Direct is to give fast, accessible health advice and information to the general public.

www.nhsdirect.nhs.uk

Personal Medical Service Pilots
A flexible alternative to the General Medical Services contract, enabling GPs and their practices to tailor services to the particular health needs of local people. Many pilots focus on particular patient groups such as older people, children, people in deprived areas, or travellers.

www.doh.gov.uk/pmsdevelopment/whatispms.htm

Healthy Living Centres
Set up in January 1999 by the New Opportunities Fund to promote health in the broadest sense and target areas and groups that represent the most disadvantaged sectors of the population. Healthy Living Centres seek to encourage community participation and complement relevant local and national strategies. Projects include health screening, physical activity programmes, community gardening, crèches, smoking cessation and crime prevention.

www.doh.gov.uk/hlc/index.htm

Teenage Pregnancy strategy
A cross-government initiative led by the Department of Health. The overall strategic goal is to reduce the rate of conceptions among under-18s by 45% by the year 2010 and to enhance support for teenage parents.

www.doh.gov.uk/teenagepregnancyunit/index.htm

Infant Feeding initiative
Provides funding for local projects to encourage breastfeeding. Midwives, health visitors, GPs and other health professionals have been actively providing mothers with information about breastfeeding.

www.doh.gov.uk/newsdesk/archive/august2001/4-naa-31082001.html

Other initiatives

New Opportunities Fund (NOF)

The New Opportunities Fund was established by the National Lottery in 1999 to fund new and innovative projects in health, education and the environment. It promotes health in the broadest sense and targets areas and groups that represent the most disadvantaged sectors of the population.

www.nof.org.uk/index.cfm

Social Exclusion Unit (SEU)

Set up in 1997 to address factors which can affect people's chances of success and good health: poverty, parenting, environment, education and employment. The SEU's work on children and young people has covered: teenage pregnancy; truancy and school exclusion; and 16-18s not in education, employment or training. The Unit's report on young people resulted in the setting up of the Children and Young People's Unit. The SEU has more recently looked at the issues of young people who run away, the educational achievement of children in care, and transport and social exclusion.

www.socialexclusionunit.gov.uk/

UK government websites

UK-wide website

www.ukonline.gov.uk/Home/HOHome/1,1031,~801b22~fs~en,00.html

UK Parliament

www.parliament.uk/

Northern Ireland Executive

www.nics.gov.uk/

Northern Ireland Assembly

www.ni-assembly.gov.uk/

Scottish Executive

www.scotland.gov.uk/topics/?pageid=1

Scottish Parliament

www.scottish.parliament.uk/

Welsh Assembly Government

www.wales.gov.uk/index.htm

Index of policies and initiatives

PART 3

Children's voices

Chapter 13

Social and cultural circumstances and health-related lifestyles – understanding children's experiences and perspectives

Dr Kathryn Backett-Milburn

Dr John Davis

Dr Sarah Cunningham-Burley

Department of Community Health Sciences, Medical School, University of Edinburgh

This chapter:

- examines research on the social and cultural circumstances and lifestyles relevant to children's health behaviours, focusing particularly on children's own definitions and perspectives
- considers how new ways of researching with children demonstrate how they play an active part in shaping their own heterogeneous social worlds
- discusses research – on child poverty, children and social capital, and on children, the body and parental controls – which has relevance for heart health, and
- presents findings from recent research on children's perspectives on social and health inequalities.

Key themes

- Children's childhoods are far from homogeneous; their experiences of health and inequality are diverse, as are their understandings and negotiations of such difference.
- Clear evidence exists that child poverty is associated with a range of outcomes relevant to health including child mortality, morbidity, neglect and physical abuse, poor housing conditions, homelessness, educational attainment, smoking, and lack of self-esteem.
- It is argued that social, emotional and physical factors in childhood are complexly related to health outcomes. Research accessing children's and young people's own perspectives on health indicates that concerns about friendships and family relationships, privacy, personal space and neighbourhoods are more salient to them than adult-defined health promotion concerns.
- It should not be assumed that children hold the same views about health and inequalities as adults; that adults treat children's health in the same way as their own; or that children define and negotiate their own social circumstances in equivalent ways to adults.

Introduction

There is widespread acknowledgement of the impact of socioeconomic inequalities on health outcomes at every stage of the life course, including childhood. Moreover, child poverty is high on the government's agenda and there is concern about social exclusion of vulnerable groups, particularly children. Recent legislation emphasises that children's voices should be listened to and acted upon by adults who make decisions concerning their lives.[1] However, ethnographic data are still lacking on how inequalities relevant to a range of health outcomes, including cardiovascular disease, impact on and are experienced and acted upon by children and their families on a daily basis. In this chapter we examine research which sheds further light on children's social and cultural circumstances and lifestyles relevant to their health behaviours and, particularly, on children's own definitions and perspectives. We begin by considering issues around researching with children and then focus on research on child poverty; children, relationships and social capital; and children, the body and parental controls. We also present some preliminary findings from our own qualitative research which was carried out in Edinburgh.

Background

Children's socioeconomic, cultural and familial circumstances are part of the pathways implicated in health and illness in adulthood.[2] Longitudinal surveys and historical and epidemiological analyses continue to suggest linkages between social class in childhood and subsequent patterns of adult mortality and to unpack the relevant variables and refine the associated indicators.[3, 4] However, these studies can only present a partial picture of causation, as contemporary health concerns and theories of causation informed both the questions asked at any one point in time and the demographic and health data historically recorded. Indeed, recent research has acknowledged this partial nature of epidemiological data by assessing the feasibility of combining it with sociological and demographic approaches to create 'family reconstitution' data. This aims to reconstruct a fuller picture of the socioeconomic circumstances of a sample of families during the course of the 20th century.[5]

In all of this work the voices of children themselves are curiously absent, and adult-defined data about health and illness continue to be accumulated. With regard to health and healthy lifestyles we are still in the early stages of understanding children's own perspectives, the interactive socialisation processes taking place, and the extent to which children play an active part in matters affecting their own health. If childhood experience is indeed creating and recreating inequalities which impact on health in later life, understanding the child's own perspective is surely one of the missing links. This was one of the main reasons for the development of a qualitative study which aims to illuminate the children's everyday experience of inequalities and the production of health variations.[6] In the first phase of our research with children aged 9-12 years, living in two contrasting areas of Edinburgh, one relatively advantaged and one relatively disadvantaged, we explored the children's experiences and perceptions of inequalities in the context of their daily lives. In the second round of interviews we addressed health issues and ideas about health variations more directly, and conducted interviews with parents. Some preliminary findings from this ongoing study are presented throughout the chapter.

Researching with children: setting the scene

There has been a burgeoning international interest in the social study of childhood during the 1990s. In the UK this was reflected in the commissioning of the Children 5-16 Programme by the Economic and Social Research Council (ESRC), but no project specifically addressing children and health was funded. However, the body of multi-disciplinary research on childhood carried out in this programme (and elsewhere) has greatly advanced our wider understanding of the social worlds of children empirically, theoretically and methodologically. Consequently, we start by briefly outlining the main perspectives underpinning research with children, since these also frame our own approach to examining the social and cultural contexts of children's lifestyles and experiences of inequalities.

Firstly, the acknowledgement that children are social actors in their own right and not simply the passive recipients of adult socialisation is fundamental. As Prout has written: "understanding children's active participation in social life is at least as important as mapping the variables that shape their existence".[7] It is important for researchers to address the methodological, theoretical and policy implications of this in contexts where previously children have been denied rights of participation and their voices have been largely unheard.

Secondly, however, like adults, children do not exist in a social or cultural vacuum and neither do their health behaviours and lifestyles. Therefore, it is necessary to understand how they make sense of their lives with and alongside adults and in their own social worlds of childhood, as this is an important part of understanding how they respond to their own social circumstances. Gathering children's accounts of their everyday practices is very illuminative of, for instance, health or inequalities in action; and exploring these with children can elicit their own understandings of structures and cultures. Like adults, children do experience inequalities on a daily basis, and it is possible to learn much about inequalities by listening to how children describe and account for the material realities of their lives, which are embodied in their everyday relationships and behaviours.

Thirdly, there are methodological implications of this paradigm shift in many disciplines[8] from seeing children as objects of study to subjects with whom we research. Researching with children particularly highlights the power relations inherent in the relationship between adults and children, which can be seen to mirror those of the power relations between researcher and researched. Not only does this demand a major attention to ethics but it is also important not to impose an adult view of the world on to the data-gathering and analytical processes; rather, the aim is to be receptive and responsive to children's own interests and concerns.[7] For some researchers this has meant developing child-friendly methods, such as drawing, vignettes and projective techniques.[9, 10] Other researchers argue for reflexive attention to what is happening in the interview setting between adults and children[11] and for a self-conscious attention to everyday ways of relating to and conversing with children.[12, 13] Many researchers, including ourselves, have found that engaging with children's descriptions of their own experiential worlds enables them to express their perceptions and concerns to a researcher more easily than if they were asked about more abstracted adult concepts of, for instance, health or inequalities. For example, an interviewer might hear the child make reference to a health-relevant issue or experience when describing his or her daily life and then work with and build upon that issue, rather than starting directly with generalised health, illness or lifestyle questions.

Finally, though, there is an existing deficit in research with children which also involves their families. Children as active social beings have been largely absent from family studies and in the UK there have been few sociological studies of family groups, of any composition. Classically, health data about all family members, including children, have been gathered from one family member, often the mother, and health issues understood through her perspective. Where data are presently being gathered from more than one family member, including the children, the conceptual and methodological apparatus for making sense of these data is in its infancy.[14] Perhaps this is particularly important in the area of inequalities where 'the family' has been seen as one of the important pathways to adult health experience in both structural and cultural terms.

Children in poverty

There is an accumulating contemporary and historical body of evidence which unequivocally demonstrates the adverse effect on health of child poverty.[15, 16] There has been a dramatic three-fold increase in the prevalence of poverty among children in the last 30 years.[17] Families with children constitute the largest disadvantaged group of the UK population, in both relative and absolute terms, and the child poverty rate in the UK is one of the highest and fastest growing among industrialised countries.[18]

This must surely be the most important 'sociocultural context' for anticipating adverse future health outcomes, including cardiovascular disease. Clear evidence that child poverty is associated with a range of health-relevant outcomes – including child mortality, morbidity, neglect and physical abuse, poor housing conditions, homelessness, educational attainment, smoking, and lack of self-esteem – has emerged from a review of available data commissioned as part of the ESRC Children 5-16 Programme.[19] These findings, alongside data concerning, for instance, diet, exercise and biological predispositions (see other chapters of this book), present powerful evidence that children in poverty have the odds stacked against them in terms of the likelihood of many health outcomes. Moreover, from the life history studies of childhood, Wadsworth[2] concluded that it is probable that social factors operate in a cumulative fashion across the life course, resulting in children from more favourable socioeconomic and educational backgrounds having better health in adult life compared with those in disadvantaged circumstances. Lifestyle factors play a part in this complex picture as do the social, cultural and environmental contexts in which health-relevant behaviours are embedded and given meaning.

It is important to unpack these 'social, cultural and environmental contexts' qualitatively, and from the child's own viewpoint, but at present we have little understanding of how health habits and knowledge interact with social circumstances and experiences during childhood. Shared cultural understandings among groups of children are further important mediators as they may reinforce or challenge biomedically-based health information. For instance, some studies of young children's views of health suggested that they might focus on particular bodily markers of unhealthiness, such as being fat or having rotten teeth, and evaluate participation in physical activity in terms of its social prestige rather than in health payoffs.[9] Moreover, in-depth interview research in middle class families found children often describing how they subverted their parents' attempts to create 'healthy' behaviours with and for them.[20] Comparable research has yet to be commissioned into working class families or those living in poverty.

Social relationships and integration are regularly cited as influencing health and health outcomes in adult life, though there do not appear to be any comparable data for childhood. For example it has been argued that positive health outcomes are more closely related to relative poverty than to absolute poverty and also to a greater degree of cohesiveness of a society.[21] Furthermore, a national survey of poverty and social exclusion in the UK emphasised that:

"People of all ages and walks of life do not restrict their interpretation of 'necessities' to the basic material needs of a subsistence diet, shelter, clothing and fuel. There are social customs, obligations and activities that substantial majorities of the population identify as among the top necessities of life."[16]

However, almost 14% of this sample, presumably including many families with children, said they were too poor to be able to engage in two or more common social activities, such as visiting friends or celebrating special events. Unfortunately, this survey only accessed parents' views of socially perceived necessities for children. Nevertheless, from their replies it seemed that about a third of British children go without at least one 'necessity', such as three meals a day, toys, out-of-school activities, or clothing.

In our Edinburgh study, children highlighted a number of different inequalities including a poverty of material resources, but they also spoke of a lack of control over their life world, a lack of care and love, and a lack of acceptance by their peer group. Preliminary analysis of their accounts suggests that children locate inequalities as much if not more so in relationships and social life as in material concerns. Indeed, most of the children challenged the notion that their lives were affected by inequalities in income. It also appeared that, in the poorer households, gifts and transactions from wider kin were softening material disadvantages for children. However, the children themselves sometimes explained that perceived material advantages (such as particular possessions or items of clothing) in other children were evaluated and experienced in terms of other markers of status such as personality, character and popularity. Relationships were only affected by material inequalities, and experienced *as* inequality, if particular children wished or allowed this to happen. This is illustrated by the following quotation where Liz discussed with the interviewer (JD) how social relationships mediated the importance of fake or real designer items of clothing:

Liz: *Well, there's this girl in ma school, she's in P7, her name's Irene and she finks, she wears fake clothes an that, an just because she's got kicker boots she finks she's the best. She says they're fake, that's fake, no that's fake an all y that an..*

JD: *So she says that to the other children? As if to say, you're no quite ...*

Liz: *You're no really cool cos you've got fake clothes on ...*

JD: *And has that got something to do, is it,... when she's saying it's fake what ...*

Liz: *It's nothin to do wi bullyin or anythin it's just what she's like.*

JD: *She's tryin to say a'm better.*

Liz: *A'm better than you cos I've got big kicker boots an that.*

JD: *Right. If one child doesn't have kicker boots and the other one has kicker boots, how does that come about?*

Liz: *Well, if it's a nice person that's got the kicker boots she just goes, well the other person would probably say tae them, 'Where did you get the kicker boots, they're nice?' and then they would just go, 'Thank you I don't know where a got them, ma mum bought me them', or something (laughs).*

Further material disadvantages in terms of unequal access to organised activities, such as sports, were initially apparent in the interviews with children from the two different areas. In line with many studies in sport and leisure, we found that children in the more affluent area attended more clubs more often than those in the less affluent area. However, more detailed investigation of these children's daily lives led to greater caution in assuming that lesser club sports participation indicated a less active lifestyle for the less affluent children. Indeed, one girl pointed out that she regularly visited her friends who lived at the top of high rise blocks where the lifts were broken and also that, though they did not play adult organised games, they played out in the fields and hills next to where they lived. Furthermore, in the more affluent area most children reported much greater levels of transportation by car and less spontaneous outdoor games, play and walking than did the less affluent children who, by and large, indicated a greater freedom to walk around their areas and to school. When we asked children more specifically about health in the final interviews, most reacted quite angrily to and challenged the suggestion prevalent in the media that British children are less fit. Indeed, based on the interviews to date, we consider that, though there were differences within and between both areas, most of the children in our sample were fairly physically active and specific reasons existed for those who were not.

Children, relationships and social capital

It is increasingly being argued that the relationships between social, emotional and physical factors in childhood and health outcomes are complex. Biomedical models of health have traditionally related individual health outcomes to what individuals choose to eat, drink, and use (e.g. drugs), their levels of physical activity, their genetic inheritance, and their use of available medical services. In contrast material explanations have argued that poor health outcomes relate to poverty and the unequal distribution of resources, for example money, employment, housing, etc. Between these two perspectives, other health analysts have attempted to link material inequalities, psychosocial inequalities and biological influences and outcomes. For instance, Wilkinson[21] argued that the way people treat each other could create stress in individuals that resulted in differential morbidity and mortality. Moreover, he suggested that widening income gaps and economic insecurity create stress in households, which leads to poor health for adults. From this perspective, health variations are related to the fact that material deprivation and anti-social processes affect and cause greater stress in those in lower income groups and such stress affects the immune system.

These arguments about psychosocial stressors, and some suggested links with childhood (e.g. effects on childhood growth[22]), have largely been developed using longitudinal data sets. However, most of these arguments and indicators are related to adult perspectives on health and not all children's experiences of stress will relate to adults' psychosocial stress consequent on economic insecurity. For example peer relational inequality between children has not yet been considered in any detail, even though qualitative research with children and young people about positive mental health regularly points to their emphasis on the importance not just of familial but also of friendship relationships.[23-25] As Armstrong et al concluded from their research with 12-14 year olds:

"Not only were they (family and friends) seen to promote positive mental health through providing feelings of comfort and security, but through their absence, be it as a result of death, arguments or peer rejection, young people experienced more negative feelings. With this in mind professional interventions need to be rooted in an understanding of the informal networks of young people…" [25]

Linked to the psychosocial perspective, it has also been claimed that positive health outcomes are associated with social relationships.[26] Trust, reciprocity, civic engagement, positive attitudes to institutions, networks, community identity and a sense of belonging are believed to promote a positive sense of health.[27] However, although the resultant social capital arguments again point to the importance of home and work-based relations, exactly how these are enacted in everyday social practices and made meaningful through particular cultural lenses, such as those of childhood, has yet to be fully explored. Moreover, it has been argued that there is an overemphasis on the parent-child relationship at the expense of understanding the importance of other influences from kin, peer group, family friends and neighbours.[28] Morrow suggested that the social capital debate was stuck in the socialisation paradigm and failed to understand the creative complexity of social life and potential benefits of cultural variety. She pointed out that:

"Young people are caught in a web of interlinked individual and neighbourhood-specific networks which are in turn embedded in material and environmental circumstances such as street, park and school; and social and family circumstances such as parents' social networks ... These sets of circumstances are likely to be experienced differently as they are mediated by gender, ethnic background and age ... Young people's 'communities' more often constitute a 'virtual' community of friends based around school, town centre and street, friends' and relatives' houses, and sometimes two homes, rather than a tightly bound easily-identifiable geographical location".[28]

Further, Morrow argued that in Putnam's case this focus on socialisation led to the entire focus being on individual parents and individual children as explanations for low social capital. This resulted in a very restricted perspective involving children being seen as 'passive burdens' on adults[26] with, for instance, large families and single parents being specifically pathologised, and complex families overlooked. Importantly this focus denied how children can play an active part in shaping their own lives by, for example, failing to appreciate that children can and do negotiate different locations and social contexts differently, notably at home and school.[28, 29]

There has been very little empirical work investigating children's perspectives on social capital issues. The exception is Morrow,[28] who employed a range of qualitative methods to explore the perspectives on social contexts and environments of 12-15 year olds attending two comprehensive secondary schools in England and to elicit the implications of these accounts for their general well-being. She found that children expressed a fear of sexual attack, vandalism, race-related violence and encounters with the police. They also bemoaned a lack of play facilities and criticised the aesthetics of areas in which they lived and went to school and the places they passed through on their way to school. Interestingly, these young people's accounts also suggested that they were troubled by lack of respect from others in their schools and neighbourhoods and by their lack of inclusion in decision-making processes at home and in school. Her findings also indicated that children appeared very capable of commenting on their social environments, appreciated the importance of school and educational qualifications and that, despite their apparent lack of feeling of self-efficacy and participation in their neighbourhoods, were not as rebellious or disaffected as depicted in much dominant imagery.

In our Edinburgh study, when talking about inequalities, children tended to focus less on material explanations but rather to talk about 'fairness' and 'unfairness' and to locate these principally in social relationships. This finding echoes other research with mid-adolescents about their own self-defined health issues, where concerns about friendships and family relationships, privacy, and personal space were much more to the fore than the adult-defined concerns of exercise, diet, alcohol, drugs, smoking and sexual health.[30] In our study, many children concentrated on poor relationships with adults and with peers, particularly bullying, as explanations of unfairness and experiences of inequality.

We found that children were bullied for a vast variety of reasons, largely centering on being seen as 'different', such as wearing glasses, clothing, age, size, gender, ethnicity, religion, wealth (children from a fee-paying school talked about being challenged on the way home from school by those from state schools), noticeable behaviour traits, or the area they lived in. One example came from Jake, who explained:

Jake: *Um, well, Joe bullies like Molly, Pat. Pat's weak and everybody says things about Molly. Like, if you touch her you get Molly disease. ... the boys are the mostly strong, I think there's one boy, well, sometimes they pick on Rob, who is the fat one.*

JD: *But it's sort of different things that they pick. It seems to be ...*

Jake: *Yeah, but I'm the most popular for battering, I think. I'm the favourite punching thing.*

JD: *And do you fight back, or... what do you do if something happens?*

Jake: *Oh, oh, oh! No way.*

Our study indicates that experiences and relationships with peers are extremely important in children making sense of inequality. Many children discussed bullying and suggested that it was usual to experience some form of bullying in schools, but indicated that whether this became sustained depended on the ability of the child to stand up for him/herself and the ability of teachers to believe the pupil being bullied. Interestingly, some children who attended fee-paying schools suggested that there was benefit to wearing school uniform. They suggested that it meant that there was not a 'trainer culture' in their school and acted as an equaliser so that children did not pick on each other for the clothes they wore. Ironically, other children from the same school suggested that there was a danger to wearing school uniform on the way home because children from state schools could identify and bully them. Thus the same artefact, a uniform, had different cultural significance depending on the settings and contexts in which the children found themselves.

Such accounts illustrate how 'unfairness' and children's experience of inequality was developed and sustained through everyday interactions and social processes involving both children and adults. Other examples of unfairness were related to adults exercising unfair power over children and not listening to them, for instance, complaining about street play, or moving children on from certain areas. From our interviews it seemed that such experience of adults having unequal power over children was keenly felt, as the following example illustrates:

Pete: *Sometimes when we play in the park, the parkie comes and tells us off. All they say is, 'If you play a game, we will just', because they can't do anything, they just take you home quite a lot of times, just for playing near, there's a, you know, what was the work site?*

JD: *Aye.*

Pete: *Well, you know down from it how there's a forest kind of down there that goes right past the back of the (exhibition place) and I was playing there one day, and there was already smashed windows and we got in trouble. They said we smashed the windows and all we were doing was walking past.*

Children also talked about positive experiences with adults which they considered to be examples of 'fairness'. Such accounts could be seen as children valuing adults who did not exercise power inappropriately. Extrapolating from children's descriptions of their daily experiences, such adults were those who treated boys and girls the same; did not shout; showed an interest in them; were funny but were also strict when necessary; or helped them when they were sick, tired or sad. Children said they valued people who listened to them, asked questions, and believed them when it was important.

Children, the body and parental control

Culturally, another important area of interest for health is how adults and children perceive the body and how it is to be managed and looked after. Here studies have suggested that ideas about body maintenance are far from shared and fixed either among adults and children, or across the life course. Qualitative studies with British adults have shown that the same health-relevant behaviours and how the body is to be looked after are evaluated differently depending on the perceived stage of the life course. For instance, behaviours which might be seen by the respondents as potentially damaging or detrimental to the middle-aged body, such as eating too much junk food or engaging in physically dangerous sports, were defined as more acceptable for younger, more resilient bodies.[31] Related findings have emerged from a study of perceived family history of heart disease.[32] In this study, both adult respondents who saw changing their own health behaviours as somewhat pointless, and those who expressed motivation to improve such behaviours, all stressed the importance of ensuring that their children took up healthy lifestyles before it was 'too late'.[33] Therefore, in order to understand the sociocultural contexts of children's health lifestyles it is important to investigate how children see and experience their own bodies and health concerns, as well as how adults see and influence children's health concerns, and to highlight points of convergence and divergence, which may have behavioural outcomes.

Prout pointed out that:

"... children's understandings of the body cannot be treated as an imperfect or incomplete version of the adult. Rather, children understand and perform their bodies in ways often different from adults." [34]

Although there are now some data on children's views about health and illness, much of this has been conducted using projective techniques, such as the draw and write technique, in the school setting.[35] Research is only beginning to focus on how children manage and negotiate health-relevant behaviours on a daily basis in other settings, notably the home, and the part played by parents or carers in these processes.[29] Moreover, previous research has often focused on children's developing understandings of illnesses and their bodies[36] which, it has been argued, has tended to be too problem-oriented and focused on the deficits in children's knowledge compared with that of adults.[37] Further understandings of how social and cultural contexts may influence health-relevant behaviour in childhood can be gained by examining work about how children relate to the body and how it is being managed and controlled in the private and public spaces of childhood.

Echoing the experiences of those working in health promotion, qualitative research on middle class families found that children, like their parents, were able to cite the headline messages about healthy lifestyles.[9] However, the precise details of exactly how health messages were to be put into operation in actual behaviour and fitted into existing behaviours and body management appeared to be much less clear. Both adults and children in this research study spoke about health and healthy bodies predominantly in terms of *immediately* identifiable and/or visible short-term physical and psychological signs and signals such as energy levels, social functioning, physical and mental activity and performance, and feelings of wellness and fitness.[20] It seemed easier for these middle class children to identify signs of *unhealthiness*; and they talked about peers who were fat, physically lazy or unfit, ate too many sweets or had rotten teeth. However, behaviours which might be defined as 'healthy' by adults were often valued by the children more for their immediate payoffs. For instance, having a fit and not fat body was valued because it led to inclusion in games, pleasure, personal credibility and peer acceptance; and these comments were qualitatively different from the more self-conscious exercising of the adult body for health and social benefits as described by their parents. These children found it much harder to identify signs of *healthiness* and were even more reluctant to identify and comment on markers of adult healthiness or unhealthiness, for instance in their parents. Christensen's[38, 39] ethnographic and observational research in schools provided further illumination of children's cultural understandings about everyday illness and bodily malaise. She found that children identified illness more by the change in everyday routines and social interactions, such as how they related to other children, whereas adults saw it more as something physically wrong with the child which needed to be fixed. This resonates with early findings from our current Edinburgh study which suggested that children found it hard to identify and name life-threatening illnesses in the adults and relatives they knew and therefore meaningfully to participate in 'adult-framed' discussion of long-term illness causation.

Just as we can learn about children's own understandings of their bodies and health through exploring how they negotiate their social worlds at home and school, so research on children and risk is illuminating how children's physical mobility and vulnerability are being shaped and constrained by culturally mediated fears at the turn of the 21st century. Issues of children's personal safety and the risks and dangers they face in the course of their daily lives have become a key social and parental issue in the UK. It has been argued that 'risk anxiety' has had demonstrable material effects on many child-rearing practices and thus on how children themselves view their worlds and themselves as social actors.[40] It has also been claimed that there have been knock-on effects on health and well-being, most notably the 'couch potato' syndrome and resultant increase in childhood obesity. However, although the greater restrictions currently placed on children's independent mobility are located in part in parental fears for their safety, there is often a disparity between the statistical likelihood of threats to children and how these are portrayed in the public discourse and the media. One study indicated that 'stranger danger' was the greatest fear of 98% of parents. However, in the UK between 1984 and 1994 less than 6 children under 14 were killed by strangers each year. Such contradictions suggest the relevance of understanding the social and cultural construction of risk anxiety and how parents translate this into control over children, their mobility and activities, as much as documenting actual dangers.

In a recently completed study,[41, 42] younger children (aged 10-12 years) perceived risk as emanating primarily from public spaces and very few of them spontaneously mentioned risks in the home. Consequently, although children described many instances of subverting their parents' controls, for instance by manipulating the times they should come home from play or go to sleep at night, or exploring places and activities forbidden by parents, overall most acquiesced in their parents' controls over their movements. Several said that their parents' restrictions over their independent mobility and the extent to which they were encouraged to take public or private transport rather than to walk, constituted evidence of caring and a concern for their safety. Thus it could be argued that cultural constructions of unsafe people and public places are providing the framework for more home-based and inactive lifestyles in children, which may have implications for future heart health.

Conclusion

Although researching with children is a greatly expanding field, there are still relatively few studies which illuminate children's own perspectives and everyday experiences of either health or inequalities. Indeed, it has only recently been acknowledged that children play an active part in shaping their own worlds within the constraints of the adult environments which they must negotiate. Importantly, children's childhoods in the UK at the turn of the century are far from homogeneous; their experiences of health and inequality are diverse as are their understandings and negotiations of such difference. Moreover, as we have discussed, it cannot be assumed that children hold the same views about health and inequalities as adults; that adults treat children's health in the same way as their own; or that children define and negotiate their own social circumstances in equivalent ways to adults.

In this chapter we have begun to map out some of the parameters of the social and cultural contexts of children's experiences of inequalities. Most importantly, the experience of childhood poverty is undeniably damaging on a number of health fronts. However, to understand fully the social and cultural mechanisms involved in the reproduction of health inequalities, it is also important to understand the production and reproduction of positive health and health-relevant behaviours and experiences. Research into children's own accounts of their daily lives has begun to illuminate what they feel is fair and unfair; how they view, experience and manage material and relational inequalities; how they view health and their bodies; and what they feel they can or cannot do. Through addressing children's own perspectives we move from considering health outcomes to be simply the consequence of individual choice or structural forces and allow for the incorporation of cultural factors. Such movement also directs attention to the production and re-creation of inequalities and exclusion at the level of everyday social processes, which are more fluid and consequently less easy to address in policy terms. However, this discussion suggests that a multi-level approach is necessary to tackle inequalities and the production of health variations in childhood; and supports the conclusion from Morrow[28] that:

"... social policies which are aimed at addressing health inequalities would do well to pay attention to children's quality of life,[43] in the broadest sense, in the present, as well as/or rather than be driven by a perspective which prioritises children as future citizens, in terms of human capital.[44]"

References

1 Morrow V, Richards M. 1996. The ethics of social research with children: an overview. *Children and Society*; 10: 28-40.

2 Wadsworth MEJ. 1997. Health inequalities in the life course perspective. *Social Science and Medicine*; 44: 850-69.

3 Davey Smith G, Hart C, Blane D, Hole D. 1998. Adverse socioeconomic conditions in childhood and cause specific adult mortality: prospective observational study. *British Medical Journal*; 316: 1631-35.

4 Brunner E, Shipley MJ, Blane D, Davey Smith G, Marmot MG. 1999. When does cardiovascular risk start? Past and present socio-economic circumstances and risk factors in adulthood. *Journal of Epidemiology and Community Health*; 53: 757-64.

5 Razzell PE, Barker D, Braham P. 2000. *Unravelling the Childhood Determinants of Adult Health: A Methodological Pilot Study. Final Report*. Swindon: Economic and Social Research Council.

6 Backett-Milburn K, Cunningham-Burley S. 2001. The socio-economic and cultural contexts of children's lifestyles and the everyday production of health variations. *ESRC Health Variations Programme Phase 2. Final Report*. Swindon: Economic and Social Research Council.

7 Christensen P, James A (eds). 2000. *Research with Children: Perspectives and Practices*. London and New York: Falmer Press.

8 Woodhead M, Faulkner D. Subjects, objects or participants? Dilemmas of psychological research with children. In: Christensen P, James A (eds). 2000. *Research with Children: Perspectives and Practices*. London and New York: Falmer Press: chapter 1.

9 Backett K, Alexander H. 1991. Talking to young children about health: methods and findings. *Health Education Journal*; 11: 2-24.

10 Williams T, Wetton N, Moon A. 1989. *A Picture of Health: What Do You Do that Makes You Healthy and Keeps You Healthy?* London: Health Education Authority.

11 Davis JM. 1998. Understanding the meanings of children: A reflexive process. *Children and Society*; 12: 336-48.

12 Mayall B. Conversations with children: working with generational issues. In: Christensen P, James A (eds). 2000. *Research with Children: Perspectives and Practices*. London and New York: Falmer Press: chapter 6.

13 Harden J, Scott S, Backett-Milburn K, Jackson S. 2000. Can't talk, won't talk? Methodological issues in researching children. *Sociological Research Online*; vol 5 (2). http//www.socresonline.org.uk/5/s/harden.html

14 Ribbens McCarthy J, Holland J, Gillies V. 1999. Multiple perspectives on the 'family' lives of young people: methodological and theoretical issues in case study research. Paper presented to the British Sociological Association Annual Conference, 'For Sociology', University of Glasgow, April 1999.

15 Shaw M, Dorling D, Gordon D, Davey Smith G. 1999. *The Widening Gap: Health Inequalities and Policy in Britain*. Bristol: The Policy Press.

16 Gordon D et al. 2000. *Poverty and Social Exclusion in Britain*. York: Joseph Rowntree Foundation.

17 Bradshaw J. 2001. *Poverty: The Outcomes for Children*. London: Family Policy Studies Centre.

18 Bradshaw J. 1990. *Child Poverty and Deprivation in the UK*. London: National Children's Bureau.

19 Bradshaw J. 2000. Poverty: the outcomes for children. *ESRC Children 5-16 Research Briefing no 18, July 2000*. Swindon: Economic and Social Research Council.

20 Backett-Milburn K. 2000. Children, parents and the construction of the 'healthy body' in middle-class families. In: Christensen P, James A (eds). 2000. *Research with Children: Perspectives and Practices*. London and New York: Falmer Press.

21 Wilkinson R. 1996. *Unhealthy Societies*. London: Routledge.

22 Blane D, Montgomery S. 2000. Workplace factors within a lifecourse perspective and their influence on health in early old age. Paper presented to the 8th ESRC Health Variations Programme Meeting, 25-26 September 2000, Lancaster House Hotel, Lancaster.

23 Hill M, Laybourn A, Borland M, Secker J. Promoting mental and emotional well-being: the perspectives of younger children. In: Trent D, Reed C (eds). 1997. *Promotion of Mental Health. 5.* Aldershot: Avebury.

24 Gordon J, Grant J. 1997. *How We Feel.* London: Jessica Kingsley.

25 Armstrong C, Hill M, Secker J. 2000. Young people's perceptions of mental health. *Children and Society;* 14: 60-72.

26 Coleman JS. 1988. Social capital in the creation of human capital. *American Journal of Sociology;* 94 (Supplement): S95-S120.

27 Putnam RD. 1993. *Making Democracy Work: Civic Traditions in Modern Italy.* Princeton, NJ: Princeton University Press.

28 Morrow V. 2000. 'Dirty looks' and 'trampy places' in young people's accounts of community and neighbourhood: implications for health inequalities. *Critical Public Health;* 10: 141-52.

29 Mayall B. 1994. *Negotiating Health: Primary School Children at Home and School.* London: Cassell.

30 Schucksmith J, Hendry LB. 1998. *Growing Up and Speaking Out: Young People's Perceptions of their Own Health Needs.* London: Routledge.

31 Backett K, Davison C. 1995. Lifestyle and lifecourse: the social and cultural location of health behaviours. *Social Science and Medicine;* 40: 629-38.

32 Emslie C, Hunt K, Watt G. 2000. 'It's a family affair'. Lay understandings of a 'family history' of heart disease. *ESRC Health Variations Programme Findings no 2, May 2000.* Swindon: Economic and Social Research Council.

33 Personal communication with K Hunt and C Emslie, 2001.

34 Prout A (ed). 2000. *The Body, Childhood and Society.* Houndmills and London: Macmillan Press Ltd: 2.

35 Oakley A, Bendelow G, Barnes J, Buchanan M, Hussain OA. 1995. Health and cancer prevention: Knowledge and beliefs of children and young people. *British Medical Journal;* 310: 1029-33.

36 Eiser C, Patterson D. 1983. 'Slugs and snails and puppy-dog tails' – children's ideas about the inside of their bodies. *Child: Care, Health and Development;* 9: 233-40.

37 Sandbaek M. 1999. Children with problems: focusing on everyday life. *Children and Society;* 13: 106-18.

38 Christensen PH. 1993. The social construction of help among Danish children: the intentional act and the actual content. *Sociology of Health and Illness;* 15: 488-502.

39 Christensen PH. 1999. 'It hurts': Children's cultural learning about everyday illness. *Etnofoor;* 12: 39-52.

40 Scott S, Jackson S, Backett-Milburn K. 1998. 'Swings and roundabouts': Risk anxiety and the everyday worlds of children. *Sociology;* 32; 689-705.

41 Harden J. 2000. There is no place like home: The public/private distinction in children's theorising of risk and safety. *Childhood;* 7: 43-60.

42 Scott S, Jackson S, Backett-Milburn K. 2000. *The Impact of Risk and Risk Anxiety on the Everyday Worlds of Children. ESRC Children 5-16 Programme. Final Report.* Swindon: Economic and Social Research Council.

43 Casas F. 1997. Children's rights and children's quality of life: conceptual and practical issues. *Social Indicators Research;* 42: 283-98.

44 Qvortrup J. Preface in: Qvortrup J, Bardy M, Sgritta G, Wintersberger H (eds). 1994. *Childhood Matters: Social Theory, Practice and Politics.* Vienna: Avebury/European Centre.

Chapter 14

Children and young people: their social context and attitudes to smoking, physical activity and diet

Adam Crosier

Freelance research consultant

Dominic McVey

Freelance research consultant

Lynne Walsh

Freelance journalist

This chapter:

- summarises key research knowledge relating to young people's knowledge and attitudes concerning smoking, physical activity and diet, and
- presents knowledge of the social – and particularly the familial – contexts in which these individual determinants of coronary heart disease (CHD) occur.

The authors would like to thank the Royal College of Physicians for giving permission to reproduce extracts from their book *Smoking and the Young*[1] for the section in this chapter on *Smoking* (pages 319-325).

Key themes

- Transition from childhood to adulthood encompasses a wide range of experiences. Many children and young people feel that adults have contradictory views on the competence and responsibilities of young people.
- Spending time with friends is very important for children and young people. They see friends as sympathetic and uncritical people who offer support and advice, and keep confidences. Peer pressure is an important factor among young people and is key to many health behaviours.
- Children and young people are important consumers, with 13-16 year olds spending £16 - £17 a week.
- Child poverty increased three-fold in the 20 years from 1980 to 2000. In 1995 the UK had the highest child poverty rate among the 13 countries of the European Union.

Smoking (page 319)

- Smoking accounts for around 120,000 premature deaths each year in the UK. Almost all smokers take up the habit before adulthood. While rates of smoking among adults have fallen over the past 30 years, there has been no reduction in the numbers of young people taking up smoking.
- The routes in to smoking are complex but include personal factors, family smoking behaviour and the degree of acceptance/rejection of smoking in society.
- Among children and young people, knowledge of the health risks of smoking is high.
- Forty per cent of current young smokers said they would like to stop smoking. Two-thirds of current smokers have tried to give up. The main motivators for giving up are concerns about health, the cost, and the desire to feel fitter.

Physical activity (page 326)

- The aspects of physical activity enjoyed by 5-15 year olds include: team games/competitions, playing with friends, being active, developing skills, and competence.

- Their dislikes include: bad experiences at school, having to play outdoors in bad weather, and having too many rules/restrictions. Negative experiences of physical education at school included: the clothes they had to wear for it, changing and showering facilities and routines, the lack of choice of activities, and the authoritarian style of teaching.

- Young people recommend that physical activity should be marketed on the basis of the enjoyment, fun and social aspects rather than the health benefits, and that there should be a focus on improved feelings of well-being.

Diet (page 342)

- Forty per cent of 11-16 year old boys and 31% of girls agree with the statement 'I just eat the foods I like and don't worry about whether they are healthy or not.'

- One-third of young people (33% of boys and 31% of girls) think they do not know enough about the foods that are good for you.

- Influences on food choices for children and young people include family, friends, and the marketing activities of the food industry.

- Nearly £400 million per year is spent by children on the way to and from school. Most of this money is within the child's control to spend, and represents a significant and lucrative market for food manufacturers, many of whom advertise high sugar, high fat products to children.

Introduction

National surveys that examine young people's health behaviours – including the Department of Health's Teenage Smoking Attitudes survey, and the National Diet and Nutrition Survey of 4-18 year olds – provide vital information on the health status of young people. While such surveys are essential for strategic planning, they contribute but one piece of the jigsaw in developing an understanding of children's behaviour. Few of the national surveys provide insights into the influences on young people's behaviours, nor indeed an understanding of their beliefs and attitudes, nor of the social world within which young people live. If interventions to improve the health of young people are to be successful, a thorough understanding of these issues is essential.

Research on children's beliefs and practices across a range of issues is fragmented and uncoordinated, making the task of assembling a picture of contemporary children's health and lifestyles difficult. It is beyond the scope of this chapter to provide a complete picture of children's knowledge, attitudes and beliefs in relation to smoking, physical activity and diet. Rather, this chapter reports on research studies which capture children's views, and provides an analysis of the context within which these views are formed. Similarly, the 'social aspects' section of this chapter (see page 308) is not a comprehensive or systematic review of research, but a synthesis of selected studies to provide background data on the social world of the child.

This chapter draws on published and unpublished academic research studies and reports, and also includes findings from commercially funded research on children's and young people's lifestyles.

Learning from children and young people

In recent years there has been growing recognition of the importance of participatory approaches to health improvement. In the past, many policies to promote health failed because they ignored the needs and the views of those they were intended to serve.

Moreover, legislative change – both nationally in the form of the Children's Act (1989), and internationally in the form of the UN Convention on the Rights of the Child (1990) – place a duty on the government to ensure that its actions are conducted in the best interests of children and young people. Article 12 of the UN Convention accords children a specific right to free expression of opinion in matters affecting the child.

There are additional factors and influences on the drive towards more participative and inclusive approaches to policy-making. These include the government's commitment to extend the practice of democracy and to modernise the way that government operates. Examples from the Cabinet Office's Social Exclusion Unit – in their preparation of policy recommendations in the areas of teenage pregnancy prevention, neighbourhood renewal and rough sleepers – serve as models for how consultation with social groups previously excluded from the policy-making process may be conducted.

The movement towards evidence-based health and social care goes a long way towards ensuring the empowerment for young people to which many service providers aspire. The best way to identify problems and work towards solutions is to ask the people closest to the issues. It is dangerously wasteful to ignore the reservoirs of expertise which children and young people, families and community groups have on health issues.

Consultation with groups in whose name policies are developed offers a number of additional opportunities:

- to 'road test' proposals – and thereby improve the viability and credibility
- to identify further gaps in knowledge
- to identify creative and practical solutions.

Finally, it is important to recognise that the needs of children and young people are multi-faceted and reflect the diversity of people assumed by the category. Children and young people are not a homogeneous population, and research efforts must be sensitive to the different interests and needs that arise not only from different age groups, but also from differences in sex, family circumstances, educational opportunity, social class, ethnicity and other social characteristics.

Social aspects

"If there is anything that we wish to change in the child, we should first examine it and see whether it is not something that could better be changed in ourselves." Carl Gustav Jung

This section examines some of the key social and economic factors which may affect the health of children and young people. It focuses on some of the hard facts which help to paint a picture for us of the circumstances in which many children and young people live. It also gives a snapshot of some of the stages on the route to adulthood.

Transition to adulthood

The transition from childhood to adulthood is fraught with difficulty, not least because of the fundamental disparity between various legal restrictions and rights which govern children's lives. Children and young people themselves point out the incongruity, and often express this in a cynical way:

"...and another thing, they keep changing when you're gonna be an adult, like on the bus, you have to be 15, in the cinema you have to be 15, but in other things like alcohol, you have to be 18 to buy it." [13]

The law may act as a restriction on children's actions some of the time, but certainly not in all cases. For example, the age of consent to sex is set at 16 for young women, yet almost one in five women aged 16-19 have experienced sexual intercourse before the age of 16. For young men, the percentage of those who have had first sex before the age of 16 is almost 28%.[14]

The law stipulates that children can get certain part-time jobs at the age of 13, yet, for example, there are many paperboys and girls under this age. Research conducted by MORI for the TUC in 1996-97 showed that a quarter of 11-15 year old children said they had a current term-time job.[15]

It may be that there has been a blurring of the boundaries between childhood and adulthood. Many children take on responsibilities at an early age, perhaps caring for younger siblings, doing household chores or running errands. Meanwhile, young adults may be in higher education for longer, and in greater number, than in previous years. Some may also still live in the parental home, or have returned to it.

There are scant data on the timing or nature of leaving the parental home, but the Survey of English Housing[16] suggested that a greater proportion of men and women aged 20-24 in England were living with their parents in 1998-99 than in 1991. Data from the British Household Panel Survey for the first half of the 1990s suggested that if a young adult (defined here as 16-30) were unemployed, this increased the

Key facts about young people

- One in 16 young people leave school each year without qualifications.[2]
- One in eleven 16-18 year olds are not in education, employment or training at any one time.[3]
- One in five 14-15 year olds spend a night away from home without parental knowledge or permission each year.[4]
- One in five 16-24 year olds experience homelessness at some time in their lives.[5]
- One in six 16-24 year olds will be the victim of a violent offence in any one year.[6]
- One in five children are growing up in workless households – a higher figure than in any other OECD country.[7]

Trends

- At the end of the 1970s, one in ten children lived in poor households. Today, it is one in three (defined by the DSS as those with a total income below half the national average, after housing costs.)[8]
- At the end of the 1970s, around 7% of children lived in households with no adult in work; by 1995-96 this number had risen to 21%.[9]
- Permanent exclusions from school have risen from 4,000 a year in 1991-92 to more than 12,000 in 1997-98.[10]

The changing shape of the family

- Four out of ten children are now born outside marriage.[11]
- By the time they reach 16, more than one in four children will have experienced the divorce of their parents.[12] (Here, divorce refers to all parental separations.)
- More than three-quarters of children living in lone parent families experience poverty, compared with less than a fifth of those living in two-parent families.[8]

likelihood of leaving the parental home. However, if they were away from home and became unemployed, they were more likely to return home.[17]

In 1998-99, almost half of young people aged 16-24 in Great Britain not living with their parents were living as couples, with or without dependent children. About one in six women not living with their parents were lone parents. (The proportion of men who were lone parents was negligible.)[15] See Tables 1 and 2.

Table 1 ***Young people in households in Great Britain: by age and type of family, 1998-99***

	Age in years			
	13-15	16-17	18-20	21-24
Living with parents*				
Dependent child	100%	66%	12%	-
Non-dependent child	-	32%	60%	45%
All living with parents	100%	98%	72%	45%
Not living with parents**	0%	2%	28%	55%

* Includes dependent children living with older relatives.
** Includes non-dependent children living with older siblings where parents are not present.

Source: See reference 15.

Table 2 ***Young people aged 16 to 24 in Great Britain not living with their parents*, by gender and family type, 1998-99***

	Males	Females
Living alone	19%	9%
One-family households		
Couple		
No dependent children	23%	31%
Dependent children**	16%	18%
Lone parent	0%	18%
Other households***	42%	24%
All young people not living with parents	100%	100%

* Includes non-dependent children living with siblings where parents are not present.
** May also include non-dependent children.
*** Includes two or more unrelated adults.

Source: See reference 15.

The diversity of children's and young people's lives raises a number of questions about the nature of the transition period to adulthood. If an 18 year old is at college but still living at home, is he more or less of an 'adult' in the eyes of the law (or of his peers) than a 16 year old who has a full-time job and is living with a partner away from the parental home?

Some young people have expressed the difference they see between 'feeling adult', 'being adult' and 'settling down'. In a study carried out by Save the Children between 1998 and 2000,[18] 108 young people aged 14-27 in Great Britain were asked for their views on making the transition from 'childhood' to 'adulthood'. What was special about this group was that they were regarded as having taken on responsibilities beyond their years: they were teenage mothers, care leavers, young workers, and those participating in youth organisations.

Many respondents said they looked after themselves at home or had experience of looking after younger siblings or did the food shopping and cooked meals. They felt that the skills they acquired helped them in maturing to adulthood. In fact, several felt these were more useful than the academic work on offer at school:

"...you don't actually need, I believe, to know what Pythagoras' theory is. You don't actually need that. You need to know how to cook a dinner. You need to know how to handle some money or whatever." 17 year old male

Most of the group said that 'feeling adult' came with experience and responsibility, whatever one's age. 'Being an adult' was associated with legislation rights and status. 'Settling down' meant that the transition was complete, and implied a happy family life, a good job and a stable income.

Some respondents said that adults seldom respected them as people rather than as children. They felt they had gained valuable experience but that this was not often recognised as making a legitimate or useful contribution to society as a whole.

A study of some 140 children in London schools[19] reported that the children found that adults held conflicting views on the children's competence, particularly in areas of trust and responsibility. At school, children may not be believed or regarded as 'reliable moral actors', yet they were also expected to carry out considerable responsibilities: for childcare, household jobs and school-related work.

What is 'youth'?

Defining the 'teenager' or 'youth' may now be recognised as an impossible and pointless pursuit. In the mid-1960s however, the demarcation lines which marked out mods from rockers, and in the 1970s, punks from skinheads, appeared clearer. These centred especially on fashion in clothes, music and language, and gave teenagers demonstrable ways in which to separate themselves from the parent culture.

In the 1970s and 1980s the term 'youth sub-culture' was applied by sociologists (notably at the Birmingham Centre for Contemporary Cultural Studies). They admitted that there were several problems associated with this notion, including the fact that youth culture shifted and changed rapidly, with boundaries always on the move.

From the late 1980s on, newer forms of music and dance culture fragmented youth culture further, with hip-hop, house, jungle and techno styles creating many and varied allegiances to different styles.

These changes are, as Dr Alan Prout, director of the ESRC Children 5-16 Research Programme, commented at the final conference, often the result of other changes in society:

"In many respects childhood is no longer what it was ... Childhood change is in large measure an unplanned consequence of wider social change – change that by and large has its origins beyond public policy. The diversification of children's lives, for example in terms of their family situation, the rise of consumerism with its heightened expectation of choice, the proliferation of sources of ideas and knowledge, and the diffusion of democratic norms – all these are creating new kinds of childhood and new varieties of children."

"The effect is the creation of a generation of children who seem to have a greater sense of their own personhood." [20]

Attitudes and behaviours

This important issue of young people's sense of 'personhood', of self-awareness and self-esteem is reflected in their views about their own bodies. In a study undertaken for the former Health Education Authority,[21] more than 10,000 children aged 11-16 were asked if there was anything they would like to change about their bodies. Almost half (44%) said they would. This was significantly higher for girls, and the likelihood also increased with age. Those who disliked school were more likely to want to change something than young people overall. The change most young people wanted was in the overall size and shape of their bodies. Girls were more likely to say this, and to mention losing weight. Boys wanted to be taller, to gain weight and to have more muscles or a bigger chest.

Children's and young people's attitudes towards smoking, physical activity and healthy eating are discussed on pages 319, 326 and 342. Behaviour related to these issues is discussed in Chapters 7-10. In terms of relationships between health risk behaviours, the HBSC study[22] found that smokers were more likely than non-smokers to drink alcohol, and drinkers were more likely than non-drinkers to smoke. Smokers and drinkers were less likely to have eaten breakfast regularly, or at all, and also tended to have eaten more snacks on the previous day. There was strong evidence in this study of links between satisfaction with one's own body and health risk behaviours: smokers and drinkers were more likely to think they were too fat.

In terms of the factors affecting teenagers' health, work undertaken by Sweeting with data from 13 year olds in Glasgow shows the impact of social position and social life. While smoking, drinking and infrequent exercise were not patterned according to class, there was clear evidence that young people from a 'manual' class were more likely to have experience of drugs and to be less healthy eaters. There were also clear links between four health behaviours – less healthy eating, experience of drugs, regular alcohol drinking and current smoking – and 'hanging around the street'.[23]

Parental attention in general is significant. Young people who report more conflict with their parents are more likely to smoke, and to have health problems and lower self-esteem. Those who spent more time with their family were less likely to smoke or to have tried illegal drugs.[24]

Peer support, peer pressure and bullying

Spending time with friends is very important for children and young people. They see friends as sympathetic and uncritical people who offer support and advice, and keep confidences. It has been noted that most UK research among young people in this area has not looked at the positive and supportive effects of group membership. Rather, it has tended to see peer influence in negative terms. Such 'peer pressure', to use the more common term, is key, however, to health behaviours:

"It's blending in with the rest of the group. If the rest of the group are wearing Nike trainers, you feel like you've gotta have Nike trainers. If the rest of the group are smoking, you feel like you've gotta smoke." [13]

Children and young people themselves report the influences of 'peer pressure', whether this is encouragement to buy the 'right' trainers or other designer fashions, or bullying due to appearance, especially due to being overweight.

Bullying is an issue which has received widespread media coverage and attention over the past few years. Although undoubtedly many of the incidents of bullying are physical in nature, it is known that many focus on verbal abuse. Children have reported extreme experiences of bullying due to their appearance, though this may generally be in cases where a child is, or is perceived to be, overweight. There is also widespread anecdotal evidence that children and young people are mocked for not having the 'right' clothes, particularly trainers.

There may be a fine line between 'bullying' and what is generally regarded as 'peer pressure'. Indeed, some of this may be unspoken and relatively oblique. Participants in the North Somerset Youth Centre's Stop the Bully Project, run under the auspices of the Trust for the Study of Adolescence, said that bullying included:

"jealousy, emotional and physical abuse, racism, nasty teasing, mouthing off, bitchiness, ganging up on people ... leaving people out, saying they are gay ... taking the mick ... piss taking ... no respect..." [25]

Children and young people as consumers

Children and young people start moving towards financial independence via a process which may start with getting pocket money, then moves on to part-time jobs from the age of 13, and then to student loans, parental contributions to further education, full-time jobs or state benefits. In 1998-99, full-time employees under 18 earned an average of £6,400 per year, including overtime and bonus payments.

Although earnings make up the majority of income for 16-24 year olds, many younger teenagers receive pocket money. Results from the Small Fortunes Survey, a small-scale survey supported by the Joseph Rowntree Foundation, showed that the average amount of pocket money received in 1995 was £4.50 a week for 13 year olds, and around £7 a week for 16 year olds.[26]

In 1999, some four-fifths of 16-24 year olds owned some sort of plastic card, whether a credit, debit, store, cheque guarantee or cash machine card. According to the British Household Panel Study (BHPS), in 1996, 42% of young people aged 16-24 saved money from their income, and the main reasons given by 16-17 year olds were to buy cars, go on holiday and fund their own education.[17]

In terms of consumer choices, boys aged 13-16 spent a third of their own personal expenditure in 1998-99 on leisure goods and services (see Table 3). Girls spent more than boys on clothing and footwear. The expenditure on tobacco and alcohol (1% in each case) is acknowledged to be under-reported.[15]

In 1997-98 the most common activity outside the home for 16-24 year olds was visiting a pub, followed by eating in a fast food restaurant. Going to discos or nightclubs was also popular (see Table 4).

Table 3 ***Weekly expenditure by young people aged 13-16 in the United Kingdom, 1998-99***

	Males	Females
Leisure goods	25%	15%
Leisure services	12%	8%
Clothing and footwear	11%	20%
Fares and other travel costs	7%	6%
Confectionery	7%	7%
Soft drinks	6%	5%
Personal goods and services	3%	11%
Leather and travel goods, jewellery and watches	1%	5%
Cigarettes	1%	1%
Alcohol	1%	1%
Other	26%	21%
Total expenditure (=100%) (£ per week)	£16	£17

Source: See reference 27.

Table 4 ***Young people's participation in selected activities away from home, Great Britain, by age, 1997-98***

	Percentage participating in the activity in the three months prior to interview	
	16-24	All aged 16 and over
Visit a public house	82%	74%
Meal in a fast food restaurant	77%	48%
Disco or night club	68%	27%
Cinema	65%	34%
Meal in a restaurant (not fast food)	63%	69%
Library	41%	40%
Short break holiday	39%	31%
Spectator sports event	31%	26%
Theme park	29%	17%
Fun fair	27%	19%
Historic building	24%	32%
Museum or art galley	21%	22%
Camping or caravanning	17%	12%
Theatre	14%	17%
Bingo	11%	11%
Visit a betting shop	9%	9%

Source: See reference 28.

Poverty

The UK is considered one of the most unequal of all industrialised nations when it comes to child health. In 1982, some 10% of the population had an income below half the national average. By 1993, this figure had virtually doubled and was running at 19%. The infant mortality rate for the poorest families is 70% higher than for those in the highest socioeconomic class.[29]

Many of the challenges and risks faced by young people come about due to changes in the employment market, family relationships and structures, social structures and attitudes. The facts and figures surrounding these complex issues are given on page 309.

Researchers at the University of York have found that child poverty specifically had increased three-fold in the last 20 years. This study, from the Economic and Social Research Council,[30] reported that this was as high as it was because social and fiscal policies had been comparatively ineffective in protecting children from the effects of social and economic change.

The number of children in households with an income below half the national wage increased more than three-fold from 10% in 1979 to 34% in 1997/98. Children in families receiving basic social assistance went up from 7% in 1979 to 23% in 1998. A third of children are now being born to mothers in receipt of income support.[30]

The European Community Household Panel Survey found that the UK (with Ireland) had the highest child poverty rate among the 13 countries in the European Union in 1995.[30]

The ESRC study found evidence that some outcomes for children had got worse in the past two decades. These included low birthweight, school exclusions, crime, smoking for girls, alcohol, drugs, and suicide in young men.

The research highlights the fact that some outcomes have 'bucked the trend' and got better, despite being associated with poverty. However, there are reasons suggested for these, such as dental health (improved by fluoride); infant mortality rates (reduced by improvements in infant care); and teenage pregnancy (recent positive benefits in reducing rates seen from sex education, contraception and abortion).

The ESRC research team stressed that the UK does not produce a routine, comprehensive analysis of the well-being of children:

"There is no systematic collection or publication of statistics, no requirement to assess or publish information on policies on children and no analysis of overall or departmental budgets to assess the amount and proportion spent on children."

The research team recommended that certain indicators could be used as a measure of success in tackling child poverty and social exclusion (in addition to those in the government's *Opportunity for All* publication[8]). It suggested that self or parental reported chronic illness, obesity, dental caries, and the data on self-esteem scores for children aged 10-15 in the British Household Panel Survey could all be used as measures of success.

Young people as agents for change

According to the Young People's Social Attitudes Survey,[31] political interest among young people was already low in 1994 and had fallen further by 1998. More than a third of young people aged 12-19 claimed to have no interest in politics at all in 1998, a rise of 7% on the previous period. A further third had 'not very much' interest, leaving only one in three teenagers saying they had any interest.

The Save the Children study mentioned earlier[18] found that some young people felt that adults should recognise the contribution that young people made to society. The Trust for the Study of Adolescence ran a project called Challenging the Image, which looked at the involvement of 14-16 year olds, from three schools in Birmingham, the north-east and on the south coast, in voluntary work and campaigning. Questionnaires were used with some 1,160 pupils and more than 100 interviews were carried out. Results indicated that significant numbers of pupils were involved in activities including: working with the Red Cross, in hospitals and schools and with the elderly, and campaigning for locally based causes – often on environmental and transport issues. The teenagers were also involved with Amnesty, Greenpeace and Friends of the Earth.[32]

There have been proposals that "there is an urgent need for children and adolescents to be explicitly recognised at all levels of health policy."[33] Encouraging and facilitating participation by children and young people is highlighted as key to the way forward. There are warnings, too, that this should be real participation rather than tokenism. This may include, for example, inviting children or young people to take part in a conference, or to sit on a panel, with adults, without adapting the proceedings, to allow them to play a proper part. Allowing them to consult with their peers would be fundamental to this.[34]

Some schools have school councils, although some pupils doubt the sincerity with which these are operated:

"I think we get played like fools, cos we have council meetings ... OK, I'm a council rep, but I say this stuff, but they don't listen to me ... they think I'm just a laugh, they don't listen, cos we say stuff, what we want, but they don't listen, they ask us what we want, then they say no, we can't have it. What's the point of asking us?" Boy, aged 10.[13]

Participation via the media can be powerful, though children are aware that they can be misrepresented, stereotyped and even mocked. Many are quite sophisticated media consumers and able to read the signs that a journalist or producer may not have taken them seriously enough. In a small international study, children and teenagers told media professionals that they did not wish to be portrayed either as 'little angels' or as 'little devils', and that they were too often shown as 'little heroes', for example when bravely battling disease. They did not wish adults to speak for them, and they did not like it when adults used their (the children's) words in order to produce a humorous response from an audience, for example in mocking the children's relative ignorance of the subject matter.[35]

We would do well to bear in mind the words of Dr Alan Prout, at the launch of the ESRC's Children 5-16 Research programme in 1998:

"Children are not future members of society. They are members now."

Smoking

Knowledge of, and attitudes to smoking

The Teenage Smoking Attitudes survey, conducted between 1996 and 1998 by the Office for National Statistics on behalf of the Health Education Authority, provides information on smoking among young people in a number of European states.[36, 37] It reported on the following issues.

Starting to smoke
Twenty eight per cent of 11-15 year olds who had ever smoked tried their first cigarette before the age of 11 (i.e. before their 11th birthday). Regular smokers were twice as likely as occasional smokers to have had their first cigarette before the age of 11 (36% compared with 17%). Boys were more likely than girls to have tried their first cigarette before 11 (34% compared with 23%), despite the fact that more girls than boys were regular smokers.

Brand of cigarette smoked
Benson and Hedges was the brand of cigarette most commonly smoked – 36% of 11-15 year old smokers smoked this brand. The next most popular brand, Lambert and Butler, was smoked by just under a quarter of smokers.

Factors associated with starting to smoke
Over three-quarters (77%) tried their first cigarette with friends. Seventy-five per cent said one of the reasons that they tried their first cigarette was that they wanted to see what it was like. Nine per cent said they started to smoke because they wanted to fit in with friends, while only 3% said they did it because they wanted to look grown-up.

Stopping smoking
Forty-four per cent of current smokers said they would like to stop smoking. There were no significant differences between regular and occasional smokers.

Two-thirds of current smokers had tried to give up smoking. Regular smokers (72%) were more likely to have tried to give up than occasional smokers (56%), and girls (71%) were more likely to have tried to give up than boys (60%).The main motivators to quit were identified as: concerns about health (52%), cost (32%), and desire to feel fitter (24%).

Views about smoking
Smokers tended to be more likely than non-smokers to perceive benefits from smoking. The survey also found high levels of agreement with statements about the effects of smoking on health. (See Table 5.)

Table 5 ***Views about smoking among 11-15 year olds***

	Percentage agreeing with the statement	
	Smokers	Non-smokers
Perceived benefits from smoking		
Smoking can put you in a better mood.	50%	12%
Smoking can help calm you down.	75%	24%
Smoking helps to give you confidence.	24%	7%
Knowledge of the effects of smoking		
Smoking can cause lung cancer.	98%	99%
Other people's smoke can cause harm to the health of others.	94%	95%

Source: See reference 38.

Health information in school

Around 70% of pupils recalled lessons in the previous year on drugs, healthy eating and smoking. The majority of pupils knew that nicotine and tar are found in cigarette smoke (91% and 82% respectively) but a much smaller proportion (40%) knew that carbon monoxide is present.

Pupils were asked which they thought was the main cancer-causing substance in cigarette smoke and which they thought was the addictive substance. Forty-one per cent of pupils knew that tar is the main cancer-causing substance in cigarette smoke. Over three-quarters (76%) knew that nicotine is the main addictive substance in cigarette smoke.

Recollection of advertising about health issues in the media

Pupils were asked if they remembered seeing adverts about various health issues in the media in the previous year. By far the most common adverts that pupils recalled seeing were about the dangers of drinking and driving (88%), followed by adverts about the dangers of drugs (80%), and adverts warning young people about the health risks of smoking (73%).

Attitudes to smoking among 16-24 year olds

Qualitative research was conducted by the University of Strathclyde among 16-24 year olds in England in 1997, to explore attitudes to smoking.[39] The research involved a broad range of young people and was conducted in 12 focus groups, six paired interviews, and 33 in-depth interviews lasting 60-80 minutes. The results are shown in Table 6.

Table 6 ***Attitudes to smoking among 16-24 year olds***

	Why they smoke	Attitudes to cessation	Attitudes to health messages
Unemployed young people	To pass the time and relieve the depression and stress caused by lack of work. Also to 'escape' and relieve the stress of a 'lack of social opportunities'. *"You're just sitting there waiting for something to happen, twiddling your fingers, so you end up lighting a tab – you don't even think about it."* Female, aged 20-24, unemployed.	Rarely questioned their smoking. When asked to consider the possibility of giving up, they were dismissive of the need to do so. They tended to be committed smokers who believed the benefits of smoking outweighed the costs. Attempts to quit tended to be unplanned or circumstantial – for example if they became ill, ran out of money, or had a new partner who might disapprove of smoking.	Tended to find health messages lacking in personal relevance and unsupportive. As a result, health education tended to be dismissed.
Students	Most were influenced by changes in their circumstances, such as leaving home and forming new peer groups, providing both the incentive and the opportunity to start smoking (or to smoke more). The students were self-conscious about the impact of smoking on their image, apparently regarding smoking as part of the stereotypical image of the 'carefree and reckless' student. *"You need to break away from the books even if it's just going outside and having a cigarette."* Male aged 20-24, student.	Most had seriously considered quitting, and many planned to stop at some time in the future. Many felt guilty about wasting scarce financial resources. Female students in particular were concerned about the effect of smoking on appearance and image. Generally, students tended to see smoking as temporary behaviour associated with their current lifestyle, and something they would leave behind when leaving college or university.	Looking for empowerment, strong positive role models and rewards.
Employed young people	To punctuate the working day and relieve the stress of oppressive and pressured work environments. The transition from school to work environment could itself provide an incentive to smoke, with the exchange of cigarettes a means of easing entry into the new social group. Workplace smoking policies had a strong effect on behaviour: some would 'binge' during breaks, while others were prompted to try to quit. *"I'm from a high pressure job where there's lots of things going on and it's very rank oriented. When they come in and start the 'blah blah blah', the first thing I do is light a cigarette."* Male 16-19, employed.	This was the group most ready to quit, especially women. Many were experiencing the negative effects of smoking on their health and, to a lesser extent, on their appearance and image. A number had already tried to stop and many were committed to making the attempt in the near future. Since many were familiar with the pressures of trying to quit, they were sensitive to the barriers and able to empathise with others going through the same process.	Receptive to positive messages offering support to quit.

Source: See reference 39.

Factors associated with the uptake of smoking

The factors that influence smoking in young people overlap and fall into two categories: personal factors and socioenvironmental factors.

- Personal factors concern the micro-environment in which the child grows up – i.e. home, friends, school, and the child's personality and self-esteem.

- Socioenvironmental factors concern the macro-environment, i.e. the influences exerted by the community (including employers, advertising and the media), and the government. These are discussed in Chapter 10.

Personal and social factors influencing smoking

- Smoking among young people is directly related to adult smoking. A significant reduction in children's smoking will occur only when the role-modelling of adults is considerably reduced.

- Young regular smokers tend to be rebellious and with poor self-image, and indulge in risk-taking behaviour.

- Parental smoking and parents' attitudes are critically important influences on whether a child will smoke. Children are seven times less likely to smoke if they perceive strong disapproval from their parents.

- In older children, the smoking habits of friends are important. Going against the group norm is difficult and refusal skills have to be learnt.

- Non-smoking teachers and strict school no-smoking policies reduce cigarette consumption both in and out of school and in later life.

The factors that influence a child first to contemplate, then initiate and experiment with smoking are not necessarily the same as those associated with regular smoking. Figure 1 indicates some of the factors that operate at different stages. However, these stages are not discrete; they form a continuous process leading towards the take-up and habit of smoking.

Figure 1 ***Stages in the development of smoking***

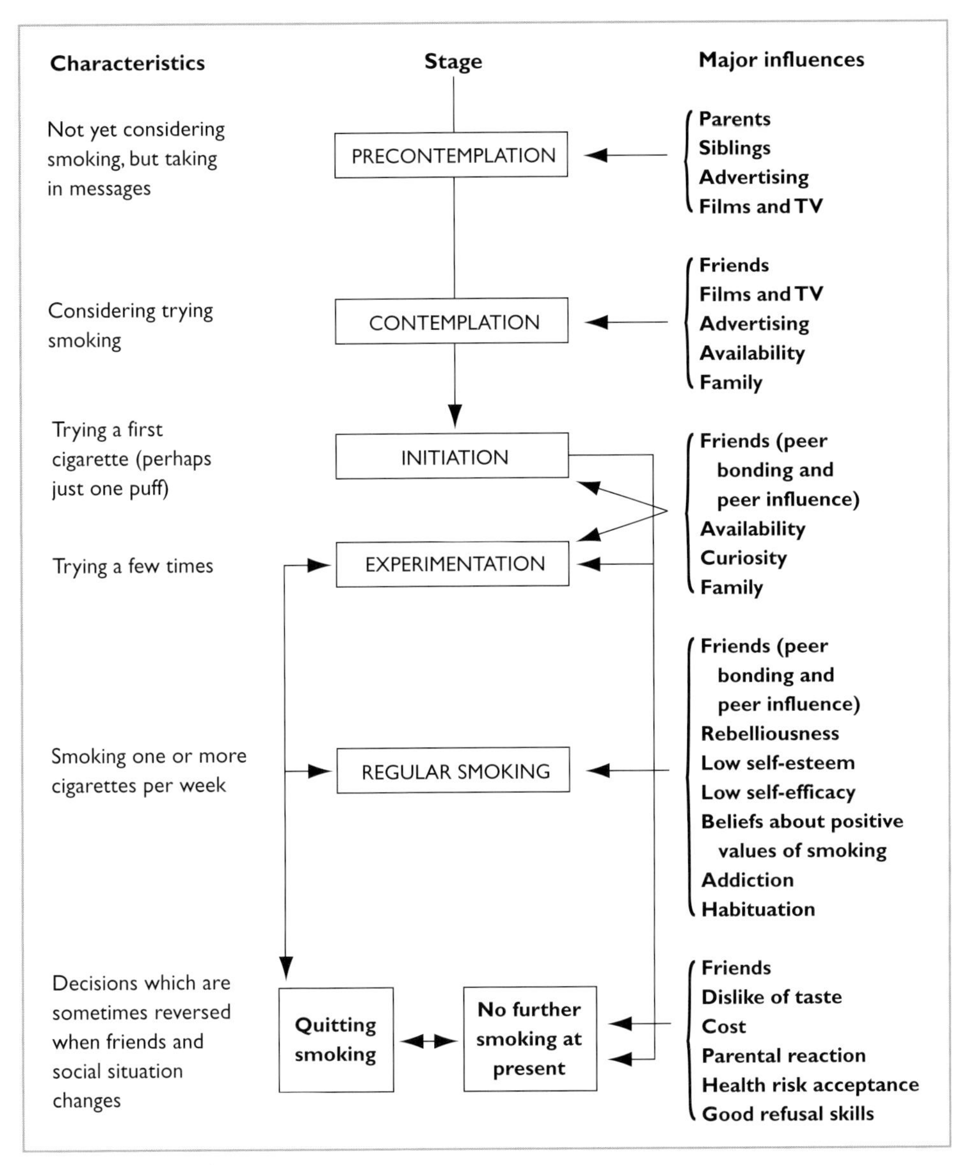

Source: See reference 1.

The young personality

Certain characteristics have been found to be related to initiation and experimentation with smoking by children. These include risk-taking, rebelliousness, and poor self-image. To these should be added the social factors discussed below. The process of 'becoming a smoker', which involves the progression from experimentation to regular smoking, retains these personal factors but is susceptible to other influences.

Transitional factors – from experimentation to regular smoking

Smokers always have good reasons for smoking, at least in their own view, and the factors affecting their behaviour must be seen in this context. Jessor[40] described smoking as one of the several problem behaviours during the developmental transition period of adolescence. He argued that such behaviour may express opposition to adult authority, provide a way of coping with anxiety, failure and frustration, express solidarity with peers, and affirm personal identity. The step from experimentation to regular smoking acts as a transition marker from adolescence to young adult status. This step suggests that smoking is seen as an adult habit. Thus, adolescent smoking is closely related to that of adults, and it might be predicted that, as adult smoking prevalence falls, so will that of adolescents. Flay et al suggest that the social reinforcements which adolescents obtain from smoking are the most important factors in the transition from experimentation to regular smoking.[41]

Risk-taking and rebelliousness have also been found to be associated with the transition to regular smoking. Young smokers are generally socially precocious, less academically orientated, have poor refusal skills, low self-esteem and believe that smoking provides them with positive gains. Transition from experimental to regular smoking can be predicted by the perception of smoking as fun, pleasant or nice and by an expressed intention to smoke. Research has shown that young 'risk-takers' in one area of behaviour tend to engage in other risky behaviours: for example, associations have been found between smoking and using other drugs.

Knowledge of the health risks of smoking

Knowledge of the health risks of smoking plays a relatively small part in a child's decision about smoking and alone is insufficient to deter a child from smoking.

Parental smoking and parents' attitudes to smoking

Parents are the source of primary socialisation and their influence is strong in the pre-school phase of children's lives. This formative period affects the child's whole life. It has frequently been shown in Britain that one or both parents' smoking is associated with smoking in their children.[1] Girls' smoking in particular is more likely to be related to that of their mother. It is not that children smoke because their parents smoke but, for a number of reasons including the accessibility of cigarettes, they are at an increased risk of taking up the habit. Parental anti-smoking attitudes are strongly influential and have been shown to carry even more weight than actual parental smoking.

Siblings' smoking

There is a strong correlation between the smoking habits of siblings. Perhaps this is because smoking is the norm in some families and not in others. Many studies have shown even stronger links between siblings' smoking than in parent/child smoking habits.[42]

Socioeconomic status

Although there is much higher smoking prevalence among adults in manual socioeconomic groups, no social class differences have been observed in the prevalence of smoking in British children and teenagers. This may be because friendships in school cross socioeconomic boundaries, or because children of manual socioeconomic groups may have less pocket money with which to buy cigarettes. When children become employed their purchasing power increases and teenage smokers have been shown to be more likely than non-smokers to have part-time jobs outside school.

Lone parent status has been shown to be associated with smoking prevalence in adults. One study showed that teenage daughters of lone parents also had an increased risk of being smokers, especially if their mothers smoked. However, studies have shown that this increased likelihood applies whether or not the lone mother is a smoker.

Children with emotional and behavioural difficulties

Children with emotional and behavioural difficulties have a very high smoking prevalence. They are often supported and encouraged in their smoking by carers, who use cigarettes as part of a reward system for improved behaviour.

Friends and social life

Although the family has the first impact on the child, as he or she grows the influence of friends becomes extremely strong. Three major studies have shown that best friends' smoking is one of the most important factors related to the uptake of smoking.[42-44] Another has shown that having a boyfriend or girlfriend is a predictor, particularly if he or she is a smoker.[45]

Leisure activities such as dancing, going to discos and parties and having friends of the opposite sex are all associated with smoking.

Physical activity

This section outlines children's and young people's physical activity levels, and also looks at their attitudes to physical activity, including the motivations and barriers. It looks firstly at children aged 5-15, using data from a qualitative study by the Health Education Authority,[46] and secondly at 16-24 year old women, using data from qualitative research carried out by the Health Education Authority in 1997.[47] (Chapter 8 looks at the determinants of young people's participation in physical activity, and Chapter 9 examines the relationship between physical activity during childhood and adolescence, and risk factors for cardiovascular disease in young adulthood.)

Current levels of physical activity

The recommended level of physical activity for young people aged 5-18 is at least one hour's moderate intensity physical activity a day. The minimum recommended level is half an hour a day.[48] The National Diet and Nutrition Survey[49] found that 61% of boys and 42% of girls aged 7-18 reached the one hour a day recommendation (see Table 7). Among 15-18 year olds, 9% of boys and 5% of girls did no physical activity at all.[49] No significant differences in measures of physical activity according to social class of head of household were found.

Table 7 ***Physical activity levels among 7-18 year olds, Great Britain, 1997***

Percentage of children and young people doing at least one hour's moderate intensity physical activity a day (recommended level)

	Age			
	7-10	**11-14**	**15-18**	**All**
Males	70%	68%	44%	61%
Females	49%	44%	31%	42%

Percentage of children and young people doing half an hour a day (minimum recommended level)

	Age			
	7-10	**11-14**	**15-18**	**All**
Males	90%	88%	71%	83%
Females	84%	76%	59%	73%

Percentage of children and young people doing no activity at all

	Age			
	7-10	**11-14**	**15-18**	**All**
Males	0%	2%	9%	4%
Females	4%	1%	5%	3%

Source: See reference 49.

Children aged 5-15 years

A qualitative survey of children aged 5-15 years, carried out by the Health Education Authority in 1999,[46] reported the following findings.

General findings

Likes and dislikes
Children liked: team games/competition, playing with friends, being active, developing skills, and competence.

Children disliked: bad experiences at school, having to play outdoors in bad weather, and having too many rules/restrictions. Some perceived activity as boring. Negative experiences of PE at school included: the clothes they had to wear for it, changing and showering facilities and routines, the lack of choice of activities, and the style of teaching, which many found too authoritarian.

Role of friends
For this age group, sport is just one feature of belonging to a group – and the friendship is more important than the activity. Boyfriends have a negative influence on participation of young women – girlfriends are more likely to spectate and support the boyfriend than participate themselves.

Role of parents
Parents can have both a positive and negative role. On the one hand, they can provide money and transport for sport and physical activities. On the other hand, many parents are concerned about their children's safety outdoors or about travelling home in the dark, or prevent their children from doing physical activity at certain times because of educational demands.

Gender
Girls are less likely to identify themselves as sportswomen than boys (and men). Sport was not considered a feminine attribute.

Ethnicity
Asian parents perceive the urban environment as more hostile and are therefore more restrictive on daughters.

Motivating factors and barriers to physical activity
After-school clubs and youth clubs were both motivating factors for physical activity.

Many children preferred other activities to physical activity. For some, transport was a problem. Other barriers included cost – especially for organised activities – and lack of facilities.

Children aged 5-11 years

Types of activity

Informal, school-based physical activity
Among 5-11 year olds, school-based physical activity included informal activity at breaks and lunchtimes. Activities included chasing games, acrobatics etc. Some schools provide balls and bats and rackets for ball games during lunchtime, and some organise dancing – for example country and line dancing. Most children are physically active during breaks, although some girls aged 10-11 preferred to sit and talk to friends. In many schools there were problems over football dominating or monopolising the space in the playground.

After school and at weekends
Activities after school and at weekends included: 'playing out' in the garden or street; football, cricket and basketball for boys; and chasing, clapping, hide and seek and skipping for girls.

Many children cycled in the local vicinity, and cycling was also used as a form of transport to meet friends. Parents set some restrictions on the distance their children could go, and which roads they could go on. Roller-blading was less popular than cycling.

Children generally had a positive attitude to walking – except in bad weather.

"I'd like to walk more really to stop the pollution. And be healthy and fitter." Male, aged 8

Organised sports, classes and clubs
Swimming lessons (for both boys and girls), football clubs (for boys), and dance classes (for girls) were the most common organised activities. Most found out about them via word of mouth, scouts, cubs and brownies.

Influencing factors

PE at school
Most primary school children viewed gym, rounders and football positively. The majority preferred competitive sports over individual sports:

"I get more confidence in a team. If I was playing alone I wouldn't. It's better to be in a team because you get more confidence and you can play well." Male, aged 11

Athletics and long distance running were considered to be boring. Boys disliked dance and movement and netball, all of which were seen as girls' activities. Girls expressed positive attitudes to dance and movement and wished to do more of these in PE. Some also wanted to play more tennis, badminton and football.

Some children disliked the methods of selection for team games:

"*I'm always picked last.*" Male, aged 9

Younger children generally considered their teachers favourably. But older children (aged 10-11) reported 'being forced into' certain activities:

"*The teachers can be annoying if you don't want to do something. They shouldn't force you to do something which you don't want.*" Male, aged 10

Some older girls (aged 10-11) stated they 'felt a bit self-conscious' about changing in front of others.

Parents
Few parents engaged in family-based physical activity sessions. Where parents were physically active, they tended to do activities on their own such as going to the gym, swimming or aerobics. Very active parents influenced and encouraged their children.

Parents had an important influence on levels of physical activity, determining whether their children walked to school, how far they were allowed to cycle, and facilitating out-of-school activities such as dancing or swimming.

The only parental restrictions on physical activities for primary children were:

- safety – not allowing children to cycle or play out too far from the home
- educational – if children had to prepare for SATs (school tests).

Friends
Friends were very important in the enjoyment of physical activity.

Gender differences
Girls felt alienated from playing football in school breaks because of the fear that it is too rough and because of the perception of not being able to play and the game being perceived as stereotypically masculine. Girls (the more active ones) who do play football tend to be seen as 'tomboys'.

"*They [the boys] don't let girls play. They let two girls play but they act like boys.*" Female, aged 7

Motivations to be active – children's perspectives
Motivations for involvement in physical activity included:

- awareness of the benefits of team membership
- increased social interaction
- enjoyment from competitiveness
- sense of achievement.

"You feel really good at the end. Once you get good at it, you feel like you're really good so you don't want to stop. So that pushes you a bit to do more things." Male, aged 11

Barriers to participation
There were few barriers to participation for this age group. Motivation and competence were not a problem, and there was a widespread belief that they would 'have a go' at an activity. Poor access or lack of transport were not considered to be an influencing factor in levels of physical activity.

The barriers included:

- lack of their own or parental time (including long working hours including shift work of parents)
- children being too busy with organised activities and clubs
- expense, including the cost of organised sports and activities.

Promoting physical activity among children
The children in the survey suggested focusing on the following motivational factors when promoting physical activity among children:

- the perception of physical activity as fun
- positive feeling while taking part in activities
- improved confidence
- enjoyment derived from social aspects of participation with friends.

Children aged 11-15 years

Types of activities
Among children aged 11-15 in the Health Education Authority survey, activity included: travel to and from school; activity at school; activity after school and at the weekend; organised sports, teams, classes and clubs; and part-time or household jobs.[46]

Influencing factors

PE at school

Long distance or cross-country running were considered boring, as was netball for some young women:

"I hate netball, most boriest game ever. You can hardly move. It's not very energetic. I don't like it so I don't bother." Female, aged 15 years

"I feel daft doing that stuff on the mats." Male, aged 12

"Games lessons are so boring that no-one bothers. Everyone would just prefer to skive rather than get changed and do something boring." Female, aged 15

"It's not a one-gender sport [rounders]. It's not sexist." Female, aged 15

Competitive sports were popular with many children, because they increased self-esteem, and gave children the sense of being part of a team.

"[I] prefer team sports because you're working together. Everyone makes mistakes." Male, aged 15

"The focus is not on you." Male, aged 11

"It boosts your self-esteem." Female, aged 14

However, some disliked competitive sports:

"If people put you down then you are not going to get the confidence to do it again. You are just going to keep on missing it." Female, aged 15

Children's criticisms of teachers focus on: lack of respect shown by PE teachers, a style that is excessively authoritarian, restricting choices, and invading privacy (especially with regard to changing).

"I think the majority of people in our school don't like PE because of the PE teachers. Because they make you do it." Female, aged 15

"Teachers come in when we are getting changed, making sure we're not up to something but I don't understand why. It would be understandable if we were making a noise or if we were all screaming and something like that. They come in and they just stand on a bench and just look and shout. And they are all looking at you." Female, aged 14

"I hate it when teachers stand and stare while you're getting changed." Male, aged 15

"He [the PE teacher] comes into the changing room sometimes when you're changing ... makes sure the girls are having showers. We were getting changed and he came in and said, 'You're late, what are you doing?' and we were just getting changed." Female, aged 13

Some PE teachers were perceived to 'pick on' less physically able students:

"Sometimes they are really horrible to people that can't do things... They don't believe them and then they embarrass them on purpose." Female, aged 15

"... like if you can't do it she'll say, 'Do it in front of the whole class' on purpose." Female, aged 15

Children disliked being forced to do certain activities, and disliked the lack of choice of activities.

Changing areas are more of a concern at secondary school than at primary school – especially for young women. Policies over showering after PE were disliked – because of lack of privacy and because it can lead to self-consciousness and embarrassment:

"You wish the lesson will run late so you don't have to have a shower." Female, aged 12

PE skirts were very unpopular with young women. They were considered to be too short. Tracksuit bottoms or jogging trousers were preferred.

Parents

Few children engaged in family-based physical activities. In particular, older groups had other priorities such as shopping. Also, there were parental restrictions on types of activity (such as rugby or boxing), and on being out after dark.

Friends

The social aspect of physical activity is very important. Doing activities with friends was considered more fun and more interesting, and provided companionship.

By the age of 15 and above, parties and discos emerge as a form of social recreation. Vigorous dancing was enjoyed in these settings. There is concern that there is inadequate provision for this age group, who are too old for youth clubs and too young for commercial (18+) dance clubs.

Young men were conscious of the importance of the sporty image in appearing attractive to the opposite sex:

"Girls normally go for the winners." Male, aged 14

The sporty image of young women does not carry the same kudos. Sporty young women are considered to be too masculine and thought of as 'lesbians':

"No, you get this image if a girl plays football, she's got to be a lesbian. So the lads won't bother." Female, aged 15

Non-sporty students were perceived negatively by both males and females, generally because of the individual's lack of effort or interest, and are associated with 'boffins' who are more concerned about 'getting an education'. These children are generally the victims of bullying:

"People take the mickey out of them a lot because they aren't any good at sports. They do sometimes get upset because it's like bullying." Male, aged 11

Gender differences

Among 11-15 year olds there are clear differences in levels of physical activity according to gender. Young women felt more negatively about PE generally and were less likely to participate in informal or formal activities. Girls reported that boys monopolised the space at school. Also, there were anxieties about appearing 'cool' to boys:

"When the lads are doing it and you know you're no good at it, you get dead embarrassed." Female, aged 12

In general, young men felt that young women did not value sports as much as the young men did.

Motivations to be active – young people's perspectives

Among inactive respondents the three main motivations to be active were:

- improved sense of well-being
- enjoyment and to prevent boredom
- weight control.

Among *active* respondents, the main motivations were:

- enjoyment and fun
- social benefits and friends
- competitiveness and being part of a team
- increased self-confidence
- sense of achievement.

Barriers to participation
Barriers to participation included:

- inertia, lack of motivation and feelings of apathy and boredom
- preference for other, non-physical activities
- feelings of embarrassment and self-consciousness about the body (women only)
- body image and body weight concerns (women only)
- maturation and bodily changes (women only)
- lack of choice and consultation in PE activities at school
- poor relationship with PE teaching staff – especially in relation to lack of privacy
- lack of time, or demands of homework
- expense, including cost of organised sports and activities
- cost of transport
- lack of access to a car
- in rural areas, poor public transport
- concerns for personal safety (women only)
- limited provision of sports facilities for preferred activities such as basketball
- limited provision of social facilities for young people to meet in, such as clubs, and to take part in activities such as dancing
- parental concerns about safety.

Maturation
For young men, levels of physical activity had increased with maturity. They had a greater freedom to go out, and also a greater range of activities on offer compared with when they were at primary school.

For young women, levels of physical activity had declined as they got older. Whereas at primary school they could play chasing games, this was now considered immature. Also, girls developed other interests – including boyfriends.

Both boys and girls felt that physical activity had become more structured as they had got older. Previously they had been active across the whole day, whereas now activity was restricted to short bursts, involving a more conscious effort on their behalf.

Young people's recommendations
Young people's recommendations for increasing physical activity included improving the choice of activities available and the facilities – but not necessarily in

school settings, since this environment would be just an extension of school and there was the fear that teachers would continue to treat them as if they were pupils:

"You can join clubs at school but then it's like going to school." Male, aged 15

They also recommended that young people should not be forced to do certain activities without consultation.

Girls felt intimidated and embarrassed about participating in physical activity with boys – and suggested that youth clubs should run single-sex sessions of the types of activity that appeal to girls such as aerobics, dance or trampolining.

Promoting physical activity

The young people in the survey made the following recommendations about promoting physical activity among young people:

- Schools were a useful resource.
- Promotional literature about physical activities and sports could be given out at half-term and school holidays.
- Activities should be marketed on the basis of the enjoyment, fun and social aspects rather than the health benefits – especially improved feelings of well-being. (The general view among this age group was that health was not an important consideration.)
- As regards role models, sports stars are already over-exposed and of limited value. Music/cultural role models are too individual to appeal to all. Young women felt that the use of slim role models should be discouraged because this was off-putting and unrealistic.

They also recommended focusing on the following motivational factors:

- enjoyment from the social aspects of taking part in physical activity with friends
- increased choice and consultation in PE activities
- more competitive and team sports
- more single-sex activities in school – especially for young women
- improving the relationship between students and PE teaching staff
- cheaper cost of organised activities
- greater provision of sports facilities for preferred activities
- greater provision of social facilities for young people to meet and to participate in activities.

Women aged 16-24

The Health Education Authority carried out qualitative research among women aged 16-24 in 1997. This included eight focus groups and 14 in-depth interviews in four areas of England.[47] The age range 16-24 is an age of transition in terms of lifestyles, opportunities, preferences and priorities, and low financial resources. It is an 'in between' stage of life marking the transition from childhood to adulthood. It is a very heterogeneous age group covering a wide span of experience.

Transitional circumstances – giving up the old and starting the new – all had effects on participation in physical activity. Transitional factors can be both barriers and incentives: for example, some give up physical activity after leaving school while others take up physical activity in response to encouragement from friends. Many young people in this age range undergo changes in friendships and financial circumstances. By the mid-20s lifestyle patterns were becoming more established.

Young people experience a range of circumstances that influence their participation in physical activity:

- attending school or college
- studying for exams
- leaving school or college
- becoming unemployed
- gap years and travelling
- attending university
- starting to live independently
- starting full-time work
- changing occupation
- pregnancy
- motherhood
- acquiring a car or a dog.

Variety in time available
Time available varied according to circumstance, but was a real constraint for students at critical moments, and for mothers. There were also competing priorities for their time.

Low financial resources

Young people aged 16-24 generally had low financial resources – especially those at the younger end of the age range. This is a barrier to using certain facilities, only partly countered by cheap access to facilities.

Transitional attitudes

Young people are concerned with 'what others would think' and about how they looked. There is also a tendency to rebellion, and opposition to anything that is presented by an 'authority' or that is instructional or 'good for you'.

In this age group young people tended to disbelieve anything that had not been proven by personal experience – perceiving, for example, that physical activity doesn't make you thin, and smoking doesn't prevent giving birth to a healthy baby.

Young people live in the present and tend not to think long term. They hold the view that illness and disease happen to others, and that they themselves are 'invincible'. By the mid-20s, there is more acknowledgement of the importance of taking action to maintain fitness and appearance.

Peer pressure is important, and so too are socialising and doing activities with friends. There is also a pervasive sense of the pressures from the media on how women should look and present themselves.

Knowledge and awareness of the benefits of physical activity

There was a high awareness of the health benefits of physical activity (both short and long term).

Awareness of the longer term benefits of physical activity included:

- for the heart: preventing heart disease or risk of heart attack
- for the lungs
- for circulation and blood pressure
- longer life
- resistance to illness
- preventing breast cancer in women
- reducing ageing.

Awareness of the shorter term benefits of physical activity included:

- body image
- appearance

- fitness
- weight loss
- muscle strength and tone
- feeling of well-being
- stress reduction
- preparation for childbirth and motherhood (becoming strong to cope with the demands of a young child, and regaining a slim figure following childbirth).

However, only the immediate benefits are likely to influence behaviour.

In general, 'instructional' messages are likely to be disregarded and to provoke a hostile response.

"If exercise is deemed that you have to do it, it's like being at school. If you're told something you don't want to do, you rebel against it." Female, aged 22-24

"I hate to be told to do anything. 'Do this' messages go over everyone's head. You open a woman's magazine and they have it all the time." Female, aged 22-24

Physical activity and smoking behaviour
Among 16-24 year olds there is a very high awareness of health education messages on the risks of smoking. Not smoking was seen as the most beneficial health action. Smoking was seen as something that would 'cancel out' the health effects of other actions. It was also seen as an effective means of weight control. Some saw smoking as a stimulus to physical activity – a compensatory behaviour for the ill effects of smoking (and similarly with poor diet).

Physical activity and diet and weight loss
There was good awareness of health education messages concerning healthy diet. However, a poor diet was sometimes used as an excuse for not doing physical activity:

"Poor diet cancels out any beneficial effects of physical activity."

Physical activity was sometimes seen as a way of compensating for an unhealthy diet:

"You burn it off."

Physical activity can be seen as a replacement activity after giving up poor eating habits:

"[If you have] success at dieting – you do physical activity too."

There was scepticism about the effect of physical activity on weight loss:

" ... *less necessary if you smoke"* (as smoking 'keeps you thin').

" ... *more an issue for older people"* (to stave off weight gain in middle age).

Physical activity was considered more effective for a fit, athletic look than for weight loss or a slim look.

Key barriers to physical activity

Key barriers for this age group included the following.

- General inertia: The allure of non-physical alternatives (TV, socialising, going to the pub, doing nothing at all).
- Lack of time.
- Lack of energy:

"You have to motivate yourself and do your own sport and keep fit but at school you had no choice." Female, aged 22-24

"It requires more effort now." Female, aged 22-24

- Low motivation: Physical activity is often perceived as boring, and reminds young people of negative school experiences.
- Requires a friend to go with you:

"It's boring on your own. It's the motivation: you need a friend to go with you to actually do it. If it's just you, you think I can't be bothered tonight, I'm just too tired. If you've got someone saying, 'I'll be round at seven' then you've got to go." Female, aged 16-24 (mother)

- The novelty wears off, and there is no quick observable effect:

"[You] lose interest after a few weeks because you don't see a result quickly enough and it doesn't seem to be working." Female, aged 16-18

- The priority is to relax in spare time.
- The strenuous image of physical activity.
- Lack of confidence about body image: Body image and lack of self-confidence applied across the age spectrum, particularly among the overweight. For many it was the key or sole barrier to physical activity. Self-consciousness or fear of exposure in front of others – of shape, size, appearance, being unfit or inept – were important factors:

"So I feel like I'm not going to fit in because I'm not thin, I don't feel pretty, I'm not tall, I'm not tremendously outgoing." Female, aged 18

"My legs put me off swimming. I'll never have thin legs. I have days when I'm conscious about my weight and days when I'm not." Female, aged 21 (mother)

"You think they're laughing at you because you're bigger than what they are." Female, aged 19-21

- Reluctance to use facilities: Facilities (centres, gyms, pools, classes) were generally considered to be alien. There was the presumption that other people would be superfit and energetic:

"See people coming out of the leisure centre – they've all got the clothes and all sporty. I wouldn't be that sort of person. I'd stand out. Look unhealthy." Female, aged 22-24

- Lack of time, or having other priorities: This was an issue, especially for mothers, and for students at critical periods:

"When you do loads of work, in your spare time you want to do something easy like watch the television – something that doesn't have to be strenuous because working really gets your mind and you're just so tired by the end that you just don't want to get up and go and pay some money for a game of badminton or do any exercise." Female, aged 16-18 (college student)

- Expense: Factors included cost of membership fees, transport, childcare costs, having other spending priorities, and reluctance to make the commitment to buy a leisure pass when commitment was likely to be sporadic.

Motivations

The immediate effects of physical activity include: appearance, weight loss, toning of body and social reasons (activities with friends, meeting people, enjoyment of team or group activities). For the very active, motivations include: enjoyment and achievement, and the challenge.

Health or fitness reasons are not a prime motivation for physical activity except in terms of appearance.

Triggers to physical activity for this age group include: as a response to an unhealthy lifestyle (smoking or weight gain), family influences (mothers with young children), influence of others (friends/boyfriends) or access to free or cheap facilities (for example at college).

Young people considered it culturally more acceptable for men than for women to be physically active – as there is greater emphasis on attributes such as competitiveness, sportiness and strength. This was reinforced by the ready availability of popular sport linked to a social scene – such as football and cricket – while there is no female equivalent for this.

Young people's ideas about how to promote physical activity

Young people felt a strong resistance to any association with 'authority' figures. Promotion of physical activity needs to be age-specific and oriented towards the key barriers. The emphasis should be on the immediate benefits rather than longer term health gain.

As regards what types of activity to promote, young people felt it is necessary to tackle young people's lack of confidence. They also recommended that the activities promoted need to be accessible to those who are unfit or consider themselves to have an unhealthy lifestyle.

Diet

There is increasing evidence that childhood diets may be particularly important in the aetiology of adult chronic diseases and therefore diet-related attitudes and behaviours developed in childhood have consequences for health throughout life.[50-52] (See Chapters 2 and 7.)

The main conclusions of the National Diet and Nutrition Survey[49] are that the nutritional health of young people is in a bad state, with children and young people eating far too much saturated fat, sugar and salt.

Children's attitudes

In the Health Behaviour of School-aged Children study, conducted by the Health Education Authority in 1995 and 1997, over 10,000 children aged 11-16 were interviewed about their lifestyles and general health and asked a range of behavioural and attitude statements.[22] This is one of the few nationally representative studies of a random sample of young people, which asks about attitudes regarding diet, nutrition and body image. Much, but not all, of the quantitative information in this section is drawn from this survey as it provides the most reliable information. The survey was conducted using protocols devised by WHO to enable comparison with similar surveys conducted across the EU. This section also includes references to other surveys, and qualitative insights into diet and nutrition are also drawn from a number of published studies including both government-funded and industry-funded research.

Dieting and worrying about weight

Two-thirds of young people aged 11-16 seem to be happy with their weight. One in ten are on a diet and one in five think they need to lose weight even though they are not on a diet. Girls are almost three times more likely than boys to be on a diet (14% compared to 5%). Of those people not on a diet, girls are more likely to be worrying about their weight. Being on a diet and worrying about weight increase as children get older up to the age of 15-16 when almost half (47%) of 15-16 year olds are unhappy about their weight and almost one in five are on a diet (see Figure 2).

Frequency of eating breakfast before going to school

Six out of ten young people ate breakfast every day before going to school, although almost one in five (18%) never, or hardly ever, had breakfast before school. Girls were almost twice as likely as boys to say they never or hardly ever had breakfast (23%, compared to 13%) and this increased for both sexes as they got older with about a third of 15-16 year old girls (31%) saying they never or hardly ever had breakfast.

Figure 2 ***Young people aged 11-16 on a diet: Are they on a diet?***

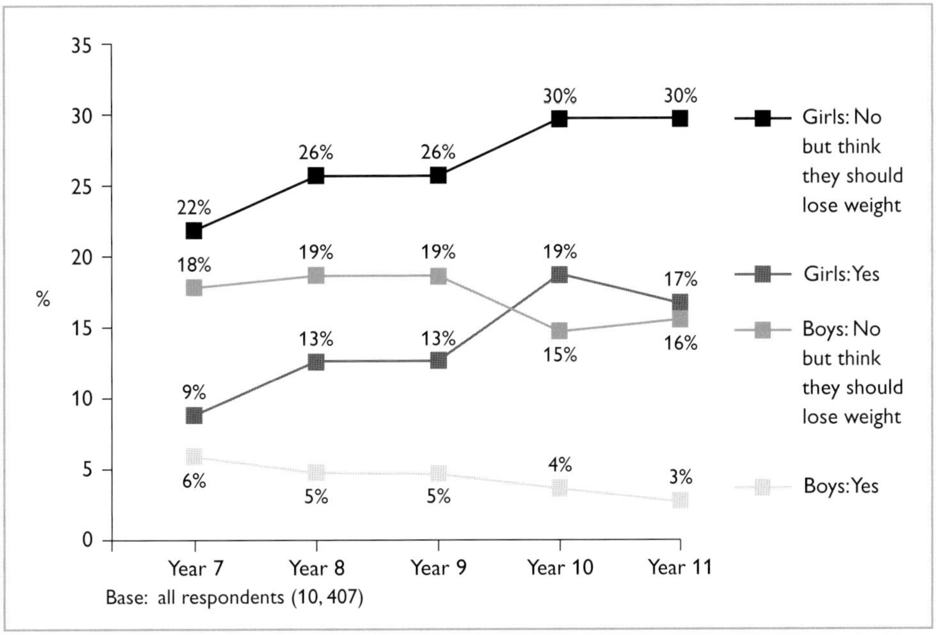

%	Year 7	Year 8	Year 9	Year 10	Year 11
Girls: No but think they should lose weight	22%	26%	26%	30%	30%
Girls: Yes	9%	13%	13%	19%	17%
Boys: No but think they should lose weight	18%	19%	19%	15%	16%
Boys: Yes	6%	5%	5%	4%	3%

Base: all respondents (10, 407)

Source: See reference 22.

Young people were also asked to describe their own health. Those who considered themselves to be 'very healthy' were more likely to eat breakfast than those describing themselves as 'quite healthy' or 'not very healthy' (73% compared to 59%).

Those who ate a greater number of 'more healthy' foods* were most likely to eat breakfast every day. Seventy per cent of those who ate a greater number of 'more healthy' foods ate breakfast every day compared to 57% of those who ate 'less healthy' food.

---

* *Definition of 'more healthy' and 'less healthy' foods*
For analysis purposes young people were asked how frequently they consumed each of several different types of food and drink and, based on their responses, they were categorised into those who eat 'more healthy' and 'less healthy' foods. Overall diet is not assessed in this survey, so for the purposes of analysis, foods for which an increase in consumption is recommended, such as fruit, pasta and bread were called 'more healthy foods'. Those which are high in fat and/or sugar and which should not be consumed too frequently were termed 'less healthy foods'. The terms were adopted for convenience of reference and because the methodology adopted cannot measure the constituents of a balanced diet. A full discussion of the methodology can be found in the published findings from the survey.

Frequency of eating snacks

Seven out of ten young people had eaten at least two snacks on the previous day, and almost four out of ten (38%) had eaten at least three. Girls were more likely than boys to have eaten snacks 'once only or not all' on the previous day. While 45% of boys had at least three snacks a day, only 31% of girls reported having three snacks. This declined slightly with age for girls but stayed fairly constant for boys.

Trends over time

Comparing the results from the 1997 and 1995 HBSC surveys,[22, 53] some encouraging trends can be observed in the attitudes of young people towards food. The percentage of young people on a diet has declined by a quarter with the greatest reduction seen among 11-13 year old girls and 13-16 year old boys. However, the proportion of 11-12 year old girls who thought they needed to lose weight has increased from 18% to 22% and the proportion of 15-16 year old boys sharing this view has increased from 13% to 16%.

Attitudes towards diet and healthy eating

In the HBSC survey, a number of statements about diet and healthy eating were put to participants, using a Likert scale. Their responses are shown in Tables 8 and 9.

"As long as you are reasonably active you can eat what you like."

A significant minority of young people agree with this statement and boys were more likely to believe this than girls (46% of boys compared to 36% of girls). Interestingly as boys get older they are more likely to agree with this, whereas for girls the level of agreement remains fairly stable as they get older at around 36%.

"I just eat the foods I like and don't worry about whether they are healthy or not."

Again a significant minority of 36% of 11-16 year olds agreed with this statement. A larger proportion of boys agreed with it than girls (40% compared to 31%). The prevalence of this attitude increased with age with a half of 15-16 year old boys and over one-third of 15-16 year old girls saying they eat what they like and don't worry about whether it is healthy or not.

"People of my age don't need to worry about the food they eat."

Fewer than one in four people agreed with this statement. There was little difference between the sexes but while this figure stayed fairly constant as boys got older, girls were less likely to agree with this statement as they got older with only 13% of 15-16 year olds agreeing with the statement.

There are many reasons for holding these attitudes. For example it may be lack of knowledge about what constitutes healthy eating, or confusion about the information provided by experts. Many children believe healthy food is boring or indeed find it difficult to get healthy food. Peer pressure to socialise and eat what their friends eat can also have an influence.

Table 8 ***Attitudes of 11-16 year old boys towards food, 1997***

	Percentage of those agreeing with the statement School year (ages)					
	Total	7 (11-12)	8 (12-13)	9 (13-14)	10 (14-15)	11 (15-16)
As long as you are reasonably active you can eat what you like.	46	40	42	50	49	48
I just eat the foods I like and don't worry about whether they are healthy or not.	40	31	36	40	46	49
People of my age don't need to worry about the food they eat.	24	25	25	27	21	24
I don't know enough about which foods are good for you.	33	30	34	34	32	33
Experts never agree which foods are good for you.	40	37	40	39	40	45
I find healthy food too boring.	35	27	33	38	38	40
Base	5,063	1,073	1,011	1,051	1,009	917

Source: See reference 22.

Table 9 ***Attitudes of 11-16 year old girls towards food, 1997***

	Percentage of those agreeing with the statement School year (ages)					
	Total	7 (11-12)	8 (12-13)	9 (13-14)	10 (14-15)	11 (15-16)
As long as you are reasonably active you can eat what you like.	36	32	38	36	38	36
I just eat the foods I like and don't worry about whether they are healthy or not.	31	22	30	32	40	36
People of my age don't need to worry about the food they eat.	22	28	28	20	17	13
I don't know enough about which foods are good for you.	31	25	28	33	35	32
Experts never agree which foods are good for you.	35	33	33	35	40	36
I find healthy food too boring.	23	18	23	23	26	27
Base	5,241	1,105	1,040	1,042	1,087	967

Source: See reference 22.

"I don't know enough about which foods are good for you."
A third of people agreed with this statement and there was no significant difference between boys and girls. Surprisingly the older children were less confident in their knowledge of healthy foods.

"Experts never agree which foods are good for you."
A sizeable minority of young people believe expert advice is inconsistent, with 38% of young people agreeing with this statement – boys more than girls (40% compared to 35%). Nearly a quarter of respondents (23%) neither agreed nor disagreed, leaving only 30% who disagreed with this statement. As children got older this scepticism increased.

"I find healthy food too boring."
Less than a third agreed with this (29%) but boys were significantly more likely to subscribe to this view than girls (35% of boys compared to 23% of girls). However as people got older they were more likely to believe this, with as many as 40% of 15-16 year old boys finding healthy food too boring.

Those who eat more healthily
Those people who eat 'more healthily' (see definition on page 343) are less likely to believe that exercise alone keeps you healthy; are more likely to believe that people of their age should be concerned about the food they eat; and generally do not find healthy food boring. However, their views about the experts tended to coincide with those of respondents who did not eat healthily; about two-fifths of both groups agreed with the statement "Experts never agree which foods are good for you."

Trends
There have been some encouraging trends in attitudes with fewer people believing that "People of my age don't need to worry about the food they eat" (33% to 23%), and fewer people believing that "as long as you are reasonably active you can eat what you like" (53% to 41%).

Children's understanding about diet

A study looking at children's ideas about fat consumption and health revealed that the relationship between dietary elements and health tends to be poorly understood other than in general terms by children aged 10-11 years.[54] Few children at this age tend to mention the heart when talking about fat and the majority of children in this study had little understanding of the structure and functioning of the internal organs of the body, including the heart.[55, 56]

The focus of children's knowledge has been on illness rather than health. A study by Backett,[57] demonstrated that the majority of children seemed reasonably well informed about foods conventionally deemed to be 'healthy' or 'unhealthy'. However, questions about individual food preferences and the effects of different foods on the body revealed contradictions and confusions. Children were more aware of the negative effects of unhealthy foods than the positive effects of healthy food.

A qualitative study by Ross[58] revealed that 10-11 year olds tend to choose food primarily for reasons of personal preference, defining food choice in terms of food liked and disliked. The health-giving attributes of foods appear to have little significance to them.

Healthy foods tend to be associated with 'proper' meals and home-made meals and tend to be valued for their rarity (not served every day) and for the fact that there tended to be family sharing with such meals. The healthy content of such meals may not be valued in itself, but is recognised by children as something important to their parents or carers.[59]

Who and what influences food choice

For children food is not a health priority

The priorities for children's health are commonly defined for them in terms of absence of disease or the absence of unhealthy behaviours such as drug use and smoking, and these issues are widely reported as the main concerns for adults and children. However, findings from qualitative studies of children's attitudes and behaviour indicate that other issues about appearance, schools, families and friendships were as important to young people.[59] Young people's priorities tend to be in satisfying family relationships and good wider social relationships with peers and adults and it is these concerns that tend to get marginalised in contemporary health promotion activities as well as in media coverage of young people.[59]

Family and friends

In the study by Ross,[58] food consumption among 10-11 year olds tended to be influenced by family and friends and the sharing of meals was seen to be an important and valued activity.

While children say that eating the same food as friends is not important, observation revealed that children do in fact eat very similar foods to their friends.[58]

In Ross's study of 10-11 year olds the health-giving attributes of food appear to have little significance to children of this age except perhaps when put forward by influential adults. Convenience and social popularity appear to have a greater influence on choice.

A Mintel report on children's attitudes revealed that children appear to have more control over decision-making, both about their own lives and aspects of the lives of the rest of their family, than before.[60] But in reality there are very few areas of their life over which they do have control. In common with other studies, this qualitative research study (conducted for Mintel by the British Market Research Bureau) revealed that among 8-11 year olds neither healthy eating nor dieting was mentioned spontaneously, and this did not seem a particular concern when prompted. For younger children the parents imposed certain food rules, which showed that however much food they ate they were being guided in the direction of healthy eating.

"*We also have a little bit of salad, at least every two days. If I don't have much on my dinner already my mum will put some on, but sometimes I just choose to have it.*" Girl, aged 8-10

"*Mine tell me to eat fruit before I have chocolate.*" Girl, aged 8-10

"*My mum says 'What do you want for supper?' and I say chips or something, and she says 'All right we'll have chicken then.'*" Boy, aged 8-10

Children in families where parental work patterns meant that children ate separately from their parents tended to be allowed to have a greater degree of freedom about what they could eat, although they were limited to what was in the cupboard or fridge.[60]

Children tended to have an aversion to foods described as 'good for you'. In a study of children and their parents by Prout it was clear from both children's and parents' accounts that children were active in shaping the family behaviours.[61] Children often had strong views about their preferences and these were in direct opposition to their parents' views:

"*I just don't like healthy foods. I don't really like many vegetables. And I like most junk food ... sausages, baked beans, beefburgers.*" Boy, aged 9-11

Children adopt complicated strategies to maintain choice. In battles over food, children develop a repertoire of tactics to create a situation where parents are compelled to negotiate the family diet. Mothers tried to persuade them to eat healthy food by bargaining over pocket money, television etc, while in return children described tactics such as 'going into a mood'.

Children lack control over school meals, which is in direct contrast to their experience at home. Ross observes that:

"*... it may be possible that the observed difference in tolerance of food restriction between home and school is a response to the children's lack of manipulation of the school environment which therefore curtails their choice and allows resentment to build.*"

Children have a clear sense that foods are valued in ways other than their perceived healthiness or unhealthiness. Prout[61] provides an anthropologist's perspective on this issue:

"What we might be seeing here is the complex reading by children of the layered and contradictory meanings of adult culture noticed by anthropologists of childhood .... Children come to their interpretations because they understand social values not only as they are explicitly told to them but also as they see them enacted and lived around them. They are therefore often acutely aware of differences between the value system as it is told to them and as it is actually lived; of course the latter is far more powerful. Attitudes to the moral qualities of food are therefore to be seen as complex and ambiguous. As James ... shows, food that is understood as 'good' in either a moral or a health sense is also seen as mundane, boring and everyday. On the other hand, food associated with celebrations (especially cakes, trifles, chocolate, confectionery and the like) is seen as highly desirable but morally bad and unhealthy. Children drew on and used these ambiguities."

The food industry – Selling to children

A survey for the Food Commission found that for every healthy product targeted specifically at children, 10 more were "nutritional disasters" and could be dismissed as "junk food" (defined as foods with: a total fat content of more than 20g; saturated fat content of more than 5g; sugar content of more than 10g; or sodium content of more than 0.5g per 100g). The report accused manufacturers of undermining children's diets by boosting the sugar, fat, additives and salt content of their food, over-processing food and removing the nutrients and dietary fibre.[62] The food surveyed included items such as cheese spreads, seedless raisins, cocoa cereals and Barbie cookies. All the products studied used cartoon characters, puzzles, gifts and other devices designed to attract children. However, foods such as crisps and confectionery were excluded from the survey as these would be well known to parents as high in fat and sugar. Of the 358 products surveyed, a third were so poorly labelled that no nutritional assessment could be made. Of the remaining two-thirds, 77% had high levels of saturated fat. Only four (1%) of the products that declared their nutritional content were low in fats, sugars and salt: these were frozen vegetables with children's cartoons on them.

Marketing and merchandising

Considerable resources are spent by manufacturers on marketing products such as toys, clothes, and food and drink to children. There is growing interest and concern about the use of sophisticated marketing techniques aimed at children, particularly where the child is manipulated by the marketing to persuade their parents to purchase products.

Recently there have been attempts by a number of EU countries to ban the use of advertising directed at children, particularly toy advertising. Sweden banned advertising aimed at children in 1991 and is trying to encourage other countries to follow. (Denmark and Greece already ban toy advertising on daytime television.) Nearly all European countries regulate advertising to children to some degree. At present guidelines in the UK forbid advertising alcohol or potentially harmful products to the young. However, much of the food advertising directed at children could be interpreted as falling into these categories.

Opponents of advertising to children believe that adverts for fizzy drinks, chocolate and toys encourage children to consume sugary, fattening foods and widen the social gulf between families who can afford the products and those who cannot.

There are few studies in this area but the increasing volume and competitiveness of the children's market means that most companies are using complex advertising and marketing strategies to gain a share of the money spent on and by children. Advertisers appeal to children in a number of clever ways, for example by making products appear to be their 'friends', using animation, celebrities or heroes (such as Michael Owen or Gary Lineker) and encouraging them to collect things and compete (for example with free gifts in cereals).

Research in this area is very patchy but a study commissioned by the Co-op and conducted by Sustain (the alliance for better food and farming)[63] revealed that 99% of the foods and drinks advertised to children during Saturday morning children's television contained high fat, or high sugar, or high salt. Cakes, biscuits and confectionery constituted 46% of advertising on Children's ITV and 53% on the Big Breakfast, compared with a combined figure of just 13% on evening television. Seventy-three per cent of children asked their parents to buy things they had seen advertised on television, and 77% of parents wanted to see a ban on this type of commercial.

Many parents and children interviewed as part of the Target Group Index survey (a regular omnibus survey used by many companies in the UK to build up a picture of the lifestyle and consumer behaviour of people in Britain), believed that merchandising was having an effect. A third of parents of 5-9 year olds believed that using cartoon characters to sell products to children was clearly making the product more attractive to the children and a fifth of children aged 7-11 stated that the cartoon or character featured in the advertisement was a factor in choosing a particular product.[60]

On the basis of their commissioned study the Co-op, in July 2000, banned the advertising of unhealthy foods and drinks targeted specifically at children, believing that such advertising 'blackmailed' parents into buying products by appealing directly to children. It also banned the use of character and cartoon merchandising on Co-op products.[64]

Sources of information

Schools tend to be a source of information about diet and disease,[54] but family members also tend to play a large role in providing health information and support.[59] The mother has a significant influence both as a source of information and as an influence on the way in which children think about food.[54,65,66]

Food and school

Views of school catering

According to a Sodexho survey carried out in 2000, the average frequency of eating a school meal was 2.84 times a week – an increase on the 1998 figure of 2.54 times a week.[67] The average amount spent on a school meal is £1.46 (compared with £1.28 in 1998). In a survey of parents commissioned by the Local Authority Caterers Association in 1999, 22% said they depended totally on schools to provide their children with a balanced diet.[68]

The average amount given by parents to children per day to spend on their lunchtime meal was £1.54 in 2000 (compared with £1.21 in 1996 and £1.35 in 1998). According to the Sodexho survey this represents £840 million per year.

The main reason for children not having a school meal is that they preferred a packed lunch (44%). Fifteen per cent said the food did not taste nice, 13% indicated that their parents preferred them to have a packed lunch, and 12% were concerned about the lengthy queues. Forty-five per cent of pupils said the queues were a problem at their school and 33% expressed concern about the crowded dining room and cramped seating.

Most parents wanted the school to provide traditional healthy lunches that are freshly prepared at school, 39% wanted mid-morning snacks, and 37% wanted the school to provide a packed lunch. Twenty-six per cent of parents wanted vending machines and 25% asked for breakfast provision.

Discussion of food in school

Sixty per cent of 8-16 year old respondents in the Sodexho study said they had discussed food and diet at school. Where there was a school food committee the figure was 79%.

Twenty-six per cent of schools had a clear policy on healthy eating but where there was a school food committee this figure rose to 62%. However, only 10% of children said their school had a school food committee.

Sixty-two per cent of pupils said what was taught in the classroom balanced very or fairly well with the food that was provided in the school dining room. Where there was a food committee this increased substantially to 81%.

Money spent on food on the way to and from school

The same survey found that children spent on average 62p per day before school: 40% bought sweets, 26% fizzy drinks, 25% chocolate, and 38% crisps. After school the average spend by school children was 57p. These figures equate to £365 million per year spent by children on the way to and from school (an increase on the 1998 figure of £257 million). Most of this money is within the child's control to spend, and represents a significant and lucrative market for food manufacturers.

In one study, researchers interviewed schoolchildren at a school where pupils regularly walked to school. For some children, this was a four-mile round trip, and would have been a healthy pursuit, but for the fact that this was along a busy road with traffic crawling into the town. Also, several described stopping at McDonald's for their breakfasts.[13] When friends congregate at McDonald's for breakfast on the way to school, part of its attraction lies in the fact that it is a separate space in which to socialise. Adults may wish to point out that burgers may not be the best start to the day, but if children as young as three are rebelling over nutritional restrictions, it is perhaps not surprising that many young people reject healthy eating advice, however well meant it may be.

References

1 Royal College of Physicians. 1992. *Smoking and the Young*. London: Royal College of Physicians.

2 Department for Education and Employment. 1999. *GCSE/GNVQ and GCE A/AS/Advanced GNVQ Results for Young People in England, 1998/99 (Provisional)*. SFR 35/1999. London: Department for Education and Employment.

3 Department for Education and Employment. 1999. Education and labour market status of young people in England aged 16-18, 1992 to 1998. *DfEE Statistical Bulletin*: 11/99.

4 Safe on the Streets Research Team. 1999. *Still Running: Children on the Streets in the UK.* London: The Children's Society.

5 Eurostat.

6 Graham J, Bowling B. 1995. *Young People and Crime. Home Office Research Study No. 145.* London: HMSO.

7 Gregg P, Hansen K, Wadsworth J. 1999. The rise of the workless household. In: Gregg P, Wadsworth J (eds.) *The State of Working Britain.* Manchester: Manchester University Press.

8 Department of Social Security. 1999. *Opportunity for All: Tackling Poverty and Social Exclusion. First Annual Report 1999 (Cm 4445).* London: The Stationery Office.

9 Department of Social Security. 1997. *Welfare Reform Focus File No.7.* London: Department of Social Security.

10 Social Exclusion Unit. 1998. *Truancy and School Exclusion (Cm 3957).* London: The Stationery Office.

11 Office for National Statistics. 2000. *Social Trends 30. 2000 edition*. London: The Stationery Office.

12 Kiernan K. 1997. *The Legacy of Parental Divorce: Social, Economic and Demographic Experiences of Adulthood. Case Paper 1.* London: London School of Economics.

13 Morrow V. 2001. *Networks and Neighbourhoods: Children's and Young People's Perspectives.* London: Health Development Agency.

14 Johnson AM, Wadsworth J, Wellings K, Field J. 1994. *Sexual Attitudes and Lifestyles.* Oxford: Blackwell Scientific Publications.

15 Matheson J, Summerfield C (eds.) Office for National Statistics. 2000. *Social Focus on Young People.* London: The Stationery Office.

16 McConaghy M. 2000. *Housing in England 1998/99: A Report of the 1998/99 Survey of English Housing Carried out by the Social Survey Division of ONS on Behalf of the Department of the Environment, Transport and the Regions.* London: The Stationery Office.

17 Brynin M, Scott J. 1996. *Young People, Health and the Family.* London: Health Education Authority.

18 Barry M. 2001. *Challenging Transitions: Young People's Views and Experiences of Growing Up.* London: Save the Children.

19 Brannen J, Storey P. 1996. *Child Health in Social Context*. London: Health Education Authority.

20 Prout A. 2000. ESRC Children 5-16 Research Programme: Growing into the 21st Century. Paper presented at a conference *Children: Making Their Future? Research and Policy for the 21st Century*, October 2000, London.

21 Speed M, Ryan H. Rudat K. 1992. *Tomorrow's Young Adults – A Survey of 9-15 Years in England.* London: Health Education Authority.

22 Haselden L, Angle H, Hickman M. 1999. *Young People and Health: Health Behaviour in School-aged Children. A Report of the 1997 Findings.* London: Health Education Authority.

23 Sweeting H. 2000. What's most important for teenage health? The patterning of health and behaviours according to social position and social life. In: Ryan H, Bull J. (eds.) *Changing Families, Changing Communities.* London: Health Development Agency.

24 Sweeting H, West P, Richards M. 1998. Teenage family life, lifestyles and life chances: associations with family structure, conflict with parents and joint family activity. *International Journal of Law, Policy and the Family*; 12: 15-46.

25 Coleman J, Richardson H, Roker D, Shepherd J (eds.) 2002. Stop the Bully Project. *Spotlight* newsletter. Brighton: Trust for the Study of Adolescence. (Accessed from: www.tsa.uk.com)

26 Middleton S, Ashworth K, Braithwaite I. 1997. *Small Fortunes: Spending on Children, Childhood Poverty and Parental Sacrifice.* London: Joseph Rowntree Foundation.

27 Office for National Statistics. 2000. *Family Spending – A Report on the 1998-99 Family Expenditure Survey.* London: Office for National Statistics.

28 The Henley Leisure Centre. 1998. *Leisure Tracking Survey*. Henley: The Henley Centre

29 British Medical Association. 1999. *Growing Up in Britain: Ensuring a Healthy Future for Our Children.* London: British Medical Association.

30 Bradshaw J (ed.) 2001. *Poverty: The Outcomes for Children.* London: Family Policy Studies Centre and National Children's Bureau.

31 Park A. 1999. Young people and political apathy. In: Jowell R, Curtice J, Park A, Thomson K (eds.) *British Social Attitudes: The 16th Report – Who Shares New Labour Values?* Aldershot: Ashgate.

32 Roker D, Player K, Coleman J. 1999. *Challenging the Image: Young People as Volunteers and Campaigners.* Leicester: Youth Work Press.

33 Aynsley-Green A et al. 2000. Who is speaking for children and adolescents and their health at the policy level? *British Medical Journal*; 321: 229-32.

34 Hart R. 1992. *Child's Participation: From Tokenism to Citizenship.* London: UNICEF International Child Development Centre.

35 Hughes L, McCrum S. 1998. *Interviewing Children: A Guide for Journalists and Others.* London: Save the Children.

36 Jarvis L. 1997. *Teenage Smoking Attitudes in 1996.* London: The Stationery Office.

37 Barton J. 1998. *Teenagers and Smoking in 1997.* London: The Stationery Office.

38 Higgins V. 1999. *Young Teenagers and Smoking in 1998. A Report of the Key Findings from the Teenage Smoking Attitudes Survey Carried out in England 1998.* London: The Stationery Office.

39 Health Education Authority. 1997. *Lighting Up: Smoking Among 16-24 Year Olds. Findings from the Health Education Authority's National Smoking Education Campaign.* London: Health Education Authority.

40 Jessor R. 1982. Problem behaviour and developmental transition in adolescence. *Journal of School Health*; 52: 295-300.

41 Flay BR, d'Avernas JR, Best JA, Kersell MW, Ryan KB. 1983. Cigarette smoking: why young people do it and ways of preventing it. In: McGrath P, Firestone P (eds). *Pediatric and Adolescent Behavioural Medicine.* New York: Springer – Verlag: pp 132-83.

42 Murray M, Swan AV, Johnson MRD, Bewley BR. 1983. Some factors associated with increased risk of smoking by children. *Journal of Child Psychology and Psychiatry*; 24: 223-32.

43 Gillies PA, Galt M. 1991. In: Winnbust JAM, Maes S (eds.) *Lifestyles and Health: New Developments in Health Psychology.* DSWO/LEIDEW. Netherlands University Press.

44 Charlton A, Blair V. 1989. Predicting the onset of smoking in boys and girls. *Social Science and Medicine*; 29: 813-18.

45 McNeill AD, Jarvis MJ, Stapleton JA, Russell MAH, Eiser JR, Gammage P, Gray EH. 1988. Prospective study of factors predicting uptake of smoking in adolescents. *Journal of Epidemiology and Community Health*; 43: 72-78.

46 Mulvihill C, Rivers K, Aggleton P et al. 2000. *Physical Activity 'At Our Time'. Qualitative Research among Young People Aged 5 to 15 Years and Parents.* London: Health Education Authority.

47 Finch H, White C. 1998. *Physical Activity: 'What We Think'. Qualitative Research among Women Aged 16-24.* London: Health Education Authority.

48 Biddle S, Sallis J, Cavill N (eds.) 1998. *Young and Active? Young People and Health-enhancing Physical Activity – Evidence and Implications.* London: Health Education Authority.

49 Gregory J, Lowe S, Bates CJ, Prentice A, Jackson L, Smithers G, Wenlock R, Farron M. 2000. *The National Diet and Nutrition Survey: Young People Aged 4 to 18 Years. Volume 1: Report of the Diet and Nutrition Survey.* London: The Stationery Office.

50 Wynder FI, Berenson GS, Strong B, Williams C. 1989. Coronary artery disease prevention. Cholesterol – a paediatric perspective. *Preventive Medicine*: 18: 409.

51 Tell GS, Tuomileto J, Epstein FH, Starsser T. 1986. Studies of atheroscelerosis determinants and precursors during childhood and adolescence. *Bulletin of the World Health Organization*; 64 (4): 595-605.

52 James W, Muir C, Tunstall-Pedoe H, Lean M, Cockburn F. Scottish Office Home and Health Department. 1993. *The Scottish Diet*. Edinburgh: HMSO.

53 Turtle J, Jones A, Hickman M. 1997. *Young People and Health. The Health Behaviour of School-aged Children. A Report of the 1995 Findings.* London: Health Education Authority.

54 Turner S, Zimvrakaki H, Athanasiou K. 1997. Investigating children's ideas about fat consumption and health: a comparative study. *Health Education Journal;* 56 (4): 329-39.

55 Carey S. 1985. *Conceptual Change in Childhood*. Cambridge, Massachusetts: MIT Press.

56 Osbourne J, Wadsworth P, Black P. 1992. *SPACE: Research Report. Processes of Life.* Liverpool: Liverpool University Press.

57 Backett KC. 1990. Image and reality: health-enhancing behaviours in middle-class families. *Health Education Journal;* 49: 61-3.

58 Ross S. 1995. Do I really have to eat that? A qualitative study of schoolchildren's food choices and preferences. *Health Education Journal;* 54: 312-21.

59 Aggleton P, Whitty G, Knight A, Prayle D, Warwick I, Rivers K. 1998. Promoting young people's health: the health concerns and needs of young people. *Health Education;* 6: 213-19.

60 Mintel and the British Market Research Bureau. 1998. *Marketing to Children.* London: Mintel International Group Ltd.

61 Prout A. 1996. *Families, Cultural Bias and Health Promotion: Implications of an Ethnographic Study. HEA Family Health Report Series.* London: Health Education Authority.

62 The Food Commission. 2000. *Children's Food Examined: An Analysis of 358 Products Targeted at Children.* London: The Food Commission.

63 Co-op Society. 2000. *Blackmail*. Manchester: CWS Ltd.

64 BBC Online news report. 6 July 2000. Supermarket bans junk food ads. Accessed from: http:/news.bbc.co.uk/1/hi/health/820319.stm

65 Mayall B. 1993. Keeping healthy at home and school: it's my body so it's my job. *Sociology of Health and Illness*; 15 (4): 464-87.

66 Mayall B. 1996. *Children, Health and the Social Order*. Buckingham: Open University Press.

67 Sodexho. 2000. *The Sodexho School Meals Survey 2000.* Kenley: Sodexho Limited.

68 Accessed from BBC Online "No worries over children's diet", 26th April 1999 about the Gallup Survey for the Local Authority Caterers Association.

Chapter 15

Giving children and young people a voice

'Give a voice to children and young people' is one of the six areas of the national plan put forward in the young@heart policy document *Towards a generation free from coronary heart disease: Policy action for children's and young people's health and well-being* (see diagram below and page 9). The National Heart Forum would like to see all the policy actions proposed in the document developed and implemented with a commitment to involving children and young people and taking account of their views so that national and local policy-making is effective, appropriate and responsive to their needs.

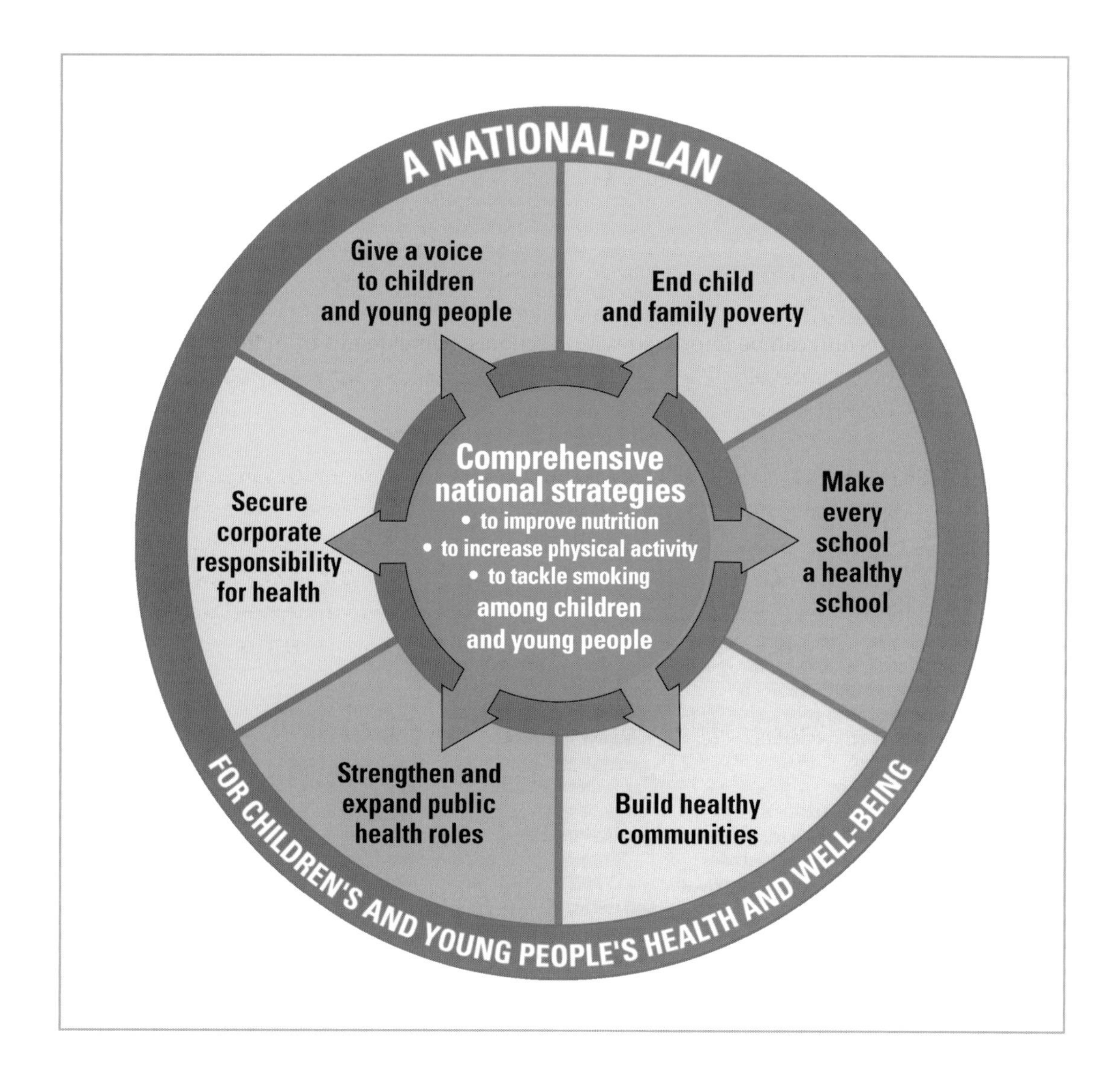

Giving children and young people a voice in the young@heart initiative

The National Heart Forum recognised the value of consulting children and young people at an early stage in the formulation of the young@heart policy recommendations and joined forces with the National Children's Bureau (NCB), an organisation which has developed expertise in finding out and acting on the views of children and young people, and which has established a set of principles and standards to underpin this work.

The NCB runs a free membership network, Young NCB, open to all children and young people. Thirty members of this network, aged 11-17 years and from all over England, were invited to a 'talkshop' in London to help the National Heart Forum produce a video. In the video, called *A Picture of Health,* they were able to speak out about what they know about health in childhood and adolescence, clarify how their knowledge and understanding of the risks translate into actual behaviour, and give their views about how work with young people on keeping healthy and reducing heart disease could and should be developed. They also gave lots of suggestions on how health can be improved within schools. Some quotes from the video are given below. (For details of how to order a copy of the video, please contact the National Heart Forum – see address on page iii.)

The video was shown at the young@heart policy summit meeting in June 2001, where it made a significant impact on the delegates and informed much of the ensuing debate. A copy was also sent to every Healthy Schools coordinator and to key government officials, together with a leaflet written by the NCB describing what participation is and giving examples of good practice in the school setting. The leaflet, which was produced as a result of the talkshop day, is reproduced on page 362.

Quotes from young people featured in the video *A Picture of Health*

"Health is, like, an important factor but it's not being dealt with properly."

"They should be promoting exercise and health issues at primary schools."

"Healthy food should be accessible to everyone."

"At school you pay about 40p for an apple. It's much cheaper to get crisps or something else."

"Not everyone just wants the junk food option."

"If we don't teach it, many people won't be healthy. That will affect the next generation."

"Young people don't have the knowledge to be able to do it [healthy eating] on their own or the motivation, so that's why they need help."

"It's not the teachers who go out to buy the food, so parents need to be targeted to know what to buy."

"You need different activities in school. We don't want just the boring stuff like basketball."

"When you're at school for like PE and games lessons, the staff from the leisure centre should maybe come to the school and help tell them about being fit and stuff."

"It's down to the environment you've been brought up in."

Government consultation with children and young people

Legislative changes, both nationally in the form of the Children's Act 1989, and internationally in the form of the UN Convention on the Rights of the Child (1990), have placed a duty on the UK government to ensure that its actions are conducted in the best interests of children and young people.

Article 12 of the UN Convention accords children a specific right to free expression of opinion in matters affecting the child and it is widely recognised that policies informed by children's and young people's views are more effective, appropriate and responsive to their needs than those developed in the absence of their views.[1]

The Social Exclusion Unit's Policy Action Team on Young People made recommendations about how the UK government could improve its approach to policy-making for young people.[2] As a result, the Children and Young People's Unit was established to join up policy-making across government departments, and to promote young people's participation in policy design and service delivery through active dialogue and partnership. The Unit has established the Children and Young People's Advisory Forum, comprising 28 members aged 11-18, to support them in their work, in particular as they develop the government's overarching strategy for children and young people.

Other areas of government are beginning to recognise the value of consulting widely on policy developments and UK Online, the government information and services website, has set up a website specifically for young people at http://www.young.gov.uk/oee/youth.nsf/sections/homepage/$file/home.htm

References

1 Lansdown G. 2001. *Promoting Children's Participation in Democratic Decision-making*. Florence: Unicef Innocenti Research Centre.

2 Social Exclusion Unit. 2000. *National Strategy for Neighbourhood Renewal – A Report of Policy Action Team 12: Young People*. London: Cabinet Office Social Exclusion Unit.

The following text is reproduced from a leaflet by the National Children's Bureau, The KOSH, and the National Heart Forum.

Giving children and young people a voice
Participation and active citizenship

This short leaflet addresses the most common questions asked at NCB about participation – what is participation? what principles should underpin it? why should we support participation? – and concludes with some examples of good practice.

What is participation?

Participation is when children and young people are involved in decisions that affect lives. This can be at home helping the family decide on a holiday through to working with fellow students and teachers to develop a school policy, or planning and developing a new national strategy with government officials.

Why should children and young people participate?

- Children and young people want to be involved. They want to tell us what they think; they want to be part of the process of creating, building and improving their school and other settings. If we want them to participate as adults we must help them to 'have a go' and get involved when young. A school culture that encourages participation provides children and young people with knowledge, skills and a positive attitude to citizenship and decision-making.
- They are entitled to participate. The United Nations Convention on the Rights of the Child underpins the rights of children and young people to participate. Children have the right:
  - to express an opinion and to have that opinion taken into account, in any matter or procedure affecting them (Article 12)
  - to obtain and make known information unless it violates the rights of others (Article 13)
  - to access appropriate information and education especially if it promotes their social, spiritual and moral well-being and physical and mental health (Article 17).
- Statutory DfES *Guidance on Participation* will be sent to all local authorities and schools in autumn 2003.
- The National Healthy School Standard (NHSS) also requires participation and provides some criteria for participation under the heading 'giving pupils a voice':
  - Pupils' needs assessment informs curriculum planning.
  - Pupils' views influence teaching and learning in PSHE and Citizenship.
  - Pupils take responsibility for some aspects of school, such as keeping the site litter-free, break-time snack sales, changing displays and the garden.
  - Mechanisms are established for involving pupils in policy development, for example through school councils and the Healthy Schools task group.
- The PSHE and Citizenship Framework also emphasises the importance and significance of active participation.

- There is a range of national and local government initiatives which explicitly support children's and young people's participation.
- Positive outcomes. Anecdotally colleagues are talking about an improved ethos of learning and improved service delivery.

How do you do participation?

Effective participation requires an ethos that empowers children and young people and encourages them to participate in needs assessment, planning, implementation and monitoring and evaluation of any aspect of their lives, school, care and youth service.

There are some key principles that underpin effective participation. Children and young people need:

- respect and trust – "not treated like children, but not expected to be adults" (quote from a young person at an NCB Talkshop);
- commitment from adults;
- information on how the school or any other setting works, its purpose and values;
- real and genuine opportunities to participate;
- to be aware of limitations/constraints before they engage in the work: e.g. fundraising may be necessary to carry out a video project that they want to do;
- continuous dialogue;
- preparation and to develop confidence;
- support (physical and emotional) which enables full participation, to fully engage and to address issues as they arise;
- proper planning of events, activities, systems and structure that promotes active and positive participation;
- feedback on the outcomes of their contributions;
- some children and young people will need specific and deliberate targeting if they are vulnerable or have special needs;
- adults who will 'rethink' how they take responsibility for decision-making.

Participation in practice

Participation is perceived to operate at different levels. Arnstein and Hart's ladder of participation* talks about a model of participation in which involvement and empowerment are acquired through different styles of participation based on varying methods of sharing or using power.

* Hart R. 1992. *Children's Participation from Tokenism to Citizenship*. Florence: UNICEF.

Continued on next page.

Initial levels of consultation maintain adult power and young people are 'used' to manipulate or decorate an event or initiative. Power is shared more when we consult with young people and ask them to tell us what they want or ask them to give an opinion about something.

Even more power is shared when young people participate, become involved and work with adults to initiate decisions based on an initial audit or needs assessment. More in-depth participation is achieved when children and young people initiate activity and choose to share the decision-making with adults.

The following demonstrates these different levels of power and actual participation within a school setting:

- The School Council is run by a teacher who organises meetings, identifies the members and asks members to ratify decisions made by the teacher.
- A teacher manages the School Council, with members who volunteer and are asked to identify their needs on a specific issue.
- The School Council has an elected membership of students and works with teachers to make decisions based on a needs assessment.
- The School Council is an elected body of students, with a budget, who identify issues that they want to address and work with teachers and other partners to make decisions to implement and monitor activity.

Some examples

- A 'healthy' primary school in Berkshire demonstrated how the School Council reviewed values in the school. All the elected members were aged 5-11 years. One 5 year old really wanted to be involved but was too nervous to come by herself so she was encouraged to bring a mentor for support. She was also a 5 year old.
- A group of girls in a 'healthy' secondary school in Suffolk carried out a survey of female pupils and physical activity. They followed this up with a detailed observation of various physical activity lessons, which they analysed and found that some girls did want to do healthy activities, which included swimming and dance. They didn't want to participate in the games. They are in the process of negotiating new ways of encouraging girls to participate in new activities in school.
- And finally a group of young people in a 'healthy' secondary school in southeast London challenged the quality of school dinners. "They were horrible" said one young man. His teacher agreed. After a detailed survey and consultation with young people, staff and caterers they negotiated the opening of a pasta and salad bar. They are working with the PSHE Coordinator to develop healthy eating as part of PSHE.

NCB Young Members meet on a regular basis and participate in occasional Saturday workshops called 'Talkshops' on key issues such as SRE (sex and relationships education), drugs education and violence. The Talkshops were 'enjoyed' by all but we felt that we wanted to get young people's voices heard beyond NCB. A partnership with The KOSH, NCB and NCB Young Members was developed. The KOSH is a theatre and film company with a great deal of experience of working with young people in an educational context.

NCB Young Members, The KOSH, NCB, Sex Education Forum, Drug Education Forum and National Heart Forum have worked together to develop three very effective and useful videos, which can be used for auditing, policy review, parents' meetings and local network meetings of PSHE coordinators.

The National Children's Bureau has learnt the following about using video in participation work:

- Young people are comfortable with video and talk with confidence and flair in a situation where video is being used.
- Young people need to be invited to be involved and understand the purpose, where the video will be shown and to whom.
- Funding needs to include a reward for young people, and adequate dissemination of the video to relevant networks.
- Young people like to receive a certificate of attendance and to have a copy of the video sent to their school, youth club or public care setting.
- This type of work is not research, but representation of diversity is important. A range of young people must be involved.
- Creating safety boundaries is essential to enable young people to express their views.
- Adults really benefit from hearing first-hand opinions and this makes video an effective tool for policy and practice development.

In the future the National Children's Bureau wants to work with young people more effectively and include them in the planning stage, train them as facilitators, and involve them in the videoing and editing.

Video is an extraordinarily powerful tool and the National Children's Bureau will continue working with The KOSH to develop this methodology with NCB Young Members.

What do children and young people think?

One of our NCB Young Members, Anna Bennett, Year 11 student from Finham Park Comprehensive School, Coventry summarises:

"Personally I think that all young people's participation would begin to increase if PSHE and Citizenship education became a more meaningful part of the school curriculum. After all, 10 As at GCSE are worthless if you are lacking in people skills. Informal discussion-based PSHE and Citizenship education lessons in both primary and secondary schools would help young people to form their own opinions and learn how to communicate these opinions. There you have it, people skills. I also think that innovations and organisations like the Young People's Parliament and the National Children's Bureau need to be promoted more through the media and through schools. We need to see the leader of the Young People's Parliament on SMTV-live; we need to read about them in *Sugar* magazine. As Tony Blair might have said, in order to improve levels of 'participation, participation, and participation' we need 'education, education, education'.

For further information please contact:

Gill Frances, **National Children's Bureau**
8 Wakley Street, London EC1V 7QE
Telephone: 020 7843 6095 E-mail: gfrances@ncb.org.uk

Young@heart policy summit meeting participants

The following people took part in the National Heart Forum's young@heart policy summit meeting in June 2001 and helped to shape the policy framework document summarised in Part 1.

Penny Allsop	Department of Health
Professor John Appleby	King's Fund
Dr Kathryn Backett-Milburn	University of Edinburgh Medical School
Dr David Batty	London School of Hygiene and Tropical Medicine
Beverly Botting	Office for National Statistics
Jackie Carnell	Community Practitioners' and Health Visitors' Association
Crichton Casbon	Qualifications and Curriculum Authority
Nick Cavill	Independent Consultant
Adam Crosier	Independent Consultant
Kath Dalmeny	The Food Commission
Niall Dickson	BBC
Andrew Dougal	Northern Ireland Chest, Heart and Stroke Association
Dr Elizabeth Dowler	University of Warwick
Dr Maria Duggan	Independent Consultant
Gillian Fine	Sainsbury's plc
Charles Foster	British Heart Foundation Health Promotion Research Group
Gill Frances	National Children's Bureau
Elaine Fullard	National Primary Care Facilitation Programme

Dr Brian Gaffney	Health Promotion Agency for Northern Ireland
John Garlick	Essex University
Peter Gaylard	Boots plc
Dr Penny Gibson	Royal College of Paediatrics and Child Health
Dr Alison Giles	National Heart Forum
Dr Paul Harker	Institute of Child Health, Southampton
Michael Harrison	Chartered Institute of Environmental Health
Joe Harvey	Health Education Trust
Marilyn Harvey	Youth Clubs UK
Dr Gerrard Hastings	Strathclyde University
Dr Ann Hemingway	Bournemouth University
Dr Melvyn Hillsdon	London School of Hygiene and Tropical Medicine
Pat Jackson	Community Practitioners' and Health Visitors' Association
Professor Philip James	International Obesity Taskforce
Professor Desmond Julian	Individual member of the National Heart Forum
Jenny Jupe	Design and Technology Associates
Dr John Kemm	Director of Public Health Services, NHS Executive
Professor Brian Kirby	University of Exeter
Jane Landon	National Heart Forum
Professor David Leon	London School of Hygiene and Tropical Medicine
Lady Sylvia Limerick	Community Practitioners' and Health Visitors' Association
Paul Lincoln	National Heart Forum
Dr Helen Lloyd	British Dietetic Association
Debbie Lye	Department of Culture, Media and Sport
Sir Alexander Macara	National Heart Forum
Tim Marsh	UK Public Health Association
Dr Alan Maryon Davis	Royal Institute of Public Health
Dr Ann McNeill	Freelance Consultant on Tobacco Control
Professor Klim McPherson	London School of Hygiene and Tropical Medicine
Dominic McVey	Independent Consultant

Dr Shanthi Mendis	World Health Organization
Margaret Mythen	New Health Network
Jane Naish	Royal College of Nursing
Barrie Neal	Lewisham Borough Council
Dr Noel Olsen	British Medical Association
Professor Richard Parish	Health Development Agency
Professor Robert Pickard	British Nutrition Foundation
Professor Roisin Pill	University of Wales College of Medicine
Charlie Powell	Sustain
Dr Vivienne Press	British Heart Foundation
Professor Peter Quilliam	Individual member of the National Heart Forum
Barry Quirk	Lewisham Borough Council
Dr Mike Rayner	British Heart Foundation Health Promotion Research Group
Lord Nicholas Rea	General Practitioner
Hamid Rehman	Ethnos Research and Consultancy
Mary Robinson	Health Promotion England
Andrew Rogers	Society of Health Education and Health Promotion Specialists
Professor Roberto Rona	Department of Public Health Sciences, Guy's Campus
Maggie Sanderson	British Dietetic Association
Amanda Sandford	Action on Smoking and Health
Louise Sarch	National Heart Forum
Imogen Sharp	Department of Health
Dame Helena Shovelton	Audit Commission
Dr Fran Sivers	Primary Care Cardiovascular Society
Hadrian Southorn	National Association of Governors and Managers
Professor Nick Spencer	Royal College of Paediatrics and Child Health
Dr Margaret Thorogood	Coronary Prevention Group
Marilyn Toft	National Healthy Schools Standard Coordinator
Chris Tudor-Smith	Health Promotion Directorate, Welsh Assembly Government

Bridget Turner	Diabetes UK
Professor Michael Wadsworth	Medical Research Council
Fiona Wheeler	Sure Start, Department for Education and Skills
Professor Peter Whincup	St George's Hospital Medical School
Nichola Wilkins	Royal Institute of Public Health
Frank Windmeijer	Institute for Fiscal Studies
Professor David Wood	British Cardiac Society
John Wyn Owen	Nuffield Trust

Policy summit meeting administration

Dan French	Administrator, National Heart Forum
Melanie Morris	Administrative Assistant, National Heart Forum
David Bebb	Profile Productions Ltd
Jo Price	Profile Productions Ltd
Simon Whitfield	Profile Productions Ltd

Index

Page numbers in bold type indicate a reference to a table or figure.

C